# THE CEREBRAL PALSY ENTITIES

# RESEARCH AND NEURODEVELOPMENTAL OVERVIEW 1994

including

Diagnostic Survey of Progressive Neurometabolic and
Neurodegenerative Disorders
Simulating CP

by

## Alexander Russell

OBE MD FRCP BHy DPH DCH

## Foreword

by

## Lord Walton of Detchant

British Library Cataloguing in Publication Data

A catalogue record for this book is available from the British Library

ISBN 1-899091 009

Typeset by InfoMed International, Maidenhead, Berkshire
Printed by Alderson Brothers, West Molesey, Surrey

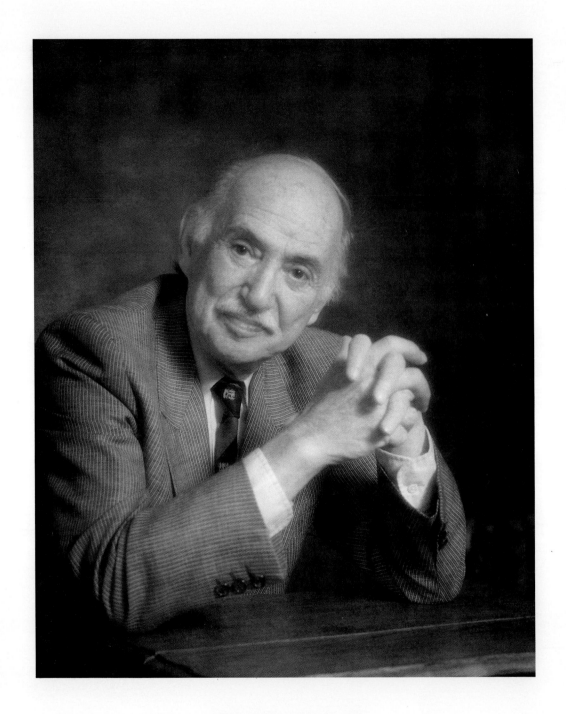

Alexander Russell

## DEDICATION

*To an uniquely wonderful wife and mother, Haya,*

*and our deeply cherished daughters, Lorna and Sharon,*

*for their very individual roles in indulging my lifelong quest*

*for truth, justice and fruition of true health in medicine*

*with*

*infinite patience, helpfulness and love.*

# FOREWORD

## Lord Walton of Detchant

**President, World Federation of Neurology,**
**former Dean of Medicine and Professor of Neurology,**
**former Warden and Now Honorary Fellow,**
**Green College, Oxford**

Alexander Russell is a most distinguished graduate of my Medical School in Newcastle-upon-Tyne, formerly a part of the University of Durham. His contributions to the field of paediatrics, not least during his tenure of the Chair of Paediatrics and Child Care at the Hadassah University Medical Centre in Jerusalem, have been outstanding and no fewer than three syndromes in the field of paediatrics have his name attached to them. During the course of a fruitful and varied professional career, he has made many original contributions to our study of neurometabolic and degenerative diseases of the nervous system and more particularly of late has turned his attention to that group of conditions generally classified under the umbrella heading of cerebral palsy. These two volumes embody much of his personal experience arising from years of study of this field, during which time he has examined innumerable affected patients. The first volume defines, describes and analyses the clinical features of the conditions falling into these groups, with particular attention to aetiology and pathogenesis. In the second volume, Professor Russell describes, with the help of his colleagues, the way in which the philosophy, principles and practice of the Petö system of management have evolved in Great Britain. In the course of his commentary, Professor Russell discusses not only medical and therapeutic applications but also pays due attention to the early developmental socio-educational integration of handicapped infants and pre-school children alongside their normal peers, a topic upon which he has written a short but persuasive booklet outlining guidelines of management.

These volumes will stand as a brilliant and lasting monument to Professor Russell's dedication to this field of study, embodying, as they do, the fruits of a very extensive life-time of experience in this field and, as such, deserve very careful attention from those working in the paediatric and neurological disciplines, as well as from those called upon to care in whatever capacity for children with cerebral palsy.

**JOHN WALTON**
**Oxford, 1994**

# CONTENTS

## Chapter 2    Definition and Classification of the Cerebral Palsy or Cerebral Dysfunction Entities

## Chapter 3    Diagnostic Neurodevelopmental and Other Criteria in Early Detection

Chapter 4    **Early Diagnostic Identification of Cerebral Palsy Components and Their Neurophysiology**

Chapter 5    **The Dystonias**

Chapter 6    **The Revolutionary Role of Advances in
             Non-Invasive Neuro-Imaging Pathophysiology**

**Chapter 7**    **Update on Neuroimaging and the Localisation of a Spectrum of Neuropathology underlying the Different Entities of Cerebral Palsy**

# SECTION II: NEUROPATHOPHYSIOLOGY

## Chapter 8   Dynamic Implications of Neuropathic Evidence and Possible Preventive Implications

## Chapter 9   Significance of Cerebral Ventricular Dilatation in relation to Periventricular Haemorrhage and Neuropathic Outcome

## Chapter 10   The Element of Ischaemic/Anoxic Damage

## Chapter 11   Vulnerability to Vascular Damage

## Chapter 12   Additional Preventive Implications: Other Possible Antecedents of Cerebral Palsy

## Chapter 13   Neuropathogenesis of Cerebral Dysfunction and Functional Recovery

# SECTION III: SIMULATION OF CEREBRAL PALSY ENTITIES BY PROGRESSIVE NEUROMETABOLIC AND NEURODEGENERATIVE DISORDERS

Chapter 19 **Syndromes Presenting with Ataxia Preceded or Accompanied by Hypotonia, or with Choreo-Athetosis Interposed**

## Chapter 20    Spasticity or Hypertonicity, and Rigidity as a Presenting or Predominant Manifestation
[Although associated with Ataxia or
Choreo-athetosis in some metabolic situations]
Infantile and Early Childhood:
Progressive Genetic Encephalopathies

Chapter 21 **Choreo-Athetosis: Definition, Diagnosis and Neurophysiology**

# INTRODUCTION

The several clinico-pathological entities of Cerebral Palsy which shall be redefined in this volume still remain the principal source of severe physical and mental disability affecting children, and still the most crippling challenge to all of us who care for them. Yet their recognition takes us back as much as one and a half centuries to its first presentation in 1843 by William John Little as a "spasmodic affection" of newborn "born in a state of asphyxia". He was to elaborate these *intrapartum* implications two decades later in 1861 before the "Obstetrical Society of London". The spasmodic rigidity of his 47 children was unequivocally attributed to asphyxia and/or trauma at birth. This view was supported and clinically adorned with the title of "Cerebral Palsy" in substitution for "Little's disease" after the famous five lectures of Sir William Osler, although with perhaps overweening emphasis upon the hemiplegias, which curiously enough have again recently shown an upswing in prevalence, predominantly in the preterm (Chapter 4). To crown this entry of a distinguished internist into the sphere of unresolved paediatric problems, both its spasticity and birth complications were first related to possible adverse *foetal* events in a monograph by Sigmund Freud then in Vienna (to be translated by Russin as recently as 1968). As much professional apathy clouded disbelief in this conjecture as there was hostility to befog initial disbelief in his more revolutionary approaches to other cerebral dysfunction. Yet today, as the tragic army of its victims within the USA alone has grown to more than 50,000, the evidence is in my view beginning to swing full circle to give credence to that early imaginative prediction of so long ago. Only recently has it come to be appreciated that the underlying cerebral damage is much more often prenatal in origin; more frequently the cause, not the sequel of so-called asphyxia at birth.

The various entities of this syndrome also include the most common motor, movement and tonic disabilities consequent upon *prematurity*. The frequency of associated sensory and mental disabilities are being highlighted by the enhanced survival of the extreme preterm which has attended sophistication of intensive care. Its underlying pathogenesis, and its possible preventive elements to be discussed, involve *several patterns of irreversible and static non-progressive malfunctioning or damage within the immature brain* leading to disorder predominantly of movement and balance as well as of tone in the majority of cases.

Whilst accepted as permanent and non-progressive in terms of the primary cerebral pathology, it remains unaltered with time, except for such changes as post-infarctive gliosis or the cystic degeneration that accompanies or follows periventricular leukomalacia. It is therefore not wholly unchanging. Some of its early clinical manifestations in any one individual may be modified during stages of developmental maturation and adaptation, so that the consequent functional disability does not necessarily remain static. Disturbance of either tone, movement or both may also be superadded. Initial and more or less transient hypotonia is thus characteristic of the ultimately hypertonic or choreo-athetoid child, so that there may be some early functional fluctuation. Likewise, intensification of their manifestations may be induced by the stress of particular postures. So that extensor postures or a degree of generalised spasticity can be sharply accentuated by stimulating anti-gravity responses, as by holding the child upright, extending his head or putting pressure on the soles of his feet.

In later childhood or adolescence, with increasing growth and adiposity, physical deterioration is possible if treatment is not reviewed at puberty, and maintenance neglected. Scrupulous monitoring will be required to avert potential problems, including contractures and those psycho-emotional, before they become irreversible. In so long term a view-point, withdrawal of services should never be acceptable, so that even the decline in physical function dependent upon normal ageing should be minimized.

It should in any case be fully acknowledged that CP represents an heterogeneous complex of entities. Moreover, the diversity but still limited definition of their aetiology will dominate the comprehensive overview in the pages ahead, with possible avenues of prevention of its different entities, hypotonic, hypertonic, choreo-athetoid and ataxic, a crucial perspective and challenge. Whilst the most prominent handicapping sequelae are of disordered movement and posture, it is also principally manifest in clinically definable disturbances of tone as well as of coordination and balance. A system of classification will later be explored in terms of their customary clinical predominance and labelling as hypotonic/atonic - very often solely as an initial phase - spasticity/hypertonicity, choreo-athetosis, and ataxia or mixtures thereof. The main clinical signs underlying these disorders of motor control and tone, therefore, are of the element of hypertonicity linked to persistent exaggeration of primitive reflexes. But hyperreflexia is also typically associated with the hypotonic state, ostensibly indicative of pyramidal localization of damage, i.e. to the upper motor neurone. Clearly separable clinical syndromes are therefore already recognizable. With the more precise localization and definition of underlying cerebral and/or cerebellar pathology that is becoming possible through new research tools, and especially via recent advances in neuro-imaging through magnetic resonance imaging, positron emission tomography, and progressive refinements thereof, especially in biochemical directions, dealt with in relation to corresponding clinical patterns in Chapter 7, an expanding mosaic of clinico-pathological syndromes is emerging, to which it is hoped this text will contribute.

There has been a noticeable change in the type and severity of cerebral palsy in the preterm population, in which it is still by far the commonest source of motor disability. In terms of preventing and treating hyperbilirubinaemia, especially in the Rhesus immunological prevention of kernicterus, the West has at least propagated a world-wide fall in the incidence of athetosis. Nonetheless, other forms of *hyperbilirubinaemia* still remain a grave threat for cerebral palsy, also as a result of kernicteric brain damage, especially in preterm infants. Intensification of preventive efforts in this direction is still required. A globally important cause today is the neonatal jaundice stemming from glucose-G phosphate dehydrogenase deficiency, which is after all the commonest enzyme disorder in human beings. At least its neonatal jaundice is readily overcome by phototherapy. Severe perinatal jaundice has in particular been recently correlated with a "globo-Luysian" group of neuropathologies (Hayashi et al., 1991), the major sites being in pallidum and subthalamic nucleus. The principal clinical manifestation is a rigidospasticity, combined with fluctuation in the athetosis. A separate chapter (5) is likewise devoted to clarifying the clinical confusion surrounding the Dystonias.

Despite vast areas of persistent poverty, malnutrition and infection, a distinct decrease in spastic quadriplegia linked to mental retardation may yet prove to derive from broader general health factors including improvements in nutrition and health care. The form of CP currently most commonly diagnosed is spastic diplegia which is also the commonest category of CP in the preterm. This would appear to stem most commonly from extension of haemorrhage, and/or hypoxic/ischaemic damage to the white matter of the internal capsule, thereby to incriminate most severely the medial corticospinal fibres subserving leg function. Only the more severe and extensive lesions encroach upon trunk and arm functions. At the same time, relative freedom from cortical damage in the premature, where the germinal matrix is the commonest focus of haemorrhage may explain their near-normal cognitive function, whereas *parasagittal cortical* infarctive lesions in the full term birth-asphyxiated infant affects the upper limb girdle, arm, face and tongue. Thus, there is more proximal distribution of motor dysfunction in the full term, whereas in the premature the primary motor defect and most severe involvement is distal or caudal. The association with mental retardation and epilepsy is especially close in the spastic tetraplegic, although by no means infrequent in hemiplegics. The significance of changing trends over the past two decades in the prevalence of these different categories of CP in the preterm and full term will be expressed in the epidemiological conclusions outlined below. With the increased survival of low and very low birth-weight preterm infants, a progressively greater proportion especially of ultimately severe spastic/hypertonic forms stems from them. Particularly is this being increasingly recognised in the "small for gestational (SGA)" infants, to which the work differentiating "birth morphologies" related to spastic CP (Blair and Stanley, 1992) must contribute.

Intra-uterine growth retardation, to which we have devoted a subsequent section is thus an important source of the increased perinatal morbidity related to CP, including that derived from the pre-eclamptic or pregnancy-induced hypertension, which has been more recently shown to be frequently responsive to the blocking of $\alpha_1$-adrenoreceptors of peripheral arterioles by maternal labetolol therapy, etc. (Cruikshank et al., 1992).

A wide spectrum of neurometabolic and neurodegenerative disorders also need to be identified as clinical although progressive analogues of the known entities of CP. In one or more phases of their natural history they may come to closely *simulate* one or more components of CP. These will be outlined in subsequent chapters of what amounts to a third section of the book under the subdivisions they functionally resemble of *Hypotonia, Spasticity, Choreo-athetosis* and *Ataxia*. Studies of cellular and molecular damage underlying the cerebral and cerebellar pathology they produce should help greatly in our understanding of the different cerebral palsy manifestations and how to alleviate or circumvent them.

In the same fashion as one specific form of athetotic CP stemming from Rhesus incompatibility and kernicterus is close to elimination in the West by virtue of a corresponding specific preventive programme - anti-D administration soon after delivery to at-risk mothers - logical avenues of research open up. These would depend upon the definition of the neuropathophysiology of other distinct syndromes within the CP spectrum. Hence a major theme of this text is the neurophysiological differentiation of such syndromes based upon genetic and other prenatal, peri and postnatal factors whereby programmes for primary or secondary prevention can be more specifically focussed. The intensive study of progressive neurometabolic disorders in the simulating CP in the third section of the book has a similar motivation insofar as their neuropathology leading to specific cortical, basal ganglia, cerebellar or other foci of damage may enhance our comprehension of the non-progressive variants of CP.

**Alexander Russell**

## References

Cruikshank DJ et al. (1992) Intrauterine growth retardation and maternal labetolol treatment. J Obstet Gynecol 12: 223-227

Freud S. (1968) Infantile cerebral palsies. Translation: LA Russin. University of Miami Press, Miami

Hayashi M, Satoh J, Saramoto K, Morimatsu Y. (1991) Clinical and neuropathological findings in severe athetoid cerebral palsy: a comparative study of globo-Luysian and thalamo-putaminal groups. Brain Dev 13: 47-51

# SECTION I

# 1

# CEREBRAL PALSY UPDATE

## Aetiological Facets

Pre- and Perinatal
Prenatal Infection and Toxicology
Congenital Rubella and CMV Encephalopathies
The Contribution of Prematurity
Selective Nutrient Deficiency: Iodine
Effects of Hyperthermia: Experimental and Human
Genetic Implications
Increased Prevalence of CP in Multiple Pregnancies
Intra-uterine Growth Retardation:  A Relevant Role in
      Cerebral Palsy including the Place of Maternal
      Hyperoxygenation in its Treatment and
      Prevention of CP

## Significance of Epidemiological Appraisals

Recent Epidemiological Assessments
Epidemiological Focus upon Prevalence of Hemiplegia
Correlationships with Socio-Biological Risk Factors: Gestational Age,
      Birth-weight, Male Preponderance and Socio-economic Factors
Prevalence of Different Entities of Cerebral Palsy

## Factors Underlying Disorders of Neuronal Migration

Developmental Neurobiology and Congenital Anomalies of the Brain
The Lissencephalies and Early Prenatal Infection with Cytomegalovirus
Foetal Metabolic and Interrelated Nutritional/Myelinational Influences
     *Zellweger Cerebro-hepato syndrome*
     *Marshall-Smith syndrome*
Interrelations between Myelination and Early Nutrition

Microcephalic and Dysmorphic Examples of Unexplained Disorders of
        Neuronal Proliferation
        *Meckel-Gruber*
        *Cerebro-oculofacio skeletal (COFS) syndrome*
        *Neu-Laxova syndrome*
Destructive Disorders of Foetal Brain: Subtotal Cortical Necrosis
Pre- and Perinatal Hydrocephalus
Prenatal Cerebral Perfusion Failure

## Perinatal and Postnatal Cerebral Palsies

Reappraisal of Immediate Prenatal and Perinatal Factors as Source of Early
        Postnatal Expression of CP
Patho-Physiological Sequences which Could Lead to Cerebral Ischaemia
Chronic Foetal Distress as marker for subsequent CP or Other Adverse
        Neurological State
Postnatal Metabolic and other Episodic Damage
Hyperbilirubinaemia as a Continuing Threat
Resultant Postnatal Categories of Motor Handicap
Preventive Implications in Postnatal CP

## *Associated* Disorders or Other Intrinsic and Co-existing Dysfunction, Disability and Handicap

Associated Cognitive Deficit
Relative Microcephaly
Craniostenoses and CP
Aberrant Spatial Perception in CP
Specific Memory Impairment in CP
Memory Dysfunction
Dyslexia or More Specific Learning Disability in CP
Awareness of the Common Apraxia and Agnosia in CP
Ocular and Visual Anomalies
Visual impairment
Hearing Impairment
        *Cochlear Implantation in Sensorineural Deafness*
        *Vestibulometry*
Language Functions
Other Communication Disorders
Non-verbal and Augmentative Communication Aids

Speech Disorder
> *Dysphasia*
> *Dyspraxia*
> *Dysarthria*

Left-Handedness in Cerebral Palsy

Emotional and Behavioural Disturbance

Sleep Disorders and Valuable Potential Role of Melatonin

Epileptiform Seizures
> *Association with Hemiplegia*
> *Association with Intraventricular Haemorrhage*
> *Association with Porencephaly*
> *Association with Focal Cortical Dysplasia*

Infantile onset Progressive Myoclonus Epilepsy

Neonatal Seizures: Prognostic Risks for Motor Disability and CP

Therapeutic Management including Surgical Intervention
> *Surgical intervention in refractory epilepsy*

Use of the SPECT Technique to Clarify Haemodynamic Pathophysiology of the
> Cerebral Cortex in Epilepsy

Silent Gastro-oesophageal Reflux in CP

Swallowing and Ventilatory Problems: Patho-physiology

Hip Subluxation

Adaptive and Orthotic Devices

Contractures

Premature Cervical Spondylosis in Athetoid CP

Odontogenesis

Submandibular Duct Diversion to Overcome Refractory Sialorrhoea in CP

Associated Hypothalamic or Neurovegetative Disturbances including Obesity

Growth Deficit

# AETIOLOGICAL FACETS

## Pre- and Perinatal

Extensive epidemiological analyses throwing light on the aetiology of the different syndromes of cerebral palsy (CP) will be interpreted in a later subdivision of this section. The *aetiological* bases of CP are still a fertile source of dispute. In the main, the consensus of belief centres upon one or more of a variety of prenatal and perinatal factors but to a lesser extent upon events around or after birth. Principally early prenatal phases are incriminated in interwoven infective and neurobiological factors, and nutrient deficiencies as well as hypoxaemic-ischaemic factors and haemorrhagic pathology also operating in later pre- or perinatal phases. The foetus and neonate is thus subject to a wide spectrum of stresses, each of which may be a relevant source of future cerebral palsy.

Recognition of the greater importance of prenatal factors is also growing in developing countries. For instance in a study of the antecedent factors in Saudi Arabian children with CP (al Rajeh et al., 1991) compared with those of a control group the following risk factors were indicated: the history of CP in a sibling, consanguinity of the parents, low birth-weight (< 2000g), gestational age less than 32 weeks, twin pregnancy and respiratory distress. In other words, prenatal factors including genetic, appear to play an equally major role in the pathogenesis of CP in Saudi Arabia.

A specifically toxicological prenatal insult has been identified, for example, in Iraq, where even prenatal exposure to methyl mercury poisoning has been incriminated in the aetiology of CP by Amin-Zaki et al. (1974).

## Prenatal Infection and Toxicology

Specific prenatal infections are still relevant, and in the case of cytomegalovirus even more so. To begin with, the commonest cause of congenital infection appears to be the *cytomegalovirus*, approaching 0.3/1000 births (Rudd and Peckham, 1988), with an especial neurobiological threat stemming from its

predilection for the earlier prenatal phases. CP has also been frequently reported in the past as a consequence of the *congenital Rubella* syndrome, the universal birth prevalence of which has dropped to about 0.03/1000 live births (Stanley et al. 1986). Nonetheless, there is a significant prevalence of CP in victims of congenital Rubella which may reach 14%. The birth prevalence of *congenital toxoplasmosis* is somewhat less at 0.01/1000. *Congenital varicella*, following upon a gestational history of varicella, is an occasional factor, not infrequently marked out by no more than one or more scars on the cheek at birth. Its incidence during pregnancy is estimated as 1.5 per 10,000 pregnancies with the risk of transplacental foetal infection approximately 25%. In addition to hemiparesis, it may be accompanied by a combination of atrophic muscular and digital changes and hypoplastic extremities sometimes unilateral with cerebrocortical and cerebellar atrophy, microcephaly and mental retardation. A combination of ocular pathology obtains, including cataract, chorioretinitis, Horner's syndrome, nystagmus and microphthalmia. Given in time, i.e. within four days of delivery, a combination of herpes zoster immune globulins, supported by Acyclovir,

may still help to curb the cerebral pathology.

Whereas the birth prevalence of congenital Rubella is likely to decline still further, *Congenital HIV* will probably become an increasingly serious consideration, especially as it rapidly spreads eastwards. The foetus and neonate can also be subjected to *maternal drug abuse* (a severe choreo-athetoid infant was a recent sequel of maternal heroin addiction), anaesthesia, prescriptive drug use, general undernutritional or specific nutrient deficiency such as iodine (the implications of which are to be outlined in the next section) as well as metabolic and genetic disorder, haemodynamic disturbances including foetal distress, and other sources of perinatal asphyxia or causes impaired blood flow or hypoperfusion in the brain of the newborn.

## Congenital Rubella and CMV Encephalopathies

Neuroimaging by MRI (with $T_2$-weighted spin echo (SE) and inversion recovery (IR) sequences has also been extended to congenital encephalopathy due to Rubella virus (two children) as well as to cytomegalovirus in at least six children (Sugita et al., 1991). Periventricular and subcortical hyperintensity were demonstrated in addition to delayed

myelination oligopachygyria (two cases) and cerebellar hypoplasia. The study also confirmed that the greater the disability the more markedly abnormal were the findings of MRI, which proved more effective in defining parenchymal lesions than CT. The better visualization of calcification by CT rather than MRI depended upon technical limitations inherent in the latter process.

## The Contribution of Prematurity

The aetiological role of prematurity in the genesis of cerebral palsy remains a supreme problem. As Vaucher et al. (1993)

have recently exposed in 150 extremely premature and surfactant deficient infants, CP developed in at least 20%. And the prevention of any underlying cerebral damage remains the great challenge which we have detailed in subsequent chapters. Volpe (1992) has led many forays in this direction, with a particular focus upon the cascade of metabolic and related events leading to neuronal cell death. Meanwhile his figures have illustrated the influence of neonatal intensive care at the highest contemporary level, with 85% of very low birth-weight infants surviving. But these leave in their wake a trail of 5-15% of "major spastic motor deficit" with an additional 25-50% exhibiting less prominent developmental disabilities, especially school failures.

The neonate, particularly the premature, is especially vulnerable to cerebro-vascular "accidents" such as periventricular or intraventricular haemorrhage, with periventricular leukomalacia as one sequel, although no less a crucial consequence of ischaemic/hypoxic damage, if this is not frequently primary. It was estimated by Nelson and Ellenberg (1986) that intrapartum abnormality accounted for 6% of CP and/or its associated mental retardation. The data of Stanley (1987) and Stanley and Watson (1988) raised this to 9%. The relationship to poor obstetric care has been assailed by Stanley and Blair (1991). Although elective Caesarian section, electronic foetal monitoring and induction of labour aimed at reducing the adverse effects of *foetal distress and birth asphyxia* have been used more frequently, the overall proportion of stillbirths and neonatal deaths in Western Australia from 1956 to 1988 has steadily fallen. The findings of neuro-imaging techniques which will be discussed more fully later, appear to more firmly vindicate

these as important antecedents of the cerebral palsy syndrome.

Numerous pathophysiological mechanisms have been invoked as possibly producing pre- or perinatal cerebral injury in the presence of circulatory abnormality. To what extent is there a common source of both the cerebral damage leading to CP and the premature birth, or that the factor(s) evoking the brain damage were instrumental in inducing prematurity, is also an important issue, with particularly crucial preventive implications. Foetal vulnerability to these factors will be considered more fully in Chapter 11.

*Intraparenchymal* haemorrhage in the premature infant is frequently unilateral so that hemiplegia results (Guzzeta et al., 1986), although blood flow throughout the hemisphere may be disturbed. However, it must be recalled that the available evidence suggests that there have been no demonstrable perinatal risk factors in the majority of CP victims (Stanley and English, 1986).

Earlier gestational phases also demand determined study, and the impact of cytomegalovirus upon the stage of neuronal migration in early brain development is illustrated by the lissencephaly associated with such intra-uterine infection to which reference is made later under "Developmental Biology". The fact that this is a serious threat can be realised from the known incidence of congenital cytomegalovirus of about 0.3/1000 births (Rudd and Peckham, 1988). It is thus the commonest cause of congenital infection, and apart from the grave impact of lissencephaly and severe mental retardation, about half of the affected children manifest CP if not psychomotor delay.

The prenatal role of cerebral maldevelopment secondary to drugs or other teratogens will be enlarged upon subsequently under the sub-heading of "Developmental Neurobiology and Congenital Anomalies of the Brain".

Interwoven factors of nutritional, immunological and neuro-hormonal basis, as well as genetic, could also operate in preconceptual and early post-conceptual phases to adversely influence brain maturation in the direction of CP. These potential prenatal factors include:

Acute foetal circulatory failure
Acute foetal hypovolaemia
> (Both of these may be a sequel of haemorrhage in foeto-maternal "transfusion")

Cerebral perfusion failure
> (This basis has been strongly postulated in a wide range of preterm and term gestations associated with pathology of the developing brain.)

Augmented foetal blood viscosity

Cerebral emboli

Chronic foetal anaemia

Chronic placental insufficiency

The neuropathological changes associated with hypoxic-ischaemic insults are divisible into those reflecting primary cellular or endothelial damage and those due to haemorrhage, although a frequent confluence of these two cannot be denied. Certainly, periventricular or intraventricular haemorrhage is the commonest manifestation of hypoxic-ischaemic injury in the preterm infant, with cortical infarction and necrosis of deep grey nuclei and brain stem, its main concomitant manifestation in the term neonate.

## Selective Nutrient Deficiency: Iodine

The impressive exploratory study led by Peter Pharoah (1976) of the long-established association between deficiency of maternal iodine and endemic goitrous cretinism have objectively confirmed several facets with important aetiological bearing on early prenatal CP. The focus of their study was in the isolated area of the Jimi River Valley in the Western Highlands Province of Papua New Guinea. Substitution of a rich crude salt source of dietary iodine by a commercial iodine-free salt had precipitated an epidemic of goitrous cretinism (Pharoah and Hornabrook, 1974). But such a human iodine deficit is endemic in many other parts of the world relatively remote from the sea, and it is estimated that over 800 million of the global population is at risk.

Severe iodine deficiency before conception or during early gestation leads to clinical goitre and the syndrome of endemic cretinism which is characterized by spastic diplegia in association with mental handicap, deaf mutism and strabismus. Deficits of growth and of motor sensory and cognitive performance ranging from the mental deficiency, deaf mutism and more subtle manifestations of speech, physical and other disturbances of memory, etc., were detectable not only in goitrous subjects but in siblings or other members of relevant pedigrees who were free from the fully fledged goitrous syndrome.

In the follow-up study of pregnant women in the area of severe iodine deficiency, there were also more stillbirths and deaths, as well as the endemic form of cretinism among the progeny. As a consequence of the deficiency of elemental iodine, there is a deficiency of synthesis of T4 with abnormally low serum total and free thyroxine (TT4, FT4) without clinical evidence of hypothyroidism, the euthyroid status being apparently maintained by a normal or possibly raised serum triiodothyronine (T3) (Pharoah et al., 1976).

If it is not a direct product of the deficiency of elemental iodine, another related thyroid factor may be disturbance of thyroid hormone binding proteins, or of thyroxal binding globulins. The iodine deficiency appears to operate in the embryonic phase of neurodevelopment, that is before foetal maturation of the thyroid follicle between the 12th and 13th week of gestation (Norris, 1916), disturbance of iodine trapping and synthesis of thyroxine (T4) late in the first trimester being the result (Fisher et al., 1977). Aberrant neuronal proliferation, migration organization and myelination will be involved. Pharoah et al. (1976) was able to confirm this timing of neuropathic operation of iodine deficiency since prophylaxis of such endemic cretinism necessitated iodine supplementation before conception.

The impairment of brain development at a critical stage is thus placed after the 13th-14th week, perhaps extending through the third trimester. Neurone and dendrite growth is mainly affected. Gliotic lesions have been identified in the globus pallidus (de Long, 1993). In what way this correlates with the proximal motor rigidity is not clear. But in classical myxoedematous hypothyroidism, a better level of intellectual, motor and hearing function is found. A second possibly independent factor in the pathogenesis of iodine deficiency is endemic cretinism.

## Effects of Hyperthermia:
## Experimental and Human

The impact of hyperthermia on the ependymal cells of the developing brain is an important consideration. Experimental studies on the guinea pig (Edwards, 1969) have demonstrated that maternal hyperthermia of 1.5°C above normal during the first third or half of gestation interrupts the growth of neuronal mitotic cells in the ependymal layer of the developing brain. The residual impact depends upon the timing, severity and duration of the hyperthermia. Elevation of 3°C or more tends to kill these cells. When the hyperthermia is induced at the time of neural tube closure, failure of closure occurs. In the period corresponding to 4 to 6 weeks of human development, severe hyperthermia (2-3° elevation for 1 hour daily) led to microcephaly with "dumb" offspring often hypotonic with microphthalmia. Hyperthermia at the equivalent of 7 to 14 human weeks led to problems in spinal cord morphogenesis.

Evidence of the association of episodes of high fever in a human has been related to neural tube defects. All the cases manifested some form of CNS deficit, and the most consistent neuromuscular abberation was *hypotonia,* with about half the patients showing correlated *hyperactive reflexes* (hypotonic diplegia).

With regard to potential dysmorphogenesis in early gestation, the majority of defects in which hyperthermia occurred between 4 to 7 weeks of gestation and may be secondary to the associated CNS involvement, for example, microphthalmia, and interference with frontal lobe growth resulting in a small midface and deficit of movement leading to micrognathia, although the cleft lip and palate and ear malformation supports the view that hyperthermia affects facial morphogenesis as well as brain development. Minor limb abnormalities and syndactyly were also produced.

## Genetic Implications

Even genetic factors appear relevant in 10%, in which other members of the family, especially siblings, are affected either with cerebral palsy itself or together with mental defect or epilepsy. The most common is inherited as the autosomal dominant form of Familial Spastic Diplegia which closely conforms with so-called hereditary spastic paraplegia or Strompell's disease. It is important to note that a progressive element is conspicuous in these hereditary cases, and that an insidious onset of spasticity may be appreciated in the lower extremities. Rare variants also occur in which spasticity is associated with other neurogenic, ocular or cutaneous manifestation, overlapping with spino-cerebellar degeneration.

There are also a few families with dominant genetic inheritance of so-called Familial Chorea, and less often of athetosis, unaccompanied by other neurological signs. Clear single-gene causation has indeed marked some cases. Several of the congenital ataxias have likewise been inheritable. The possibility of genetically-determined *predisposition* to cerebral palsy also remains a significant challenge.

In this context, some fundamental findings have emerged (Goldblatt et al., 1989) in relation to the genetic aetiology of X-linked spastic paraplegias (HSP), most forms of which are inherited as autosomal conditions. Inheritance as an X-linked recessive has already been defined in several pedigrees. In one such, linkage was demonstrated between HSP and genetic markers on the distal long arm of the x-chromosome ($X_q$). Another showed linkage to loci in the $X_q$ 21-22 (central) region of the long arm of the X-chromosome, including DXYSi (pDF34) and not to the distal $X_q$ loci. Another pedigree, this time within India, revealed X-linkage associated with nystagmus, optic atrophy, mental retardation and mild ataxia of the arms.

There is substantial *clinical heterogeneity* of the X-forms of spastic paraplegia. Whether this can be reduced to *molecular heterogeneity*, with various mutations at one locus responsible for such phenotypic variability as is observed, remains to be elucidated.

In many cases, the onset is in infancy with delay in walking, although the onset may even be deferred in extreme cases until the seventh decade. Cardinal symptoms are spasticity of the legs, a stiff-slow gait, and inability to run. Toe-stepping and easy tripping are characteristic.

Pes cavus appears in one fourth, and accompanying the spasticity, hyperreflexia, clonus and positive Babinski signs.

Impairment of vibration and position sense sometimes follows with the EMG showing distal denervation. The legs become weak subsequently. Initially normal, the arms may later show increasingly brisk reflexes, and even some distal muscle wasting particularly in the hands, with the EMG showing denervation of the distal limb muscles. Somato-sensory evoked potentials are small or unobtainable, probably as an expression of the dorsal column degeneration.

MR imaging would clarify the differential diagnosis which would require exclusion of a range of causes of other slowly progressive myelopathy. These include cervical spondylosis, intraspinal tumours, arteriovenous malformation of the cord, multiple sclerosis and amyotrophic lateral sclerosis.

Experimental exploration in mutant mice of a genetic basis for spatial learning may also have exciting relevance as a source of a recently identified CP anomaly of spatial perception which is described later in this Chapter.

## Increased Prevalence of CP in Multiple Pregnancies

Indeed it is held that CP is four or five times more frequent amongst children born as a result of twin pregnancy. The importance of this fact should be measured against the high proportion of twin pregnancies in the general population of 12 per 1000 live-births. The higher prevalence of CP in multiple pregnancies is a challenging source of the recent study of genetic or interrelated genetic and

environmental factors by Laplaza and colleagues (1992) in a series of 1217 children with CP. Eighty-six CP twins were found, the rate of CP in twins being shown to be *six times higher than in singletons*. The distribution of the different CP entities was similar to that in singletons, although according to Pharoah (1992) diplegics constituted a somewhat higher proportion, at 46%. A significantly higher prevalence of

CP in twins was clearly established, monozygotic twins having a higher risk of CP than dizygotic twins. This increased incidence of CP as a product of twin pregnancy especially affected mothers less than 24 or more than 34 years of age. This greater prevalence in twins had also been confirmed by Leon Root (1988) who identified 86 twins in his series of 1217 children with cerebral palsy. A genetic basis was not supported. The prevalence of CP in this study was 7.1% and in the study of 86 twins, the rate was six times higher than in singletons. Associated prematurity is an added factor, as was illustrated back in 1960 by the data of Illingworth and Woods who found that 35.9% of their children with CP were born prematurely in comparison with the far higher level of 78%, arrived at by Russell (1961) amongst CP children who are products of twin pregnancies.

The enhanced multiplicity of births - and possibly of congenital anomalies including Down's syndrome (Sharav, 1991) - related to delayed conception beyond the 15th day of the menstrual cycle, and the consequent aging gamete may have a bearing upon this association of increased prevalence of CP with multiple births. In other words, this may be one common early prenatal or rather post-conceptual aetiological factor accounting for a proportion of CP. Other data supporting a common prenatal factor is higher incidence of foetal loss either prior to or after the pregnancy associated with CP. It has been estimated (Nelson, 1988) that the mothers of child subjects of CP suffered 35% more foetal loss in previous pregnancies than in the general population. In other studies even 47% has been cited (Hall et al., 1989). The greatly augmented preterm prevalence in twins may be another reflection of a common aetiological factor, even stemming from the gamete itself.

Indeed the rates of preterm and very low birth-weight (<1500g) infants expected in twin pregnancies are 60 and 12% respectively (McCarthy et al., 1981; Morales et al., 1989). The distribution of the different entities of twin CP is similar to that in CP singletons, although diplegics constitute the somewhat higher proportion of 46% than is revealed in the large CP population of the Mersey Region surveyed by Pharoah (1992). The lowest birth-weights in the twin CP series (mean 1430g) in fact characterized the hemiplegics. The 13% rate of congenital malformations in this group also overshadows the 3% rate expected in twins (Little and Bryan, 1986) and adds weight to the above hypothesis and the circumstantial evidence favouring early prenatal factors in the aetiology of CP. Likewise, this is supported by the higher monozygous (MZ) dizygous (DZ) ratios for CP, i.e. that MZ twins have a higher risk of CP, and the higher concordance for CP amongst DZ twins.

# Intra-uterine Growth Retardation:
# A Relevant Role in Cerebral Palsy including the place of
# Maternal Hyperoxygenation in its Treatment
# and Prevention of CP

It has also been hypothesized by Blair and Stanley (1990), and others, that the phenomenon of *intra-uterine growth retardation* may be of greater relevance to the aetiology of CP than preterm birth. Recent data from case control studies have indicated a strong relationship between it and CP arising in infants of over 34 weeks gestation. It has been presumed that it may stem from a cause common to both the CP and the growth retardation. It remains probable that damaged or defective cerebro-cortical maturation can lead to poor growth in utero, even attended by considerably reduced foetal movements. Nevertheless, none of over 80 personal examples of the intra-uterine growth syndrome first identified by Russell (1954) and ascribed to interwoven facets of embryopathy and placentopathy, have shown any element of CP. Its relatively normal head size, even leading to the term "pseudo-hydrocephalus" in the original French literature, may contribute to this freedom from brain damage and impaired brain growth.

Whilst the numbers of surviving very low birth-weight infants or those small for gestational age (SGA) have increased, the incidence of CP in those groups has increased by the same proportion. IUGR has thus come to be related to the increased incidence of CP (Illingworth, 1985). The changing prenatal and gestational pattern with increasing numbers of SGA infants, dictates more basic research into the causation of intra-uterine growth retardation, its more precise detection during gestation, and the possibility of effective treatment in-utero.

A strong relationship has emerged between IUGR and CP in infants of over 34 weeks gestation, again possibly both generated by a common cause. One such possible factor may be the defective or damaged motor area of brain *per se* leading to poor overall growth of the foetus, with the reduced foetal movements characterizing IUGR possibly being one causative component. The series of Uvebrant and Hagberg (1992) embracing 519 child subjects of CP born between 1967-1982 were compared in relation to intra-uterine growth retardation with a control series of 445 children. There was a significantly increased risk of CP in small-for-gestational age infants in term and moderately preterm infants. The highest proportion amongst CP infants born at term was in tetraplegics, and a lesser proportion in diplegics and dyskinetic forms of CP. Bearing in mind that so many SGA infants including the syndrome reported by Russell (1954) appear to escape cerebral brain damage, their overall conclusion appears too far fetched. Not only that SGA primarily reflects early prenatal brain damage, it mediates prenatal risk factors comparable with foetal deprivation, and may also potentiate subsequent adverse effects of birth asphyxia and neonatal hypoxia.

A more precise definition of foetal growth retardation is called for. At present, it ranges from absolute size in terms of low birth-weight (>2500g or 1500g), relative size (SGA) or <3rd or 10th centile or to <2 SD below population mean for gestational age and sex. An overall foetal failure to attain its growth potential is implicit, excluding confusion with factors connected with premature gestation, let alone the embryonic or foetal effects of intra-uterine virus infection or other congenital malformation. Making appropriate allowance for such variables (Teberg, Wallher and Pena, 1988), there is a sixfold risk of neurodevelopmental disability at one year of age.

But the term IUGR has been somewhat loosely extended to include any infant with a low birth-weight for gestational age, although a morphological definition has been pursued whereby the birth-weight is below the 10th percentile, the ponderal index also under the 10th percentile and with evidence of skeletal disproportion in crown-heel length to head circumference. Certainly a particularly high prevalence of CP in this increasingly large group of infants cannot be denied. In Blair and Stanley's large series of 171 spastic white subjects (1990), birth-weights are recorded as having been significantly lower than median births of their comparable population, 22% being below the 10th percentile of the comparable population and weight distribution. They demonstrate a strong statistically significant association between spastic CP and poor intra-uterine growth in 134 cases born at more than 33 weeks gestation, whilst Kyllerman added data regarding a CP incidence of 13.5% with birth- weights <2.5 SD below the mean in term infants (>37 weeks) and 7% in preterm.

In the first place, it is apparent that there are differing entities of such growth retardation, quite distinct from that first reported in five children as "intra-uterine growth deficiency recognizable at birth" by the author. In specifically drawing attention to its distinction from prematurity, he initiated the conception of "Intra-uterine growth retardation" especially in their very low birth-weight of 1 to 1½ kg *despite postmaturity*. They were also associated with sluggish growth of the uterus, relative foetal immobility as well as *episodes of prenatal bleeding* in the mothers of three of these five infants. Placental pathology and presumptively placental "bed" and utero-placental insufficiency, was furthermore supported by their disproportionately small and multiply infarcted placentae which were ultimately revealed after delivery, but could perhaps now be defined by *Doppler* or *ultrasonography* to be referred to overleaf or *other more refined exposure of the "micro-placentae"* or their *impaired vascularity* and *infarction*.

Corresponding histo-morphological pathology of the placental bed has recently been more clearly defined in other variants of intra-uterine growth retardation (Joachim et al., 1992) by Doppler sonography with a pulsed Duplex system of the ACUSEN 128 (3.5 Mhz sector scanner). This technique is capable of identifying clinical, morphological and doppler sonographic signs of utero-placental insufficiency with utero-placental perfusion disturbance even in cases without hypertension. The small size and multiple infarction of the placenta initially stressed by Russell in relation to his category of IUGR could be effectively identified by such sonographic techniques.

*Biopsy of the placental bed* is carrying such histo-morphological study a stage further. A correlation has been tentatively suggested (Hohenhauer, 1980) between blood flow rates and the histological signs of malperfusion. It was claimed that after recognition of an underweight foetus by "ultrasound foetometry" pathological flow parameters were detectable in all examples of foetal growth retardation ostensibly playing a significant role in its pathogenesis. It is true that the presence of the impaired growth and infarction of the placenta could well be the source as well as the product of foetal malnutrition. A major mechanism could be the increased resistance to blood flow and perfusion due to the infarction. In my view, a prenatal cine scanning of the foetal movement pattern may one day establish whether and how early some prenatal expression of cerebral palsy may arise. Hypertonicity may be implied by conspicuous restraint of limb movement, whereas floppiness linked to sparsity of movement could reflect underlying hypotonia. Intermittent *tremor* of hand and arm in reaching out movements may be the first recognizable expression of early atactic involvement.

Furthermore, the grid of Doppler shifts can provide a two-dimensional outline of placental vessels, so that a particular vessel can be picked out for study. Integrity of the trophoblast as the intima of such vessels can be gauged by the uterine artery Doppler. Resistance to flow can also be specifically

assessed as well as the absolute velocity of flow as an indication of volume of flow. In the foetal Doppler, moreover, the falling $PO_2$ levels in the foetus can be measured, and anticipated, with foetal hypoxia likely to be induced by any decrease in foetal oxygenation below the normal level wherever arterial $PO_2$ in the foetus is 25-33% of the arterial $PO_2$ in the adult. Such a decrease may be followed by a reduction in the $PO_2$ of umbilical venous blood (hypoxic-hypoxia).

*Chronic intra-uterine hypoxic-hypercapnia* has been described in association with acidosis, hyperlacticaemia and erythroblastosis. Another expression of the latter as an index of chronic intra-uterine hypoxia was reflected in a study focused on the prediction of perinatal brain damage by umbilical cord plasma levels of erythropoietin (Ruth et al., 1988). A high level characterized infants born after pre-eclampsia regardless of outcome. But asphyxiated infants with a clearly abnormal outcome were all attended by high erythropoietin values (33 to 137 mU/ml). The conclusion reached was that such high values after normal pregnancy but not after pre-eclampsia, pointed to an increased risk for CP - or death.

When chronic foetal distress might be a relevant factor, electronic foetal monitoring of the foetal heart rate pattern could provide a significant index, recognizing that the risk of ultimate CP appears to increase with the duration of abnormal patterns.

The underlying hyperlacticaemia has been ascribed to a combination of factors including an increased placental site of lactate hyperproduction, impaired foetal gluconeogenesis and inadequate oxygen supply (Nicolaides et al., 1989). Pragmatic efforts to decrease the associated foetal morbidity may be better directed towards more comprehensive and intensive antepartum care, bearing in mind in any case that antenatal complications are commoner in infants later showing neurodevelopmental retardation, etc. (Hall et al., 1989; Scott, 1992). For example, one goal should be the earlier detection of IUGR and the protection of the foetus from added hypoxic insult in the hope of reducing foetal morbidity (Niswander et al., 1984).

Other practical aspects in *the prevention of preterm delivery* are concentrated within Chapter 12 entitled "Additional Preventive Implications: other possible antecedents of cerebral palsy".

Trials of maternal hyperoxygenation in the treatment of IUGR have thus been launched (Brown et al., 1990). Foetal blood is sampled at the entrance to the study by cordocentesis for immediate blood gas analysis. In the former, 36 pregnant women were studied between 26 and 34 weeks of gestation. To achieve long-term maternal hyperoxygenation, humidified 55% oxygen was administered continuously at the rate of 8L/min via an MC face-mask (Nicolaides et al., 1989). A significant difference in the Doppler flow patterns was achieved alongside a complementary modification in foetal blood gases. The reduction in foetal mortality was significant with an incidence of 29% and 68% (p <0.01) stemming respectively from treated and untreated groups. Even more convincing on the positive side was the improvement in the

maternal oxygenation status with maintenance of foeto-placental oxygenation. The foetal blood gas concentrations is modified and consequently the chemo receptor-mediated vascular reactivity. The brain sparing effect is reversed, and notably restored on anaerobic metabolism resulting in decreasing incidence of foetal death and neonatal complications.

In the series of Brown et al (1990) 21 pregnant women were evaluated with sonographic evidence in each of IUGR without other obvious abnormality. Maternal oxygen transport was assessed by blood cell 2,3-diphosphoglycarate, haemoglobin oxygen affinity, haemoglobin, pH and PCO2. An important finding was the relationship between the IUG characteristics of foetal and maternal RBC oxygen delivery systems, the RBC 2,3-diphosphoglycerate /Hb molar ratio and the P50 being related significantly to intra-uterine growth.

*Pre-eclampsia* or pregnancy-induced hypertension, a disease of primigravidae, is associated with both a reduced utero-placental flow and IUGR (McGillivrin). According to McIlwaine et al. (1979), it accounts for a perinatal mortality of 1 to 1.5/1000 live births or 7.5-9% of all perinatal deaths, but IUGR is the main cause of the associated increase in perinatal morbidity and mortality. Cruikshank and colleagues (1992) in particular emphasized the relationship between the labetolol treatment of eclampsia and intra-uterine growth retardation. The labetolol operates by blocking the α1-adreno-receptors of peripheral arterioles, thence diminishing peripheral resistance. Utilizing placental scintigraphy, the reduction of vascular resistance can be visualised in the materno-placental circulation.

So-called symmetrical growth retardation which these groups represent appear to be associated with the onset of growth failure at <30 weeks of gestation. Its precise identification, and its timing, still remains the diagnostic and therapeutic challenge already emphasized. In the main, *measurement of utero-foetal growth - and its deceleration or interruption* - remains the critical clinical parameter with confirmatory monitoring by ultrasonography to follow.

The most valid guide to intra-uterine growth insufficiency thus depends upon foetal measurement by ultrasonic means. This can begin early in pregnancy, between 6 and 12 weeks, by measuring the crown-rump length, the length of the foetal back from the crown of the head to the rump. The head-width (or maximal transverse diameter) could then be so measured between 13 to 20 weeks, the abdominal circumference to follow at 32 weeks. Russell, Deter and colleagues have initiated a system of such measurement by computerising the results obtained when high frequency sound waves are beamed at the foetus -without biological hazard. Tanner (1989) has estimated that if applied to the screening of all babies, it could detect even 90% of all small for dates babies, with a negligible number of false positives.

The challenge facing us in this context is whether we can reduce foetal morbidity and especially its CP component, by earlier detection of IUGR with immediate protection of the foetus from added hypoxic insult.

Oxygen is thus one factor readily alterable in the maternal environment and its augmentation by supplemental maternal oxygen can increase placental oxygen transfer and foetal oxygen tension (Netzar et al., 1979) and thereby enhance foetal growth as well as survival (Vilensis, 1985).

The initial enthusiasm of Nicolaides for maternal hyperoxygenation (1989) has been tempered by his realisation (1993), although without scientific confirmation, that exposure of the nutritionally disadvantaged foetus to increased oxygen concentration may have paradoxically adverse effects. These could be the result of heightened oxygen concentrations producing secondary or conditioned nutritional deficiency of already low placento-foetal nutrients.

Limitation of blood flow to the pregnant uterus restricts availability of all potential metabolic substrates both to the placenta itself and subsequently to the growing foetus. The first premise is that basic *maternal* nutrition is adequate. Secondly, adequacy of maternal oxygenation is crucial, as has been clearly illustrated by experimental ligations of the uterine artery (Moll, 1973), although allowance must also be made for a parallel limitation of substrate supply. Inadequacy of oxygen supply to the utero-placental bed will profoundly influence metabolic functions with both placenta and foetal tissue. For example, hypoxia would play a vital role in suppressing fatty acid synthesis in foetal tissue. Likewise, hypoxaemia has long ago been shown to reduce the placental capacity to transfer glucose (Lumley and Wood, 1967) or amino acids (Longo et al., 1973), both contributing significantly to the pathogenesis of foetal growth retardation in pregnancies complicated by utero-placental insufficiency. To what extent this effect is secondarily reinforced by diminution of hypothalamic and other release of growth promoting factors in most entities of IUGR remains to be clarified. In the specific Russell-Silver version, this may well be a primary factor, although the superimposition of the unilateral shortening could well suggest disturbed control of preceding factors of growth regulation *above* hypothalamic levels.

Other such factors may include transforming growth factor ($\alpha$(TGF$\alpha$), a 50 amino acid peptide, and epidermal growth factor (EGF) which act through the same 170 kd tyrosine kinase receptor for signal transduction, both having been implicated as *autocrine* or *paracrine* regulators of cellular function.

If severe *maternal malnutrition* is an aetiological factor, a reduction in energy intake would be one factor leading to pathological foetal growth.

Relatively mild *maternal alcoholism* can be another risk factor for foetal growth retardation with the risk increasing progressively with the number of drinks consumed. The risk of growth retardation are augmented at least five-fold by opiate addiction.

The risk is doubled in the presence of proteinuric pre-eclampsia alone, but quadrupled if superimposed on pre-existing hypertension.

A raised maternal serum $\alpha$ foetoprotein in the first half of pregnancy also carries a foetal risk of growth retardation. A positive predictive value for foetal growth deficiency of 30-50% attends assays of human placental lactogen, oestriol and Schwangerschafs protein-1.

The contribution of maternal smoking to foetal growth retardation may reach 40% in developed countries (Carlson, 1988), infants born to such mothers being 250 g lighter (Nicolaides et al., 1989). It has also been shown that forfeiting both smoking and alcohol in the first half of pregnancy has objectively improved foetal growth.

**Prediction of IUGR**

More precise prediction can be achieved by Doppler ultrasound using recordings from both the uteroplacental and foetal circulation. A study by Campbell et al. (1986) of uteroplacental waveforms in 126 pregnancies at 16-20 weeks demonstrated that abnormal waveforms could predict 68% of pregnancies with foetal growth retardation. Umbilical artery Doppler recordings (Marsal, 1989) can even effectively predict subsequent foetal asphyxia.

**Monitoring Foetal Growth**

Serial ultrasound recording is feasible as a screening procedure in a small proportion of women obviously at risk (James, 1990). In the evaluation of Villai and Belizan (1983) the sensitivity varied from 43-94%, specificity from 84-92% and the positive predictive value from 20-70% and were not dissimilar figures from measurements of fundal-symphysial length.

### Assessment of Foetal Health

Biophysical testing has largely replaced biochemical methods. When exposed to chronic asphyxia or hypoxia, parallel changes may be recognizable: reduction in amniotic fluid volume consequent upon renal dysfunction, and upon cerebral dysfunction, foetal tone, movements, breathing and variability of heart rate.

Perception of foetal movements has long been accepted as an index of foetal health although the use of kick charts in a study of about 70,000 pregnancies showed no reduction in the rate of foetal loss (Grant et al., 1989).

The presence of meconium in the liquor has long been accepted as an ominous sign. Its absence linked to normal foetal heart rates are evidently indicative of foetal well-being during labour, but there is a growing need for well-planned prospective studies aimed at more precise methods of concurrently and continuously assessing the health of the foetus.

### Foetal Heart Rate at Rest

Its measurement at rest proved to have a sensitivity of 50, a specificity of 90%, and a positive predictive value of 40%.

Doppler recordings from foetal vessels appear to be sensitive indices of the foetal circulatory state. Absence of end diastolic recordings in growth-retarded foetuses whether in the umbilical artery or descending aorta or both (Marsal, 1989) relates to a *high incidence of foetal hypoxaemia*, and of *subsequent perinatal asphyxia*. Foetal blood gas tensions can be measured by cordocentesis.

### Management or Treatment of IUGR

One must bear in mid that it is often impossible to distinguish the foetus suffering pathological growth from the foetus constitutionally or genetically small. Investigation must follow to both confirm the diagnosis and identify the aetiology. Further ultrasonic recording of growth may be helpful in the pathologically growing foetus whose growth (especially of the abdomen) will divert from expected trajectories. After carefully weighing the risks that are justifiable, aetiological exploration could include placental biopsy to permit rapid karyotyping, and *umbilical cordocentesis* for both karyotyping and viral serology. Specific measures may be advisable when the foetal abnormality is known.

There is already some evidence that not only can *aspirin* prevent foetal growth retardation, it may also limit or improve it once it exists.

The haemodialysate solcoseryl has also become an important therapeutic consideration. It may improve foetal growth by a combination of effects upon foetal metabolism and upon the maternal circulation. One study of its use recorded a *ten-fold lower incidence of babies small for gestational age.*

# SIGNIFICANCE OF EPIDEMIOLOGICAL APPRAISALS

## Recent Epidemiological Assessments

Recent *epidemiologic studies* at first served to introduce some complex and contradictory evidence, but these are gradually resolving into significant directions. To begin with, one will try to adhere to a uniform use of the term prevalence rather than "incidence" which is sometimes regarded as inappropriate in reference to the cerebral palsies. Mainly this is because they are aetiologically heterogeneous, arising in different phases of foetal and infant development. Prevalence represents the number of cases present during a certain time period, and for CP, this is usually calculated as an age-specific prevalence rate.

Whilst there had been a dramatic fall in the prevalence of cerebral palsy in Sweden from 2.24 per 1000 live births in 1954-58 to 1.34 in 1967-70 (Hagberg et al., 1975) mainly in spastic and ataxic diplegia, it almost simultaneously increased in Western Australia between 1956 to 1975 to an overall rate of 2.5 per thousand live births (Blair and Stanley, 1982) with 90% of those CP children manifesting its spastic or hypertonic form. The proportional prevalence of diplegia in the first five years of this study was only 8%, but rose to 25% during its last five years. The Australian figures of Atkinson and Stanley (1983) concurred with a rate in the region of 2.6 per thousand live births. The prevalence rate in Japan proved to be somewhat lower at 1.9 per 1000 live births (Suzuki and

Kedama, 1991), who also cited the "incidence" of severe mental retardation as 1.0 per 1000. This was confirmed by Suzuki and Iso in 1992 at the slightly higher level of 2.2 per 1000 for a small suburban population of Tokyo.

The Australian figures from 1972 to 1975 were strikingly heightened in low birth-weight infants. Indeed, the relative risk for low birth-weight infants had risen from 12-fold to 26-fold between 1961 and 1975. In several different geographical situations, this uniformly clear trend has emerged, with the prevalence of neuro-developmental disorder rising as the birth-weight declines. Conversely, in what might be called the 3500 to 4500g safe range, prevalence figures may fall as low as 1.6 per thousand live births, whereas they increase more than 100-fold within the very low birth-weight group (<1500g). The analyses of Nelson and Ellenberg (1985 and 1986) carried this even further, indicating that infants of a birth-weight below 1500 grams have a 90% chance of incurring cerebral palsy, contrasting with only 0.3% for a term infant weighing more than 2500 grams.

Applying differences in birth-weight-specific rates using live births and neonatal survivors as denominator, the rate of cerebral palsy per thousand survivors, weighing less than 2000g at birth in the study of Stanley (1979) had reached 20.9 per thousand, whilst the rate per thousand live births of the same weight equalled 14.1 g. With birth-weight reaching lower extremes, it has been repeatedly confirmed in widespread studies that the prevalence rate of CP is strikingly heightened. It varies from 2 to 5% where the birth-weight is below 1000 to 1500g. Below 800g, prevalence even reaches 6 to 24%. Nevertheless, infants of very low birth-weight account for less than one quarter of the total CP incidence in infants. Very similar trends have also been reported from Finland and Ireland. At the end of the earlier Swedish phase already mentioned (Hagberg et al., 1975), however, an expected parallel improvement in the survival of premature infants, hopefully linked to advances in their intensive care, did not materialize. It was moreover galling to learn that the promising trend in Sweden had really undergone some significant reversal between 1971 and 1978.

As thus expressed in the various forms of cerebral palsy, an overall prevalence still abtains in Sweden of 1.5 per thousand live births whilst several texts have arrived at an estimate for Great Britain ranging between 2 and 3 per thousand live births.

We can also turn to the more precise studies led by Pharoah (1987) based upon the Mersey region. They analyzed the rates of CP from 1966 to 1984 as a function of birth-weight. During this period, the prevalence rate of CP in very low birth-weight infants (<1500g) increased to a striking degree from 13 to 14 to over 64 per thousand live births. During the study (Pharoah, 1992) the relative proportions of CP that are of low birth-weight altered from 30% to 65%. As in Western Australia, the risk of CP rose as birth-weight fell. Likewise, a significant rise in the prevalence of CP in the region of Turku, Finland from 1968-1972 to 1978-1982 (Riikonen et al., 1989) from 1.6 per 1000 live births to 2.5 per 1000 live births was attributed to an increase of CP in low birth-weight children (p=0.0002). That this was due to increased survival is an interesting view that has been challenged elsewhere. On the other hand, many more low birth-weight infants survived who did not manifest CP. The prevalence for low birth-weights between 1501 and 2500g rose much less, with a peak of approx. 4 per thousand live births, whilst that for more than 2500g remained constant between 1 and 2 per thousand.

## Epidemiological Focus upon Prevalence of Hemiplegia

The epidemiology, aetiology and developmental outcome of the apparently steady increase in the prevalence of hemiplegic CP were subjected to analysis in a retrospective population-based survey in south-west Sweden (Uvebrant, 1988). The earlier birth-year phase from 1969 to 1978 was covered. This was an especially good

example of the opportunities for correlation with neuroradiology which the new imaging techniques now invite. First of all the prevalence at ages 6-15 years has reached 0.66 per 1000, with postnatally-acquired forms, mainly post-infectious, iatrogenic or post-traumatic, comprising 11% thereof. Of the term children, the prenatal aetiology consisted mainly of cerebrovascular and maldevelopmental factors. The rate of preterm birth amongst these congenital cases was 24%.

Clinical follow-up differentiated 152 cases into 50% of mild motor dysfunction, 31% moderate and 19% severe, the total handicap in the latter being highest amongst postnatal cases.

In the exemplary study of spastic hemiplegia in 1048 low birth-weight survivors (Powell, Pharoah, Cooke and Rosenbloom, 1988) 16 were clinically identified from 42 cases of CP. The increased prevalence was found to be associated with previous reproductive loss, breech vaginal delivery, later birth order, prolonged second stage of delivery, emergency Caesarian section and low Apgar score. It could be calculated that such variables could identify a higher or lower estimated probability of hemiplegia. There was also an association of hemiplegia with prolonged respiratory disease and intraventricular haemorrhage.

Impairment of the stereognostic sense, so often characterizing CP, was elicited by Uvebrant (1988) in 44% of his series, extending to astereognosis in 20%. It is also important to note that ultrasonography of the hemiplegics exposed unilaterality of the ventricular dilatation in 36%, and cortical/subcortical cavities in 20%. There was a strong correlationship between the CT findings and the degree of severity and magnitude of the associated handicap. A normal CT scan implied mild disability, whilst moderate disability was related to unilateral ventricular dilatation with severe

handicap - extending to mental retardation and epilepsy - proving to be closely related to cortical/subcortical cavities.

It is technically of considerable interest that in 25 hemiplegic children subjected to single photon emission computed tomography (SPECT) using N-isopropyl-p-1-123-iodo amphetamine (Hamano et al., 1991), *crossed cerebellar diaschisus* (CCD) was demonstrated in five (20%). Seven of these 25 were diagnostically labelled as CP, whilst in the others hemiplegia appeared to be the sequel to a brain injury acquired between ten months and fourteen years of age. CCD was not detected in those with prenatal CP, although ipsilateral cerebellar diaschisis was definable in two cases of postnatal CP.

The focus, however, was specifically upon small-for-gestational age (SGA) infants in relation to CP. In the recent analysis of 104 cases of spastic CP by the outstanding Australian workers, Blair and Stanley (1992), they attempted to vindicate an hypothesis that such subjects of CP differed in their birth morphologies as defined in terms of weight, length, head circumference, ponderal index and length to head circumference ratios from that of the normal liveborn population. Dimensions were considered in terms of percentile ranges of the appropriate populations. Their previous studies have consistently confirmed a highly significant association of spastic CP with low weight for gestational age (SGA) in infants of over 34 weeks gestation. They have now gone on to demonstrate that such abnormal measurements defined as associated with extreme risk contained 44.4% of cases of spastic CP in excess of the proportion in the total population, more than half of those excess cases who manifested more severe clinical forms presumably of hypertonicity being short for their gestation, size deficits postulated as originating before the third trimester. In contrast, a "milder" degree of spastic CP in a further excess of 7.4% was associated with a head circumference above the 90th percentile. The source of this was not clarified.

*In school-age children*, the prevalence in British and USA surveys (Nelson and Ellenberg, 1978) ranged between 1.4 and 3.0 per thousand. In their analysis between 1959 and 1966, covering 54,000 pregnant women, an overall 5.2 per thousand children were still alive at the age of seven years. If the mildly affected were excluded, this figure fell to 2.6 per thousand. Spastic diplegics constituted 32% of these, and hemiplegia 29%. Their conclusion at that stage was that there was no evidence of a decrease in the incidence of total congenital cerebral palsy and/or of spastic diplegia. On the other hand, contemporary figures for Great Britain should soon emerge, when

conclusions are reached on six regional surveys of CP, including that of the Mersey Region (Pharoah et al., 1990) outlined above, which in all cover more than 330,000 children (Alberman, 1991). Meanwhile, a remarkable consistency of prevalence rates throughout the Western world still shows minimal fluctuations around 2.0 per thousand live births.

School age populations have also been used as the denominator. During the two decades mainly referred to above, there has been increasing awareness that minor degrees of motor disability whether or not linked to developmental delay may be associated with clumsy, uncoordinated or awkward behaviour which may not amount to overt cerebral palsy. Such borderline disorder of brain function, estimated to affect about 4-5% of the school population, has been glibly embraced by the term "minimal cerebral dysfunction" although "maximal cerebral confusion" of the professionals too readily prone to this diagnosis, might be more aptly applied.

## Correlationships with Socio-biological Risk Factors: Gestational Age, Birth-weight, Male Preponderance and Socio-Economic Factors

The most common relationship reported between birth factors and the cerebral palsies is that between birth-weight and gestational age. In respect of birth-weight, specific prevalence in different countries displays a striking consistency (Childs and Evans, 1954; Russell, 1960). Nonetheless, the association with gestational age may be of greater significance, even if mainly

documented in retrospective studies. The important differences between risks of CP amongst preterm births compared with the "intra-uterine growth retarded" have been acknowledged (Alberman, 1963; Stanley et al., 1981). The relationship between birth-weight, gestational age, and the spastic syndromes - which predominate among all cerebral palsy populations - was studied by both the Stanley group and Eva Alberman. Davies and Tizard demonstrated what we have already stressed, i.e. that spastic diplegia confined to the legs (paraplegia) arose more often amongst infants who had been preterm. Evans had previously drawn attention to the contrast between infants with congenital spasticity, for whom prematurity had been the commonest finding, and athetoids for whom a stormy birth, often instrumental, had been commonly succeeded by severe neonatal asphyxia and convulsions.

But a more detailed study by Childs and Evans (1954) has revealed a subdivision, within both spastic diplegia and paraplegia into cases premature by birth-weight and those of more normal birth-weight, suggesting even different aetiological bases. In spastic diplegia it was concluded that there was a bimodal distribution of birth-weight (Churchill, 1958; Russell, 1960). Moreover the low birth-weight group tended to be of a more mixed clinical pattern with a higher proportion of other handicaps and mental retardation. It later became apparent (Alberman, 1963) that whilst some syndromes were especially related to gestational age, others were particularly related to foetal growth rate.

The birth prevalence of spastic diplegia, for example, increased sharply with diminishing gestational age and falling birth-weight. Other types of CP showed no such relationship with gestational age. The cohort study of Ellenberg and Nelson (1979 and 1981) applied to 54,000 children between 1959 and 1966, acquired follow-up data on 40,000 children aged 7 years. A very significant association with birth-weight was confirmed; the risk amongst infants weighing less than 1501g at any gestational age was 27 times that for those weighing 2500g or more, and born at term. Males had a higher risk than females in nearly all categories.

## Male Preponderance

This higher risk of CP amongst males was a consistent biological association. Whilst probably directly related to the presence of the Y chromosome, the precise mechanism accounting for the higher incidence in the male foetus and infant of such "brain damage" (Neligan et al., 1976; Stanley, 1979) and in general, of their greater vulnerability from conception onwards, remains to be clarified. One recent example (Largo et al., 1990) was a cross-sectional study of 249 preterm children, with 97 preterm and 93 term children as controls. Neurological outcome at 5-6 years of age showed that 15% of the boys and 9% of the girls in the preterm group had CP. Mild spastic diplegia was most often observed. A small but consistent sex difference in neurological outcome in favour of the term and preterm girls was identified. It also appears to be equally applicable to examples of spastic and other syndromes of CP where brain damage has been regarded as of *post-natal* aetiology.

## Socio-economic Factors

Their importance have not received adequate attention in previous studies. A survey undertaken in Cape Town, South Africa (Arens and Molteno, 1989) compared the relationship of three ethnic groups to the prevalence of postnatally-acquired CP, the main causes of which were documented as cerebral infections (particularly meningitis), cerebral trauma, and cerebrovascular accidents. In the so-called "white" group considered to occupy the highest socioeconomic stratum, the percentage was 13,2, in the coloured (of mixed ancestry) it was 24.0 and in the black group occupying the lowest socio-economic stratum the figure was 36.1%.

A large group of 289 cases of CP born in the Eastern Health Board area of the Republic of Ireland provided the setting for a study aimed to examine the influence of social class on the prevalence of CP (Dowding and Barry, 1990). Principally, a clear social class gradient was defined in the overall prevalence of CP, but also solely in the individual syndromes of hemiplegia and diplegia. The social class gradient evident solely in these entities suggest an important aetiological role for environmental factors. Intra-uterine growth retardation, on the other hand, seemed to be equally a factor in CP across all social class groups. The prevalence of CP of significant severity ("severe enough to prevent walking by the fourth birthday"...) clearly increased with socio-economic disadvantage.

## Prevalence of Different Entities of CP

Changes in the relative proportions of the major categories of CP are also worthy of note. For the normal birth-weight infants, the proportions of hemiplegia, diplegia and quadriplegia had remained fairly constant in the West. But in very low birth-weight infants, particularly during recent years up to 1993, there has been a distinctive increase in hemiplegias with the proportion even reaching 31.2%. The proportion of spastic diplegias has declined but still constitutes about one-third, with a disproportionate survival of severe quadriplegias. Unhappily, this also exposed an increasing proportion of severe mental retardation. But in a large Indian series of 544 cases of CP (Srivastava et al., 1992), 497 or 91.4% are still described as of spastic type, although 28.7% of these are hemiplegic with tetraplegics at 34.9% constituting the highest proportion. Of the remainder, the proportion of hypotonic, ataxic and athetoid CP categories were 5.5%, 1.5% and 1.3% respectively, mental retardation being already associated in 47.2%. In a recent Japanese report (Suzuki and Ito, 1992), of 100 children with CP (56 boys, 44 girls), spastic cases totalled 71% (tetraplegia 36%, diplegia 20%, but hemiplegia only 15%). It was associated with other severe handicaps in 70%, the commonest being epilepsy in 35% followed by deafness, speech disorders and blindness in that order.

Such figures firmly draw attention to the need for a continuing appraisal of the net effects of improved intensive care. It may even be suggested that the figures of increased prevalence amongst very low birth-weight infants stem from advances in *perinatal* care, leading to improved chances of survival, even though with increasingly severe or extensive brain damage.

# FACTORS UNDERLYING DISORDERS OF NEURONAL MIGRATION

## Developmental Neurobiology and Congenital Anomalies of the Brain

Congenital cerebral anomaly may still be causative of CP, and may even remain the greatest source of infantile neurological handicap in the view of outstanding perinatal pathologist, J.S. Wigglesworth (1989). Cerebral cortical dysgenesis, secondary to disordered neuronal migration, probably accounts for almost one third of CP in term infants. Clinical and neurogenetic understanding of them has been especially opened up by their recognition during life through high resolution MRI.

More than one anomaly may co-exist in a single brain, especially of migrational anomalies leading to a polymicrogyria or to lissencephaly, clinically characterized by spastic tetraplegia, decerebration, microcephaly, severe mental retardation, seizures and *even a CP pattern of "atonic diplegia"*. A spectrum of anomalies can be defined as stretching from the lissencephalies at one end (Aicardi, 1991) to periventricular nodular heterotopias at the other. Indeed it has long ago been seriously suggested that lissencephaly, diffuse pachygyria and generalized heterotopias may be the expression of variations in severity of the same process (Friede, 1989). Even if the initial diagnosis is made by ultrasound, it is now worthwhile to confirm it by magnetic resonance imaging (long TR MRI scans). Cystic lesions may warrant an additional modality such as injection of radionucleotide or contrast material into subarachnoid, ventricular, or cystic spaces. It also appears that ultrasonography is superior to CT at visualizing cyst walls which interrupt the speed of communication with ventricles.

The morphogenetic developmental events which ensue embody the following:

1. *Primary neurolation/dorsal induction.*
2. *Ventral induction.*
3. *Neuronal proliferation* followed by neuronal migration, neuronal organization and neuronal myelination.

The central nervous system evolves through two broad sequences of complex cellular processes. *Firstly*, events that are completed during the first half of gestation, that of cytogenesis and histogenesis initiated with the formation of neuroblasts and many glial cells in a specialized columnar epithelium lining the ventricular cavities: the ependymal matrix or periventricular germinal zones (Fig 1). *Thence their migration or failure of migration to specific cortical positions*, with concurrent development of primary neuritic processes contributing to dendritic fields and axon fascicles. The overlapping processes of proliferation and migration begin about the 6th gestational week and extends to mid-gestation. *Secondly* comes the differentiation and growth of neurons, the elaboration of

## Embryonic Neural Tube

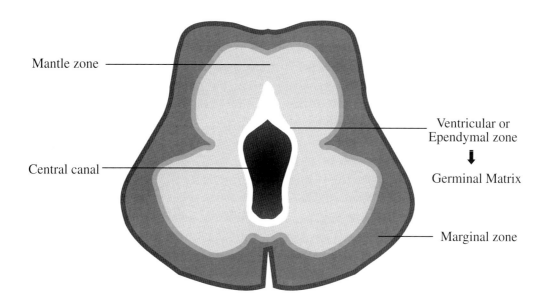

Mantle zone

Central canal

Ventricular or
Ependymal zone

⬇

Germinal Matrix

Marginal zone

terminal dendritic and axonal arborizations. During migration the neuroblasts are closely attached to radial glial fibres which serve as guides for the ultimate neuroblast distribution and positioning into specific ontogenic columns and layers within cyto-architectural areas of the cortex. This is preceded by progressive detachment from these fibres, presumably as a result of reduced biophysical affinity or derangement of molecular mechanisms responsible for neuron-glial interactions. That this cyto-architectonic cortical positioning is pre-empted in a stem-all "proto map" source within the periventricular germinal matrix has been convincingly postulated by Rakic (1988). The eventual laydown occurs in the well-known "inside-out" fashion, the first cells to migrate ending in the deeper cortical positions. If the above detachment should

fail, subsequent migrating neuroblasts could not pass and would lead to a residual heterotopia. Parallel pruning of the organisation of circuitry linked to regressive changes, probably add to the potential of the developing CNS to adapt to injury. Within the cerebellum on the other hand, a subpially treated generative zone gives rise to the granular cells, interneurons of the molecular layer and glial species of the cerebellar cortex.

**Pathogenesis of Migration Derangements**

Several forms of diffuse or generalized migration defects may arise following arrest of such migration at different levels or stages along their centrifugal path.

The possible pathogenic factors accounting for such disturbed migration

(Friede, 1989) could include damage to the radial glial fibres by hypoxaemia or ischaemia around the 16th week of gestation. The expected outcome would be subcortical heterotopia position for the associated neuroblasts. Another possibility in more diffuse disorders of abnormal gyration like lissencephaly would be a diminished initial number of proliferative units in the periventricular germinal matrix, or damage thereto. The damaging influence would therefore be timed even before the onset of migration, i.e. before the 6th week of gestation. An overall smaller true cortical area as a result is in fact demonstrable in diffuse pachygyria and lissencephaly.

On the other hand, if the total or partial migration is *selective*, some glial neuronal pathways would be obstructed and some would not. The timing of the damaging influence, the extent of the consequent glial radial fibre injury, and the site of involvement along these glial guides could each contribute. In the "double cortex" syndromes the site of maximal damage would be distal, with heterotopic close to the cortical mantle. Much more proximal damage could account for diffuse laminar heterotopias in a periventricular position. Where pathology is patchy or discontinuous, the heterotopias would tend to be nodular, or in discontinuous laminar abnormality typifying the double cortex syndrome (Palmini et al., 1991).

Structural abnormalities of the developing brain stemming from a multiplicity of factors disrupting such neurobiological processes, are an important source of cerebral palsy. They constitute a significant proportion of the gross malformations which mar 3-5% of live births. These cerebral malformations take three basic forms: *true malformation*, *tissue deformations* and *tissue destructions* which have remained unexplained in life until high resolution MRI investigation was prompted by intractable seizures. Whether those most relevant to cerebral palsy interfere firstly with the growth and differentiation of neurons peaking during the second half of gestation, remains to be resolved. For instance, in lissencephaly associated with the absence of sulcation, the major insult and interruption of neuronal migration is believed to occur before the end of the third month of gestation, succeeding waves of migrating neurones being thereby prevented from reaching the cortex. There is thus a morphological association with various grey matter heterotopias or macrogyria - which produce a similar clinical pattern as in lissencephaly - micropolygyria, disturbed cortical lamination as in the "double cortex" or even schizencephaly - with clefts extending from the cortex to the ventricular cavity. There is also the view of Menkes that the primary teratogenic stimulus may strike *after* the 30-day induction period and before the onset of primary sulcation at 60 days. Recent work in both primates and humans (Rakic, 1988) has indeed confirmed that both the proliferation of neuroblasts at the periventricular germinal matrix and then migration to the cortical mantle begin *around the sixth gestational week,* extending thereafter until mid-gestation.

*Disorders of cerebral gyration* are amongst the most conspicuous of abnormal outcome. Typically, they derive from disturbances already mentioned in neuronal migration from the pseudostratosphere of germinal cells lining the ventricular cavities. The timing of this process is important, that of gyrus formation on the medial cortical surfaces being before 20 weeks, and that on the lateral aspects after 24 weeks, with microgyria and polymicrogyria being the especially dominant defects. But most of the viable brain defects affecting gyration derive from *subtotal necrosis* of the cortex which marks the second half of gestation (Evrard, 1989). And most of the microgyria appear to arise *after the end of neuronal migration* and before the establishment of cortical gyration between 20 and 30 weeks. Foetal accidents or infections appear to induce polymicrogyria during this same period.

These and other related anomalies such as pachygyria, subcortical laminar heterotopia or the "double cortex" syndrome, and periventricular laminar heterotopia appear to represent stages along a continuum of migration defects. High resolution MR imaging is naturally being focussed more and more upon the clarification of this whole neurobiological issue. Studying 10 patients between 6 and 23 years (mean age 14 years 5 months) Guerrini et al. (1992) detected bilateral macrogyric-like maldevelopment of the insulo-opercular regions. An anatomo-clinical syndrome was indeed defined comprising the bi-opercular gyral anomaly linked with pseudo-bulbar palsy (cortical or central) and mental retardation. The associated epilepsy varied greatly in age at onset and severity, diffuse EEG abnormalities and intractable seizures especially marking five of these, relief being achieved by anterior callosotomy in one case. Epilepsy may indeed emerge

relatively late in these particular malformations. Apart from infective pathogenic factors to be discussed, a possible genetic basis should not be overlooked. In particular, this is suggested but not proven in the familial cases of lissencephaly reported by Dobyns (1989) or of bilateral perisylvian micropolygyria documented by Andermann et al. (1992).

That *early prenatal infection*, in particular with *congenital cytomegalovirus infection*, may play a highly relevant role in causing such basic disorder of neuronal migration has been recently documented by Hayward et al. (1991). Their work was in relation to five multiply-handicapped children in whom lissencephaly-pachygyria was unearthed. This gives added point to the outline below of the more important illustration of such disorders of gastrulation, and neuronal migration, etc. Evidence has grown that such defects even limited to "*minor* cortical dysgenesis", may lead to functional disturbance ranging from minimal learning disabilities to major motor and cognitive handicaps, possibly even constituting the unexpected bases of forms of dyslexia, or of autism as well as partial epilepsy.

The organogenetic period from the 3rd to the 8th weeks of pregnancy encompasses the period of *gastrulation* ranging between 15 and 19 days post-conception. This first major developmental phase in the normal morphogenesis of the nervous system is crucial to the induction of some of the common malformations of skull and brain, such as those related to chromosomal defects, particularly Trisomy 13 in which *rigidity* is clinically characteristic, especially affecting the hands to produce the classical "fisting". Arrhinencephaly and holoprosencephaly are included, apart from maldevelopment of the pituitary. CT scanning by Shanks and Wilson (1988) revealed that a spectrum of an holoprosencephalic malformation complex may present with spastic diplegia.

## The Lissencephalies and Early Prenatal Infection with Cytomegalovirus

The early prenatal role of cytomegalovirus (CMV) in the aetiology of CP is at last being confirmed as long suspected. The correlation between CP and prenatal CMV infection confirmed by serology and virus culture in the neonate was clearly defined in 9 of 10 affected children studied by Boesch et al. (1989). Severe mental retardation accompanied the CP, which in one patient was of the ataxic form, and also attended by deafness. The MRI visualization was of particular interest, all nine showing evidence of destruction or atrophy in the shape of dilated lateral ventricles and a dilated subarachnoid space in eight. A vital aspect in this context was the oligopachygyria in 8, as well as delayed/pathological myelination in 7, paraventricular cysts adjacent to the occipital horns of the lateral ventricles and solely separated by a thin membrane in what may become to be a specific sign of the prenatal impact of CMV in 6 with intracerebral calcification only in one. The evidence of oligopachygyria is especially significant, since it may be a reflection of the underlying lissencephaly attributable to interruption of neuronal migration which was so dramatically identified in a subsequent report (Hayward et al., 1991) as a product of congenital cytomegalovirus consistently leading to tetraplegic CP.

The brain is therefore characteristically marked by absent or poor brain sulcation. Both CT and MRI scans clearly confirmed evidence of migrational CNS defects characteristic of the nineteenth century term Lissencephaly, literally meaning "smooth brain", a cortex resembling the smooth two to four month foetal cortex (Fig 2). In the cases reported by Hayward and colleagues (1991), related anomalies were added typical of pachygyria, colcephaly, incomplete opercularization, thickened cortical mantle and sparse arborizing white matter with especially abnormal periventricular white matter linked to ventriculomegaly. With CT scanning, it was also possible to reveal degrees of its classical periventricular calcification. Two relevant clinico-pathological entities have been identified. Congenital CMV infection was considered present if urinary culture for CMV is positive during the first week of life or anti-CMV immunoglobulin (Ig)M or G is raised at birth. Neonatal jaundice accompanied by hepatomegaly were also early warnings, clarified in this instance by raised CMV-specific immunoglobulin M or viral isoeatin from urine. Spastic tetraplegia, severe psychomotor delay and seizures characterized all five *Type I*, or the Miller-Dicker syndrome as first described in 1963 (Jones, 1988).

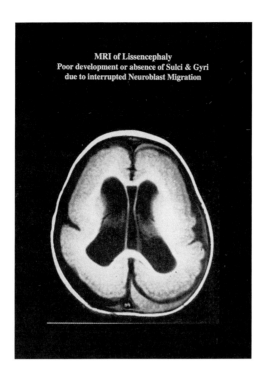

MRI of Lissencephaly
Poor development or absence of Sulci & Gyri
due to interrupted Neuroblast Migration

The cortical surface is smooth with broad gyri and areas of pachygyria and heterotopias interspersed. The corpus callosum is absent as well as frontal and temporal opercula. There is failure of migration of the first generated neurones destined for cortical layers V and VI, but these cases furthermore represent extremely severe examples of the effects of CMV on neurological growth, maturation and development. *Bitemporal narrowing* marks the microcephaly of clearly prenatal onset together with a high forehead, small nose with anteverted nostrils, and the micrognathia. There may also be clinodactyly.

Type 2 Lissencephaly or Warburg syndrome, first recorded in 1971, showed agyria, pachygyria, cerebellar hypoplasia, occipital encephalocele or Dandy-Walker cyst, and obstructive hydrocephalus microphthalmia. Principal dysmorphic failures apart from the microcephaly with bi-temporal narrowing relate to the eyes including megalocornea, cataract and retinal dysplasia.

Congenital cytomegalovirus (CMV) infection imposes an increasingly grave universal problem. Fatality early in life or serious neurological and/or perceptual organ damage is the outcome in over 10% of CMV infected infants. The pre-existing maternal antibodies to which we have referred may be protective (Fowler et al., 1992) but not consistently or adequately. Transmission of CMV to the foetus during pregnancy may follow recurrent infection (Peckham et al., 1983). Resulting congenital infection in consecutive siblings (Embil et al., 1970; Ho, 1991) has been reported.

In a recent such example (Nigro et al., 1993), fever during the fifth month of pregnancy was attended by high levels of CMV specific IgG antibodies. CMV infection was confirmed by viral isolation from urine and saliva, accompanied by IgM and IgA antibodies detected by enzyme immunoassay. The infant's complement fixing titre was 1:32 (same as her mother). Subsequently, intermittent urine and salivary CMV excretion was associated with persistently high levels of CMV specific IgA antibodies. During the mother's next pregnancy three years later, an infected neonate was delivered despite negative findings, including CMV culture or CMV/DNA detection in urine and serum or CMV-specific IgM and IgA antibodies. Conversely, a positive CMV culture in urine and high levels of CMV-specific IgM and a complement fixing titre of >1:128 were found.

Diagnosis of foetal CMV involvement mainly depends upon culture and detection of CMV-DNA in the amniotic fluid. The practical issue is whether specific diagnosis can be achieved in time for termination of pregnancy. Methods more sensitive than culture and detection of CMV-DNA or CMV-specific antibodies are likely to be required to expose recurrent CMV infection in pregnancy. Amniocentesis for this purpose in pregnancies following initial CMV infection would appear to be justified.

The role of *congenital CMV* can thus be a serious pathogenic and cerebro-destructive source of CP, with MR imaging making it possible to recognize in life the severe migrational abnormalities of neurones, and the nature and extent of gyral and white matter abnormalities that may ensue. It is probably an underestimate that it occurs in only 0.5 to 2.4% of newborn in the USA. In my study of antenatal blood samples of pregnant women in Jerusalem (Ashkenazi, Russell and Zadik, 1976), 46% showed positive antibodies to CMV. Its incidence is probably even higher in situations of heavy overcrowding and poor hygienic conditions elsewhere in the world. Neuro-developmental handicaps in a minority of those infected also include hearing loss, and learning, cognitive and behaviourable disabilities recognizable in later childhood. In a significant minority symptomatic at birth and displaying a characteristic triad of systemic manifestations, thrombocytopenia, jaundice and hepatosplenomegaly, subsequent neurodevelopmental sequelae were severe in 15 to 75% of this group.

## Foetal Metabolic and Interrelated Nutritional/Myelinational Influences

Hypotheses concerned with such cerebral malformations have recently postulated disturbance of molecular species distributed on cells determining affinities with interacting cells as underlying distortions in the overall timing and rate of cell migration. In parallel, there may be *interference with fibronectin and the neural cell adhesion molecule* (NCAM), a stabilizing substance limiting "shear", or relative movement.

Malformations such as polymicrogyria, pachygyria, olivary dysplasia, as well as other defects of neuronal migration may also be linked to *myelin breakdown*, or with gliosis or accumulations of lipid in glia. These may compound a disorder described as *Sudanophilic leukodystrophy*. This clinico-pathological situation also characterizes *Zellweger's cerebro-hepato-renal syndrome*, known to be characterized by defective formation of peroxisomes due to *lack or absence of hepatocellular and renal tubular peroxisomes*. Structural and chemical abnormalities in mitochondria have also been associated.

The formation of hepatocellular peroxisomes is also defective in *neonatal adrenoleukodystrophy* which may also be marked both by especially profound demyelination and clinically by severe hypotonia and seizures. *A third disease, embodying defective formation of peroxisomes in hepatocytes*, underlies Refsum's syndrome, wherein *cerebellar ataxia* may emerge in its first or second decade of life. Involvement of the cerebellum, with heterotopia and olivary dysplasia, also marks the Zellweger entity. Considerable overlap has been identified between these syndromes which are also characterized by dysmyelination as well as defective neuronal migration. Plasmologens are particularly important in myelin membranes and if not synthesized in the peroxisomes, hypomyelination ensues. But cerebellar ataxia is also a feature of

cerebrotendinous xanthomatosis attributed to deficiency of the mitochondrial enzyme, 26-hydroxylase.

## Zellweger Cerebro-Hepato Syndrome

This is outlined again under the heading of progressive disorder simulating CP in Chapter 19. It is ascribed to lack of a paroxysmal enzyme, although the interrelationship between defective enzymatic function and the anomaly of neuronal migration is not yet known. *Microgyria, polymicrogyria* and incomplete white matter myelination are the principal CNS outcomes.

## Marshall-Smith Syndrome

*Macrogyria* appears in this instance to be comparable to that in the Lissencephaly associated with cytomegalovirus infection, likewise in the presence of cerebral atrophy and absent corpus callosum. The cranium is long, the forehead prominent, the orbits being shallow with prominent eyes. The accompanying acceleration of growth and maturation is another unusual feature.

*Excess of pipecolic acid*, believed to be a principal product of lysine in the brain, is typical of all these disorders of peroxisomal biogenesis. Pipecolic acid is recorded by Takahama et al. (1982) as competing for the receptors of GABA (gamma amino butyric acid) in such a pathway as that from lysine to pipecolic acid. It may be a major cerebral pathway competing with that for GABA. Furthermore in one study in the experimental animal, *injection of pipecolic acid induced profound hypotonia*.

# Interrelations Between Myelination and Early Nutrition

This neurogenic process is the most vulnerable to undernutrition in both animals and humans. The deficit of myelin synthesis so induced by nutritional deprivation is irreversible. Essential fatty acid deficiency which alters myelin formation and turnover, is a particularly relevant aspect of undernutrition. Disturbances in the profile of PUFA's can alter the functioning of membrane enzymes, disturb the interactions between receptor and legand, disrupt intercellular interactions and even upset the correct functioning of the organ.

Up to 50% of the ultimate mass of cervonic acid in the infant brain accumulates after birth. It must be taken into account that large quantities of dietary linoleic acid (18:2n-6) could inhibit the transformation of linolenic acid into cervonic acid in the liver, thus causing suboptimal cervonic acid nutritional status.

Furthermore, it has also been recently confirmed that early undernutrition can selectively reduce the concentration of certain gangliosides in the human brain. If ganglioside concentration reflects the number of dendritic arborizations, then it may be presumed that the process of dendritic branching may be retarded by early undernutrition.

# Microcephalic and Dysmorphic Examples of Unexplained Disorders of Neuronal Proliferation

Three *microcephalic, multifocal* and *profoundly dysmorphic* disorders *presenting with hypotonia* are representative:

**Meckel-Gruber** (Jones, 1988)

The microcephaly (head circumference more than 1.5 standard deviations below the norm) is complicated by dorsal encephalocele, sloping forehead, and underlying cerebral and cerebellar hypoplasia. Micropththalmia, micrognathia plus cleft lip and palate, slanting eyes and hypo- or hypertelorism coexist, whilst a short neck, polydactyly and both cardiac and renal defects may also appear.

**Cerebro-oculofacio Skeletal (COFS) Syndrome or Neurogenic Arthrogryposis** (Jones, 1988)

*Hypotonia* is marked, and is accompanied in this COFS syndrome by hypo- or areflexia, which in part may be explained by the severe flexural contractures. A reduction of white matter underlies the cerebral defect, and the associated microcephaly is linked to bilateral microphthalmia and cataracts, with the prominent root of the nose accentuating the ocular depression.

**Neu-Laxova Syndrome** (Jones, 1988)

In this disorder of granulation, the *hypotonia* is also associated with *flexion contractures and short limbs*. Underlying the microcephaly, microphthalmia (but eyes protruding without lids), hypertelorism, flattened nose, cleft lip, micrognathia and short neck, is the atrophy of cerebellum and pons, together with *absence of corpus callosum and olfactory bulbs*.

# Destructive Disorders of Foetal Brain:
## Subtotal Cortical Necrosis

*Destructive lesions* causing subtotal necrosis of the cortex may be responsible for disordered gyration. When this disturbance prevails before 30-35 weeks the cortex becomes anomalously thin and hyperconvoluted: the so-called polymicrogyria. Most prenatal perfusion failures associated with microgyria appear to occur *after the end of neuronal migration,* and before the establishment of cortical gyration between 20 and 30 weeks. This abnormal finding can be identified soon after birth by CT scanning or NMR imaging. So monitored by prenatal sequential ultrasound or other imaging, most foetal accidents or infections already exemplified lead to polymicrogyria during the same period, thus confirming the neuropathic dating.

Functionally, the most viable brain defects derived from destructive processes mark the second half of gestation (Evrard, 1989) leading to neurological defects and consequent dysfunctions ranging from minimal learning disability or motor defects, to major motor and cognitive handicaps. The nascent field of developmental imaging is more recently exposing these, as well as other relatively minor cortical dysgeneses, and quantitative cytoarchitectonic disturbances arising from defective neuronal growth and differentiation. It is important to realize that these have been found to be the *unexpected bases of some examples of dyslexia, of autism, as well as of partial epilepsy.*

More severe destructive processes lead to larger defects in the cerebrum such as underlie hydrancephaly or porencephaly, especially if they operate before the stage of glial maturation at about 30-35 weeks. Cortical laminar destruction augments prenatal growth differences between inner and outer cortical layers. A reduction of the wavelength of the cortical folding with multiplexation of the convolutions is the outcome.

# Pre- and Perinatal Hydrocephalus

Pre- and perinatal hydrocephalus is being increasingly suggested as a prenatal *source, if not an association*, of CP especially in spastic diplegia. It is certainly correlated with one form of ataxic cerebral palsy, and it may also be secondary to prenatal post-haemorrhagic consequences, to infections, and to resorption of damaged nervous tissue producing obstruction of the cerebral spinal fluid pathway. Membranous stenosis of the aqueduct of Sylvius may be the sequel, for instance, of intercurrent infections, especially mumps during the last trimester. Similar aqueductual stenosis is also a frequent sequel of the lesions mentioned above, obstruction resulting from brain tissue resorption especially marking both holoprosencephaly and hydranencephaly, which can be readily excluded by a halo of greater than 3.5 cm on transillumination. The aqueductal stenosis reinforcing the familial X-linked hydrocephalus of the Bicker or Adam type is instead attributed to prenatal compression by the dilated lateral ventricles of the mesencephalon.

Although the association of hydrocephalus with CP is by no means always a clear-cut issue, its exclusion in epidemiological surveys does not appear justifiable in the light of the circumstances cited above. In the valuable analysis of the epidemiology in Sweden and long term outcome of infantile hydrocephalus (IH) by the Hagberg team (Fernell, Hagberg, Hagberg, Hult and von Wendt, 1988), it was found that the hydrocephalic children with associated brain parenchymal defects had the poorest outcome. In other words, amongst the 68 children studied, the most important factor determining an adverse outcome of the IH was the presence of associated primary brain damage or maldevelopment.

## Prenatal Cerebral Perfusion Failure

*Prenatal cerebral perfusion failure* in the second half of gestation has increasingly been appreciated as a vital pathophysiological factor associated with, or producing ischaemic disturbance. This adversely influences prenatal development of the central nervous system to become responsible for foetal brain damage.

Statistical data is limited, but other clinico-pathological and patho-physiological evidence in this area is growing. According to an analysis of our own data in the past (Ornoy et al., 1976), uterine haemorrhage had marked the pregnancy of one third of mothers ultimately delivering newborns with brain abnormalities, a much higher proportion than in the control population. In most cases, the circumstances indicated perfusion failure within the foetal brain or

foetal malnutrition, data which calls for confirmatory replication and further exploration.

It has thus become clearer that such cerebral perfusion failure is a frequent cause of viable malformation, and probably responsible for a major portion of neurodevelopmental disturbance marking the last two trimesters of pregnancy. There is moreover evidence of its foetal genesis in a range of maternal disorders, beginning with maternal shock and hypoxia. Maternal hypo- and hypertension may also play a potent role. In addition, there is foeto-maternal and foeto-foetal transfusion together with premature placental separation or excessive infarction. Sequential ultrasound studies were carried out in several examples in the recent

Multicentre Collaborative study from the time of the prenatal perfusion disorder until birth. And these sufficed to confirm that this as a significant pathogenetic mechanism (Evrard et al., 1984).

An important influence of eclampsia and pregnancy-derived hypertension in substantially reducing the risk of germinal matrix and intraventricular haemorrhage (GM/IVH) was confirmed in the prospective epidemiological study of 449 babies of birth-weight less than 1501g (Kuban et al., 1992). Of 72 of these babies who developed GMH/IVH, only one (or 2.5%) was the progeny of an eclamptic mother, whilst 71 (17.8%) of the non-eclamptic mothers were delivered of babies who developed GMH/IVH.

A vital facet was that GMH/IVH in 6 of 107 (or 5.6%) babies from mothers with hypertension (including 4 of 69 or *6.8%* of

mothers with pregnancy-induced hypertension) could be contrasted with 66 of 352 or *18.8%* from mothers who did not suffer hypertension. Figures also worthy of recall were those emphasizing the low incidence of GMH/IVH in 5 of 89 or 5.6% in the progeny of mothers who suffered both hypertension and proteinuria, instead of the 63 of 333 or 19% babies from mothers who lacked both.

An additional challenging observation was the significantly reduced risk of such haemorrhage following treatment with magnesium sulphate - even in those who did not have eclampsia. To what extent reduction in maternal hypertension can influence or stabilize autoregulation of cerebral perfusion or more specifically prevent sudden increase of intracranial blood pressure, invites intensive experimental research.

# PERINATAL AND POSTNATAL CEREBRAL PALSIES

It should also be recognized that each of the cerebral palsies can stem from a brain-damaging influence at any stage of development and maturation of the foetal or infantile brain, of course including those arising perinatally. In more precise definition, perinatal or postnatally acquired cerebral palsy could be considered to encompass a non-progressive motor handicap arising in an infant or child born sometimes apparently free of identifiable brain damage but *in the course of whose subsequent development* neuropathic damage

incurred during labour or postnatally is clinically and developmentally expressed. On the other hand, there is still a strong school of thought in support of postnatal developments as largely a milestone in "the continuum of reproductive casualty", the expression of a pre-existing or prenatal condition bringing about susceptibility to the stress of birth, whether it be normal or abnormal.

Nevertheless, the postnatal proportion of cerebral palsy was as much as 14% in

Chicago where an over-representation of black children (32:100 black to white ratio compared with 10:100 black to white ratio for congenital cases) was especially linked to meningitis at low socio-economic levels. A lower level of 11% has marked both New York and Western Australia (Stanley and Blair, 1984). In the latter series, the postnatal rate per 10,000 of neonatal survivors born between 1956 and 1975 was 2.4 (Blair and Stanley, 1982). They also clarified a special relationship to racial factors, if not of social disadvantage, insofar as aboriginal children were over-represented (22% compared with 5% of all live births) with 31% of them derived from infections including gastro-enteritis and consequent dehydration.

The Australian perinatal estimate for related intrapartum asphyxia had subsequently levelled at about 8% of all their series with spastic CP, i.e. 15 examples in 183 children (Blair and Stanley, 1988), whilst in the Irish study of Cussen et al. (1978) the estimated prevalence for perinatal factors again reached 10%, in striking accord with that in other developed countries. The typically objective study of Hagberg et al. (1975), however, led Sweden to the lowest figure of 6%. In contrast, the analyses in two less affluent settings rose to 25% of total cases in both South Africa (Arens et al., 1978; Molteno et al., 1980) and India (Garg and Srivastava, 1965). The higher incidence of *perinatal* morbidity than in the general neonatal population *amongst the postnatal cases* of CP in the Western Australian study, cannot be overlooked. As much as 14% had been admitted to special or intensive neonatal units compared with 6.5 of all live births over the same period. The level of

respiratory distress in these infants (3%) was distinctively higher than in the total live birth data (1.3%). Likewise, abnormal central nervous system signs were significantly more prominent than in liveborn controls: Convulsions in 8% (compared with 0.4% of all liveborn and 0.2% of neonatal survivors), "cerebral irritation" in 4%, marked drowsiness in 4% and initial difficulties with sucking in 14%. In contrast, only 1.4% of neonatal survivors manifested any "cerebral signs".

This relative excess of such expressions of neonatal morbidity may have reflected the increased vulnerability to infections, etc., of infants who had been small or sick. Nonetheless, the subsequent brain-damaging influences may be related in some way to a problem initiated at birth. Thus this postnatal series, and perhaps others, do not precisely conform with Blair and Stanley's own acceptable extension of a definition of postnatal CP, that "it was unrelated to any perinatal cause". But the connection with significant perinatal cerebral involvement cannot be so easily dismissed. The classical causes incurred in labour still include especial difficulties in labour, breech and other complex presentation, apart from prolapse of the umbilical cord.

In all three studies in Chicago, New York and Western Australia, the majority of so-called postnatal CP had, however, been attributed to infections (67, 47 and 63% respectively). In New York, 40% of these were believed to be viral, measles encephalitis in 5%, 30% bacterial and 30% unknown, whilst tuberculous meningitis was thought to account for 8%. Viral infections were cited as representing 50% in the Western Australian series, with measles encephalitis again an important cause, with bacterial agents mainly being the meningococcus, haemophilus influenza and pneumococcus.

It is thus gradually being accepted in the West that birth trauma is a rare primary cause of perinatal death, at most arising only once in every 1000-2000 births. But as the source of brain damage and subsequent handicap, one needs to *dissociate such birth injury from concomitant effects of asphyxia, intra-uterine growth retardation or preterm delivery*. It is suggested that trauma may nonetheless be implicated in a few examples of CP and severe mental retardation. Breech delivery and related perinatal trauma has thus been related to a higher incidence of so-called minimal brain damage syndromes.

## Reappraisal of Immediate Prenatal and Perinatal factors as Source of Early Postnatal Expression of CP

Recent evidence, especially encompassing that of the important 1990 report of Sinha and his colleagues, calls for a serious reappraisal of *immediate prenatal and perinatal* factors as the source of early *postnatal* expressions of CP. They emphasize the relevant implications of common complications arising *before or during birth* which may produce ischaemic brain lesions and periventricular haemorrhage. Included to begin with is *maternal* antepartum haemorrhage, of which a subplacental clot may be significant evidence. In the baby, perinatal hypoxia, hypercapnia and acidosis may play a part. A fall in systemic blood emerges again, in my view, as an important factor *precipitating ischaemic brain lesions* particularly in the presence of *birth asphyxia, recurrent apnoea*, or even septicaemia.

The sequences of these pathogenic factors were highlighted in their study of 232 neonates of <32 weeks gestation. Ultrasonography shortly after birth, daily for the first week and twice weekly thereafter, exposed periventricular echogenicities in nine babies within two hours of birth (early onset) from which evolved convincing evidence of ischaemic lesions such as leukomalacia (PVL). In 30 other babies, similar lesions developed subsequently. These *late onset* cases were linked to hyaline membrane disease, whereas in early onset cases, intra-uterine growth retardation and early recurrent apnoea were mainly represented.

*Spastic diplegia* was the outcome, alongside the typically associated disabilities of sensorineural hearing, of vision and of developmental delay, in four of six survivors with early onset PVL. The underlying PVL appears to stem mainly from infarction in areas especially prone to lowered perfusion, such as "watershed" areas divided between what Pape and Wigglesworth (1979) had labelled as ventriculofugal and ventriculopetal branches of cerebral blood vessels. Apart from the impact on a fall in systemic blood pressure, a rise in intracranial pressure as a result of oedema caused by hypoxia may reduce cerebral perfusion.

Intra-uterine growth retardation appears to have become an increasingly important basis in its association with:

(a) impaired uteroplacental blood flow, as measured by the Doppler technique, probably leading to *foetal hypoxia*, and

(b) reduced glycogen cardiac reserves (Adlard et al., 1973) which could account for the drop in cardiac output during hypoxia, and impaired ability to maintain its blood pressure.

It is suggested by Sinha et al. (1990) that blood pressure readings soon after birth could enhance the recognition of poor cerebral perfusion. *Using plasma and inotropic drugs to maintain blood pressure* may prove to be a vital programme for improving cerebral blood flow and preventing PVL.

The effects of *recurrent apnoea*, sometimes severe enough to necessitate respiratory ventilation, in accentuating hypoxic-ischaemic encephalopathy would be worsened by declining heart rate (Perlman, McMenamin and Volpe, 1983). Further progression to PVL would ensue in the arterial border zones most susceptible to damage.

In some babies showing ultra-sonographic features of ischaemia but without a history of late foetal heart rate deceleration or of a low Apgar (<5 at 5 minutes), it may be presumed that the brain lesion is prenatal: arising before birth.

## Patho-Physiological Sequences which Could Lead to Cerebral Ischaemia

*With potential for prevention in mind*, it might be opportune at this point to list the various possible *patho-physiological sequences* already touched upon which could lead to ischaemic brain injury:

(1) Hypoxia inducing cerebral oedema → rise in intracranial pressure accentuating reduction in cerebral perfusion.

(2) Intra-uterine growth retardation associated conditions leading to:

impaired utero-placental blood flow
↓
Foetal hypoxia
+
↓ cardiac glycogen reserves
↓
progressive fall in cardiac output
↓
limitation of ability to maintain blood pressure
↓
reduction in cerebral blood flow

Treatment aimed at maintaining blood pressure, including plasma and inotropic drugs, may improve cerebral blood flow and perfusion. For example, in ischaemic brain damage of late onset in babies of *approximate growth* for their gestational age, there is a relationship with hyaline membrane disease. Its relationship with periventricular haemorrhage with subsequent leukomalacia is well established. It has been suggested that contributory pathogenic factors may include:

1. Fall in $CO_2$ pressure during mechanical ventilation (Dubowitz, Bydder and Muskin, 1985).

2. Reduction in systemic blood pressure from blood loss from haemorrhage or intracerebral haematoma (Volpe et al., 1983).

It is inferred from this series that in a third of the babies with disability, including CP in later childhood, the ischaemic brain damage may have already occurred by the time of birth. Optimal obstetric management related to the highest level of foetal monitoring should be planned for optimal timing and mode of delivery.

The situation which bears these greater perinatal risks also includes too large an infant for gestational age, breech delivery and multiple birth. In the case of breech delivery, however, adverse prenatal factors may be reflected rather than birth injuries. There is thus ample room for competent preventive handling.

Convincing data on the importance of other perinatal factors derive from the recent MRI exploration in 30 survivors of severe perinatal asphyxia by Steinlin and his Swiss colleagues (1991) which revealed unchallengeable cerebral injury relatable to a perinatal hypoxic-ischaemic lesion. In early MRI (i.e. 1-4 days of age), *severe cerebral necrosis* was interpreted on the basis of $T_2$ hyperintensity of the white matter, and blurred limits to the cortex. The necrosis was established at 3 months of age. The tragic sequel was confirmed in 11 children revealing this pattern, 8 showing severe CP and 3 of moderate degree on subsequent examination. Although none of the 13 children with normal late MRI scans developed severe CP or marked mental retardation, 2 children showed focal ischaemic lesions and of intracranial haemorrhage in 4, although none leading to CP, thus consolidating the prognostic value of MRI.

## Chronic Foetal Distress as Marker for Subsequent CP or Other Adverse Neurological State

The relationship of several significant perinatal events to the subsequent development of CP was carefully studied by Shields and Schiffrin (1988) in 75 infants. Association of CP with acute intrapartum asphyxia occurred in 8%, a figure identical to that of Blair and Stanley in an Australian setting (1988). CP was also linked to traumatic delivery in 11%. An important observation was that 35% of cases were associated with chronic foetal distress. This was identifiable by an unique foetal heart rate (FHR), a pattern embodying "a normal baseline rate with persistently absent variability and mild variable decelerations with overshoot" (Shields and Schiffrin, 1988). This pattern has often been found in combination with postmaturity, meconium staining, intra-uterine growth retardation and neonatal seizures.

Twenty-seven percent of the cases involved a combination of chronic foetal distress, acute intrapartum foetal asphyxia and/or traumatic delivery. Their challenging conceptualization was that *antenatal intermittent umbilical cord compression* -secondary to oligohydramnios - results in *repetitively transient ischaemia* of the CNS with the consequent FHR pattern and neuropathy.

The important point is that chronic foetal distress and the unique foetal heart rate may be firm markers for CP and other adverse neurological outcomes.

## Postnatal Metabolic and Other Episodic Damage

*Neonatal hypoglycaemia* still appears to play a continuing aetiological role in the immediate postnatal period. Debate upon the possible continuing neurological impact in the neonate of moderate or asymptomatic hypoglycaemia was refocussed by the multicentre study of Lucas, Morley and Cole in 1988. In 661 preterm infants, moderate hypoglycaemia (plasma glucose concentration less than 2.6 mmol/l) was a common complication occurring in 433 (in 104) on 3 to 30 separate days. Indeed the number of days on which it occurred proved to be "strongly related to reduced mental and motor developmental scores at 18 months (corrected age). When hypoglycaemia had appeared on five or more separate days, mental and motor developmental scores at 18 months were significantly reduced by 14 and 13 points respectively, and the incidence of CP or developmental delay was increased by a factor of 3.5 (95% confidence interval 1.3 to 9.4). Therefore, the neonatal management of hypoglycaemia must be adjusted to recognize that serious neurodevelopmental sequelae are to be expected.

## Hyperbilirubinaemia as a Continuing Threat

So-called toxic insults or even bilirubin encephalopathy or kernicterus may still be important sources in the developing world, although no longer the dominant factor that it was in the Western world before immunization against the Rhesus factor became routine prophylaxis. For example, in Foley's recently reported series (1992) of 219 cases of dyskinetic and dystonic forms, kernicterus had still been the aetiological background in 57. But other forms and degrees of hyperbilirubinaemia still remain a serious threat. Our preventive duty dictates that we focus more practical and research attention upon hyperbilirubinaemia.

The prospective national survey of this aspect in 1338 preterm and small for gestational age infants in the Netherlands (Van de Bor et al., 1989) rightly emphasized a convincing relationship between the maximal serum total bilirubin concentration in the neonatal period and the neurodevelopmental outcome at the corrected age of 2 years. In 831 children at that point, a consistent increase in the prevalence of handicap consisting mainly of CP was correlatable with each 50 umol/L (2.9 mg/dL) increase of the maximal serum total bilirubin. The typical evolutional sequence of CP in hyperbilirubinaemic encephalopathy ranges from rigidity to athetosis and other ataxia (Kalizhnwik, 1989). On a multiplicative scale, the risk of handicap increased by 30% for each 50 umol/L (2.9 mg/dL) increase of maximal serum total bilirubin. There proved to be an undoubted causal relationship for CP between the maximal serum total bilirubin and the neurodevelopmental outcome.

The continuing aetiological incrimination of hyperbilirubinaemia, particularly in the preterm, was also vividly illustrated in another recent European study by Ikonen et al. (1992) of 103 preterm infants with a gestational age less than 33 weeks. There was a correlation with the duration of hypocarbia (PCO$_2$ <on = 30 mmHg) during the first 72 hours. This and the hyperbilirubinaemia at three days of age proved to be independently and significantly related to periventricular leukomalacia (PVL), but not directly to CP although this is convincingly contraindicated by many other studies. The only perinatal variables that could be so related were periventricular leukomalacia and ventriculomegaly. In addition to hypocarbia, it still remains clear that hyperbilirubinaemia may still play a significant role in the pathogenesis of periventricular leukomalacia and hence of CP in preterm infants.

In the context of hyperbilirubinaemia, it must be appreciated that a *globally crucial cause* of neonatal jaundice stems from *glucose-6-phosphate dehydrogenase deficiency* - the most frequent enzyme disorder of human beings. The secondary haemolytic jaundice may lead to kernicterus and death, or spastic CP. The subsequent life-threatening haemolytic crises because of interaction with specific drugs and with fava beans, also dictate a preventive educational campaign. At least the neonatal jaundice can be successfully overcome by phototherapy, which is after all cheap and simply enough for universal application.

Amongst iatrogenic factors for postnatal CP is a single report of the apparent impact of human leucocyte *interferon*. At a dosage level of 2 million units every two days administered to a 2-year-old boy for recurrent juvenile laryngeal papilloma, an upper motor neuron lesion exhibiting *spastic diplegia* inexplicably emerged after seven months of treatment.

Studies by Hansen et al. (1985) on brain hippocampal slices have focussed on the specific effects that bilirubin may have on aspects of neuronal cellular function. He demonstrated interference with electrical activity in brain slices in culture as a reversible phenomenon. Schiff et al. (1985) studying neuroblastoma cells clarified suppressive effects upon DNA synthesis and mitochondrial function.

The toxic effects appear to follow the areas of intensified yellow staining in various cerebral nuclei: globus pallidus, subthalamic nuclei and hippocampus in particular. Neuronal loss, gliosis and gradations of demyelination leads clinically when bilirubin levels exceed 20 mg/dL to *hypotonia, lethargy, poor sucking reflex, hypothermia, opisthotonos and seizures.* Survivors reveal high-tone deafness, as well as severe choreo-athetosis and mental retardation.

Newer technology such as the measure of auditory evoked brain stem potentials pioneered by Sohmer can identify more subtle effects (Perlman, Sohmer et al., 1983) including those depending upon demyelination (Sohmer and Russell).

The responsibility fell upon accidents and particularly upon skull trauma in about one fifth of all postnatal and acquired neuropathies in these three series, mostly stemming from the malevolent iatrogenic plague of motor vehicle accidents but also represented in the no less universal malevolent scourge of child abuse (Diamond and Jaudes, 1983). Probably a better term for these neuropathic sequelae is static encephalopathy rather than CP.

An exponential fall with increasing age in the frequency of brain damage marked both sexes, the majority or 66% affecting infants under 12 months of age. Their especial vulnerability to skull trauma is believed to include immaturity and weakness of blood vessels, and the critical rapidity of growth and development of the brain. Even fatal motor accidents in the USA (Baker, 1979) occur at a higher rate in infancy than in the preschool period. With regard to infections, specific vulnerability would be linked to immaturity of the immunological system following upon the gradual decline of passive immunity from maternal antibodies, especially to viral sources. A striking illustration was drawn by Finlay (1958) in the relation to age of the neurological damage secondary to Western equine encephalitis. 56% of neonates were so afflicted, 41% of infants between one and two months of age, and only 22% of those between two and three months.

Hypoxia secondary to near-drowning, suffocation and cardiac arrest are other postnatal factor underlying grave cerebral damage. It would again be logical to identify this consequence as "static encephalopathy" rather than cerebral palsy.

## Resultant Postnatal Categories of Motor Handicap

In the New York study, almost three quarters (73.4%) of the postnatal cases were spastic and 12.5% ataxic, whilst 7% were of mixed type and 3% exhibited what was called rigidity and only 1% were athetoid. There was especial severity, in the shape of tetraplegia, in nearly half of these (47.5%). In the remainder, hemiplegia predominated

(46%) with paraplegia in only 5%. Likewise spastic hemiplegia was strongly represented (50%) in the Chicago series, with 77% overall being spastic. In a recent large Indian series of 544 cases (Srivastava, Larsram and Srivastava, 1992), 497 or 91.4% were of spastic type with hypotonic, ataxic and athetoid types represented in the following proportions: 5.5%, 1.5% and 1.3% respectively. Of the large spastic group, tetraplegia constituted the highest proportion (34.9%), diplegia 21.9%, whilst hemiplegia reached 28.7%, approaching the relative proportion in the Chicago series. Mental retardation was also high at 47.2%, with speech impairment affecting 37%.

In effect, the principal difference of postnatal CP from CP of perinatal origin is this higher proportion overall of spastic CP, and especially of hemiplegia, and the correspondingly lower proportion of spastic diplegia. Accidents, epilepsy and cerebrovascular complications also proved to be more likely to result in hemiplegia than in diplegia or tetraplegia in the Australian study. All of those ascribed to anoxia (other than epilepsy), however, had developed spastic tetraplegia.

Non-motor neurological handicap were also a significant product of postnatal CP. Less than 70% of the Western Australian cases and 41% of the New York series were intellectually retarded. Epilepsy was represented in 36% of those CP children from North Australia, and in 18% of those from New York. The incidence of associated handicaps such as those of vision, hearing and speech reached 20% in Western Australia, but climbed to as much as 57% in New York.

## Preventive Implications in Postnatal CP

The postnatal category of CP constitutes the most preventable of all cerebral palsy groups. A worldwide educational campaign to alert everyone to the implications of the world's commonest enzyme defect of glucose-6-phosphate dehydrogenase illustrates the potential. Its consequent neonatal jaundice which may lead to kernicterus and death, or CP, is at least easily and cheaply treatable by phototherapy. With regard to infections as another common source, immunization against relevant organisms, especially measles and pertussis, remains one proven barrier. And at least there is a reasonable chance of totally eliminating the cerebral sequelae of measles encephalitis. Where no appropriate vaccine is available, some reliance must be placed upon parental education in the vulnerability of their small infants, recognition of the early signs of infection and the urgent need for diagnosis and effective therapy.

The increased virulence of infection superimposed upon pre-existing malnutrition was unequivocally illustrated in the aboriginal cases of the Western Australian study, amongst American black children (Ellenberg and Nelson, 1979), and South African coloured (Molteno et al., 1980), and brings to the fore the desperate need for the developed world to combat and avert malnutrition in their neglected minority child populations.

It is also the duty of the paediatrician and his child-caring colleagues to lead a world campaign against motor vehicle and road accidents. The legislative compulsion to instal and use seatbelts - and cot or other strapping restraints for infants - in the rear of cars has already shown to significantly curb the incidence of head injury (Steele and Little, 1983) and is one clear and enforceable step in the right direction.

# *ASSOCIATED* DISORDERS OR OTHER INTRINSIC AND CO-EXISTING DYSFUNCTION, DISABILITY AND HANDICAP

The outlook for the cerebral palsied child is not only determined by the severity of the predominant primary motor disorder, but may also be strongly influenced by the associated disability. Typically, one or more associated disorders of a non-motor category are commoner in CP where the cerebral disorder is relatively diffuse, as in spastic diplegia, hemiplegia and ataxia (where damage may also extend beyond the cerebellum), whereas they are less evident in athetosis where pathology is likely to predominate in or be confined to the basal ganglia. These are many and varied, and their appraisal or management tailored to whatever disability may be found to be associated, should be given much more consideration in depth. These co-existing problems, for example of mental retardation, epilepsy, or vision, were already firmly emphasized by Sigmund Freud in the classic volume he devoted entirely to cerebral palsy in 1893 (translated in 1968). Sensory impairments, particularly visual and auditory, necessitate careful exclusion as do perceptual and praxic deficits. Speech disorder, epilepsy and mental retardation are commonly conspicuous. These defects - as well as individual strengths - must be seen in full and interrelated perspective when viewing the whole child. Furthermore, the neglect of diagnosis and appropriate treatment of sensory defects of hearing, vision or other associated problems will naturally limit the responsiveness of the individual CP child to an habilitation programme particularly dependent upon his full and independent participation, such as the Petö system.

Apart from its influence upon the outcome of therapy, the interwoven pattern of impairments is significant in itself, reflecting as it probably does a continuum of central nervous system dysfunction. Indeed, the associated defects may reveal more about the severity of handicap, and the probability of various outcomes, than does the primary diagnosis. Such other effects of the more or less diffuse cerebral damage underlying CP may well tend to overshadow the impact of the basic motor disorder, at the same time limiting the ability of the child and his motor impairment to respond to therapeutic intervention. The list would include:

1. Cognitive defects mainly compounding a high rate of severe overall learning difficulty apart from more specific learning disabilities.

2. Relative microcephaly and craniostenoses.

3. Emotional and behavioural disturbance and attentional problems.

   Either as secondary to the above or as specifically coexisting primary disorders of social maladjustment and personality aberrations, and of other deficits in areas of human interrelationship.

4. Aberrant spatial representation and perception.

5. Dyslexia or more specific learning disability.

6. Visual impairment.

7. Hearing impairment.

8. Central visual and auditory processing problems, e.g. apraxia and agnosia in CP.

9. Language dysfunction.

10. Other communication disorders.

11. Speech disorder.

12. Left-handedness.

13. Memory impairment.

14. Neonatal seizures and epilepsy.

To what extent each individual impairment stems from a common source of cerebral, ischaemic or vascular damage or from its perhaps preventable extension or from separate and discrete localizations of such encephalogenic lesions remains to be more clearly defined. Is the disability an avoidable or an unavoidable consequence of the primary and basic disorder? For example, is dysarthria an inevitable secondary disability resulting from spastic incoordination of oral speech musculature accentuated by intention - or from the irregular involuntary incoordination more typical of athetoid or dyskinetic CP? Dysphasia or dyspraxia may well instead derive directly from more basic although related cerebral pathology.

Involvement of the cortex, especially of its connections with Broca's area, may well be a specific source of the speech disorders characterizing CP. It is presumed that separate and more specific precentral and other cortical areas are involved in the high percentage of CP children who manifest epileptiform seizures.

Likewise the presence of audiological or vestibular impairment may constitute a specifically discrete source of cerebral pathology. Loss of memory, emotional and behavioural disorders may also have a predominantly primary source rather than secondary.

Meanwhile, until a clearer clinico-pathological delineation is achieved, it is not surprising that the whole existing complex of disorder of movement and posture is often complicated by other expressions of neurological and neurosensory involvement as well as interference with intellect, or of speech in the broadest sense, and of emotional development. In about 5%, however, the child may be ataxic; and in another 5% the limbs are atonic. Whilst the latter is a static condition, it is important in the differential diagnosis to remember that progressive improvement in tone during the first five years indicates other non-CP syndromes, such as Downs, Riley-Day, Prader-Willi or the so-called "benign hypotonia", or a situation with underlying metabolic disorder, such as homocysteinuria.

# Associated Cognitive Deficit

Associated cognitive impairment or "the learning disability" of today, sufficient to impede certain tasks of learning, memory and the processing of information has been estimated to exceed 50% (Robinson, 1973), even reaching 75% in some estimates. According to Nelson and Ellenberg's studies (1978), about 50 to 65% of children with CP score within the mentally retarded range on psychometric evaluation, with tetraplegia producing the highest percentage of intellectual deficit. Severe mental retardation marked up to 35% of cerebral palsied children in the surveys of Paneth and Stark (1983) and Pharoah et al. (1987), and in the Indian series of 544 cases of CP in 1992 (Srivastava et al.), the proportion reached 47%. The Merseyside survey in 1992 (Pharoah et al.) also incorporated a computerised register of CP in this region totalling more than 1500 cases, and produced some disturbing figures of the changes in the relative proportion of mental retardation. Linked to CP in very low birth-weight infants in recent years, with a significant rise in hemi- and tetraplegia but corresponding diminution in diplegia, there had been a definite increase in the proportion of cases with severe mental retardation. Breaking down this apparent trend into more specific relationships, Pharoah and his team (1992) have first demonstrated that differing proportions and severity of mental retardation could be related to *diplegics* of differing birth-weight. Thus, of those in the low birth-weight group under 1500g, *14% showed an IQ of less than 50*, 10% with an IQ between 50 and 69, but with *76% with an IQ above 70*. In the higher birth-weight group above 2500g, however,

an IQ of over 70 was also found in a relatively high proportion of 50%, whereas severe mental retardation occurred in a higher proportion than those in the low birth-weight group - approx a third, 32% to be precise, and double that in the low birth-weight group. In the tetraplegics, stemming as they do mainly from low birth-weight infants, i.e. <1500 gms, the very low IQ proportion was less, i.e. only 20%, with 40% representing the moderately severe IQ levels of 50-69, and 40% above 70. In a study of 419 survivors of a neonatal intensive care unit in Bufalini Hospital, Cesena, Ciotti et al. showed in 1990 that CP was identifiable in 26%. Of these, 13 proved to have an IQ less than or equal to 70. The more precise serial evaluation of 153 consecutively discharged very low birth-weight infants in the Australian study of Tudehope and his colleagues reported in 1989, first of all showed that the sensitivity of cerebroventricular haemorrhage for CP was 76.8%. Even more serious is a sensitivity of as much as 70% for severe intellectual handicap.

This CP group is therefore visualized as making up an increasing proportion, recently almost one-fifth, of the overall prevalence of severe mental retardation (Nicholson and Alberman, 1992) with Down's syndrome near to one-third, whilst "X-linked mental retardation, single gene defects, and encalformation syndromes" each produce about one-tenth of the overall prevalence. But even the remainder whose global intellectual capacity may appear to be within the normal range may be considered at high risk for learning disability. Even vaguely defined "problems in reasoning and perspective" have been invoked as a residual characteristic.

The correlation with periventricular leukomalacia as revealed on CT scanning or MRI is proving to be significant. In a retrospective analysis of CT scans in 76 cerebral palsied children by Schouman-Claeys et al (1989), the cognitive and intellectual sequelae were more severe in 45% of the 88% consisting of preterm infants in whom there was CT evidence of this abnormality.

Every such child is entitled to a genuine clarification of this component during the serial developmental examinations to monitor his course which present-day standards of management should demand. Results of such testing are nonetheless to be interpreted with caution. Infants with motor dysfunction may score low on standard tests because success in many adaptive skills requires motor competence. A low developmental quotient may thus simply reflect the motor handicap rather than cognitive deficit. Conversely, the severity of the physical handicap may sometimes mask cognitive functioning. Qualitative clinical analyses of performance by a paediatric neuro-developmentalist is always advisable. So is parallel evaluation by a psychologist specifically experienced in differentiating cognitive deficit in handicapped children, helpfully in collaboration with functional as well as general assessment by a Peto-inspired and trained conductor. A more balanced appraisal of ultimate potential is the objective.

Related to the category of CP, subnormal intelligence appears to be less common in the athetoid, where cerebral damage is predominantly of basal ganglia components, although more frequent in the mixed group where spasticity co-exists.

In pursuing research into the prevention of this commonly associated element of CP, it is also vital to put any associated prematurity in objective perspective. For, after all, a normal range of intelligence marks the premature infant, although the mean appears to be shifted downward slightly. When the IQ distribution of very low birth-weight preterms and their parents were compared (Stewart and Reynolds, 1974), their ranges and mean IQ were not significantly different. So that study of the pathogenesis of the vital correlationship of cognitive impairment with CP should by no means be confined to prematurity or its degree, which does not appear to be a significant factor in this respect.

When testing at school age, disorders of abstract reasoning and disturbances in specific learning skills, become the main diagnostic problems. On the other hand, the influence of behavioural difficulties also becomes an important factor. By the late 1970s from 13 to 32% of all children were found to show aberration in school performance, behaviour and emotional patterns.

# Relative Microcephaly

This is defined by a head circumference as measured around the glabella and the occipital protuberance, of more than two standard deviations below the mean for age, sex, race and gestation. In other words, apart from the result of craniosynostosis involving premature sutural closure, this diminished size of skull reflects a small brain. The primary form is the outcome of anomalous development of brain during the first seven months of gestation, whereas secondary form follows an insult incurred either during the last two months of gestation or the perinatal period.

## Primary Forms

Transmitted as an autosomal recessive trait, the brain weight may liken that of a 3-5 month foetus. Anomalies that are frequently associated are especially those of migration, including lissencephaly, schizencephaly, macrogyria, micropolygyria and agenesis of the corpus callosum. Grey matter heterotopias co-exist and defective cortical lamination may show grouping in columnar blocks of the cortical neurons.

Irradiation may be a factor, especially exposure to ionizing radiation during the first two trimesters, especially between 4 and 20 weeks of gestation.

## Clinical Expressions

Functionally, trainable mental retardation appears to be invariably associated, and a direct linear relationship between intelligence and the severity of microcephaly was long ago confirmed (Pryor and Thelander, 1968; Martin, 1970). Attention or behaviour disorder and mild spasticity may accompany deficits in fine motor coordination, and visual defect. Seizures appear in about one-third.

All the aetiological factors below are time-specific insofar as they must *operate during the period of induction and major cellular migration*:

1. Infective causation, intra-uterine cytomegalovirus, toxoplasmosis and rubella are major factors characterized by microcephaly.

2. *Chemical factors*
   The following have been incriminated as leading to microcephaly: cortisone, sulphadryl enzyme inhibitors, aminopterin, tri ellylene melamine, and nitrogen mustard.

3. *Chromosomal sources*
   Karyotype abnormalities including trisomies, deletions and translocation syndromes are often associated. Over 20 dysmorphic syndromes linked to microcephaly do not as yet reveal such karyotypes. These include the more extreme Seckel syndrome or the Cornelia de Lange, and Hallerman Streiff syndromes.

## Secondary Forms

During the latter part of the third trimester, the perinatal period and early infancy , infective, traumatic anoxia or metabolic insults may be responsible. The outcome may include cystic areas of degeneration or porencephaly, if not encephalomalacia. Postnatal brain growth is interrupted and sutures close prematurely.

but the cerebral anomalies characteristically associated with primary microcephaly are absent. The cerebellum is the exception, with sometimes cerebellar grey matter heterotopias and hypoplasia.

One must also keep in mind that the associated circumstances of the small-for-gestational-age premature leads intrinsically to a higher risk of morbidity, including neurological lesions with significant delays in development (Gross et al., 1983), or even of brain and/or skull growth. It is suggested that severe substrate deficiencies in the intra-uterine environment may effect significant impairment of brain growth (Gross et al., 1983). Although in the Russell syndrome of "intra-uterine growth deficiency", probably embryopathic or derived from placental pathology with multiple infarction of their small placentae, both head and brain size are typically normal.

Therefore, the small size of the head relative to linear growth should be included in any analysis of neurological outcome. *Premature craniostenosis* should be especially excluded as a source of ongoing microcephaly, with deceleration or arrest of increments in head circumference being carefully monitored. Genetic or familial factors or chromosomal, and classical dysmorphological syndromes are to be considered in causation, in addition to intra-uterine infections.

## Craniostenosis and CP

This can still be a preventable source of CP and mental retardation. In outlining the results from 1973 to 1986 of linear craniectomy and extended craniectomies according to Schut or Epstein on 50 infants with sagittal synostosis, Kaiser (1988) recorded the epidural pressure intraoperatively as high as 200 mm $H_2O$ in 60% of the last 20 examined. The mean cephalic index had been 67 ± 4. Associated clinical features in 35.5% were CP and psychomotor retardation. Epstein's method, and to a somewhat lesser degree, Schut's method, have been confirmed to be superior to linear craniectomies mainly because they serve to maximally increase the breadth or space available during the period of greatest postnatal brain growth. In addition to its influence upon the neurocranium, the extended craniectomies contribute to normalization of the cranial base, contrasting with the natural history of scaphocephaly. Earlier surgical intervention, prior to 4-6 months of age, can avert the disadvantage of any residual skull defects.

Most infants need these more complex approaches of skull reconstruction in addition to resection of the affected sutures. Craniosynostosis reflects the premature fusion of one or more of the cranial sutures. Upheaping of the sutures is a frequent result, with growth of the cranium mainly at right angles to the suture, being impeded. Primarily, various abnormalities of cranial shape result, with biparietal narrowing of the skull - scaphocephaly - following premature fusion of the sagittal suture, and a tower-skull (turricephaly) being the sequel of coronal synostosis although the bicoronal synostosis of Crouzon's and Aperts' necessitates a highly coordinated multidisciplinary approach to achieve reshaping of frontal bone, supraorbital ridges and of a proportion of the lateral orbital wall, and effective remodelling of cranial vault and facial deformity. Monitoring of skull growth and of the head circumference is essential to avert the risk of its premature arrest together with premature closure of the fontanelles and gradual restriction of brain growth affecting the infant's neurodevelopmental progress. Parallel problems include airway obstruction, hydrocephalus, craniovertebral anomalies, abnormalities of movement and exposure, maxillary hypoplasia and difficulties in feeding.

How vital is early diagnosis is illustrated by the need for surgery in sagittal synostosis as early as 6 weeks to achieve the best results, with poor results if the intervention is deferred for 3 months. All children suspected of craniosynostosis should be immediately referred to one of the 30 regional craniofacial centres.

## Aberrant Spatial Perception in CP

The processing of visual and verbal information is a fundamental function. Whilst that of verbal input is relatively efficient, that of visual information often appears to be impaired. Characteristically affected is the ability to analyse and synthesize relationships between objects in the environment as is embodied in *spatial perception*. It must be appreciated by their teachers that comprehension of geometry and comparable areas of mathematical ability, for example, encompassed by diagrammatic visualization, may be impeded. Peto appeared to be well aware of this facet of cognitive function in CP.

Some recent experimental exploration in mice of a genetic basis for *spatial learning* may have exciting relevance to this particular CP anomaly of spatial perception. Mutant mice studied by Tonegawa and Sasumi at the Howard Hughes Medical Institute of Massachusetts, lacked the ability to relate their location within a maze to objects visible *outside: the type of memory termed spatial learning.*

*Loss of spatial learning ability or of memory had been exposed as a sequel of cerebral damage or disease in earlier experiments. The missing gene effects synthesis of a protein abundant in parts of the brain: a-calcium calmodulin dependant* kinase II or CaMKII. Drugs blocking this protein enzyme have led to a loss of spatial learning, possibly with analogous effects upon the process of memory or spatial memory which has been vividly portrayed as "a cascade with many steps...". These studies may offer a clue to the source of aberrant spatial perception consequent upon the neuropathogenesis of CP.

Impairment of spatial learning may also extend to perception of depth. When gazing through water to the bottom of the "therapeutic" pool, there is typically a panic reaction because they cannot sense the distance to the bottom, i.e. they cannot appreciate the shallowness of the pool. Climbing up two or three steps at a later stage, fear may be vividly portrayed when they look down, especially if through perforations in the steps themselves.

The thrust of Piagetian concepts in this context, so neatly reflected in his late infantile test of cognitive function in respect of "object constancy", was applied by Peto in several directions. In respect of spatial perception there may be a relative organic relationship to cerebral lesions linked to sensorimotor or spatial "neglect" syndromes (Robbins, 1991). In man, *right parietal lobe damage* has been associated, or in animals they have followed damage to homologous regions of the cortex and to basal ganglia components. In addition to disturbance in motor action and selective attention, there is a more or less specific component of *impaired spatial representation*. Unilateral lesions to different neural structures have been implicated in such dysfunctions of spatial representation and perception. These include a number of interrelated areas in the parietal and cingulate cortex, the frontal eye-fields, parts of the thalamus, the dorsal striatum, substantia nigra and superior colliculus.

In assessing spatial abilities, the possibility of adapting the available tests to the cerebral palsied child, remains to be fully evaluated. The WISC Block Design including embedded figures is one example. In clarifying lateralization abilities, dichotic listening involving phoneme identification is also used. Younger subjects often fail to exhibit a significant dichotic listening response or varied discrepancies are elicited. Indeed late maturers typically perform better than early maturers in tasks demanding spatial ability. Can we attribute this to the influence of slower maturation in strengthening interhemispherical differentiation, which is believed to be essential for the development of good spatial skills?

In respect of basic cerebral function, clinical and experimental evidence has been adduced to show that spatial perception in various tasks may be disrupted by damage to the right parietal lobe. This may also touch upon the goal of delineating the neural substrate of neurohumoral influence upon cognitive abilities.

## Specific Memory Impairment in CP

We have already referred in the previous section to the possible pathophysiology of impaired spatial learning or spatial memory, but that of more diffuse aspects of memory in CP is worthy of careful analysis.

In 10 patients constituting 67% of his CP material cited by Axel Landeman as suffering from severe impairment of memory, this association was also linked to obesity in six. Whilst cranial damage appeared to be incriminated in *nine of these,* a relatively specific syndrome is indicated in their association in seven of them with motor symptomatology, as well as with either ataxia or ataxia plus spasticity, and brain-stem attacks in the acute stage of eight of them. Impairment of forward and backward memory per se was also confirmed in testing the spastic diplegias associated with deaf-mutism and mental deficiency in endemic cretinism attributable to maternal iodine deficiency during the first trimester of pregnancy if not before conception.

In efforts to localize the general cerebral pathogenesis of CP, Scoville and Milner (1957) have hypothetically ascribed bilateral hippocampal lesions as the specific source of this component, other mental functions remaining intact.

## Memory Dysfunction

In the evaluation of intellectual function in CP which has just been discussed, memory and language are of course included. But insufficient attention has been paid to a possible primary disturbance in various facets of memory function that may be specific to CP and to the probable role of the limbic system, hippocampus in particular as yet another associated disability.

Not only is memory the substrate for the higher mental functions, it is an essential prerequisite for learning and adaptation upon which implementation of the whole Petö system depends and without which the child cannot progressively advance in overall adaptive behaviour regarded in the Petö perspective as an essential prerequisite for progress from dysfunction to orthofunction. If not broadly delayed, the information processed for longer retention, wherein the engrams are stored by categories rather than by temporal sequence of arrival, may be held in this mode for minutes to years.

The limbic system as a whole has an established relationship to memory storage. It also mediates the visceral sensation of olfaction and is the centre of emotional or affective behaviour, a close correlationship attesting to their common phylogenetic origins. Stimulation or destruction of limbic structures leads to potent abberations in mood, affect and behaviour overcast by strong feelings of rage and withdrawal or pleasure.

Its key role in the process of memory is of major clinical importance. This function embodies an interaction of neurophysiological and neurochemical processes involved in the encoding information processing and retrieval. It has even be appreciated that the engrams are stored by categories rather than by the temporal sequence of arrival.

Although quantitatively in the experimental animal, loss of memory can be shown to be crudely proportional to the amount of cortex ablated in both hemispheres, other cerebral structures play a major role in phases of memory. Perhaps the principal one is the hippocampus in the floor of the temporal horn of the lateral ventricle. Loss of the hippocampus of both temporal lobes leads to profound loss of recent memory. Conversely, its direct stimulation can evoke vivid memory when seizures arising in this area produce stereotyped recall patterns upon which function there is evidence of hippocampal responsibility although widespread cortical areas come to be involved in later stages of memory.

Some understanding is growing of the associated physicochemical influences at a synaptic level. Transient changes at this level are attended by modified electrical activity of abnormal calcium concentrations may underlie this together with attendant ionic conductances, modifiable by serotonic, dopamine or papliden like oxytocin. the associated time courses resemble some of the memory processes. But basic changes in molecular configuration are more likely, either in the membrane of established synaptic connections or via formation of new synaptic communications.

The turnover of ribonucleic acid (RNA) in neural tissue increases after electrical stimulation, and appears to be correlated with learning. Conversely, interference with its synthesis impedes learning. Whilst Puromycin, an inhibitor of protein synthesis, can eliminate established memory, calcium also irreversibly increases the number of receptors for glutamate on telencephalic synaptic membranes by activating a proteinase that exposes the otherwise occluded receptors.

Quite another biochemical facet is the major cholinergic input of the limbic system. Scopolamine, a cholinergic antagonist, when given subcutaneously reduces the brain's capacity to store new information, lowering the performance IQ but not the verbal IQ.

The function of the temporal lobe in this context is illustrated by severe impairment of the power to retain recent memory effected by removal of the medial aspect of even one temporal lobe. In Korsakoff's psychosis, with gross defect of recent memory often compounded by disorientation in space and time, the essential pathology again appears to involve the hippocampus as well as medial thalamus.

The role of the frontal lobe is also concerned with special memory functions involved in past experience influencing adjustment of the personality as a whole to future contingencies. The prefrontal regions are involved in investing foresight, imagination and the perception of self with emotional connotations. This is presumed to operate through association pathways, again linking the hippocampus and cingulate gyrus with the prefrontal gyrus on the one hand and with thalamus and hippocampus on the other.

Its integral components are arranged in a ring or loop deep on the medial surface of the brain. It includes the cingulate gyrus, the hippocampus gyrus-fornix, mamillary bodies and anterior nucleus of the thalamus. The cingulate gyrus immediately above the corpus callosum is connected by the long association pathway of the cingulum with the orbital frontal cortex and hippocampal cortex. Axons in the cingulum pass posteriorly and inferiorly to the hippocampal gyrus in the medial temporal lobe and the underlying hippocampus. The fornix, one of the major efferent pathways of these telencephalic limbic structures, arises from the hippocampus and looks anteriorly and inferiorly to the mamillary bodies. These limbic cortical areas thus form a ring of interconnected function around the corpus callosum. They receive input from olfactory and other cortical areas and have their outflow through the hippocampus which has an undeniably integral role in all these anatomical and functional intercommunication concerned with memory.

My own attention was somewhat belatedly drawn to the possibility of a significant impairment of memory processes in CP by a recurring observation in a number of MRI scans of CP children which have curiously enough not earned comment. Typically, these have been of severe examples in preterm infants of germinal matrix/intraventricular haemorrhage especially when linked to periventricular leukomalacia. A typical laconic statement follows: *sclerosis of the hippocampus*, neither the specific genesis of this pathology nor its functional outcome. But it is my hypothesis that direct involvement of its basic memory functions is the most likely result, with associated damage to the limbic system not only accentuating an associated deficiency of recent memory storage alongside interference with other aspects of memory from encoding, sorting to retrieval. It is also possibly responsible for the primary behavioural emotional disorder in CP, bearing in mind its central influence in the control of emotions and affective behaviour, including the affective quality of sensations. There is also ample evidence of an important limbic function in transferring acquired verbal and non-verbal sensory experiences, concepts and sensorimotor behavioural patterns.

## Dyslexia or More Specific Learning Disability in Cerebral Palsy

The nature of the learning disability, as distinct from that attributable to cognitive defect, may be more or less specific to the brain damage underlying CP. Albeit difficult, such identification of this disturbance of learning capacity could have important implications for the general management of the child, particularly for their response to the conductive learning of the Petö system. Even where a "global" cognitive deficit has already been defined, it should be worthwhile to make professionally experienced efforts to unearth an additional learning incapacity of possibly specific character analogous to that found in CP children despite normal cognitive function.

I am not aware of studies in cerebral palsy focussed on an aspect of learning disability of which there is only recent awareness in the general population of children and teenagers, and young adults, that is in respect of sexual abuse. American studies have indicated that between one in three and one in four teenagers and young adults with learning disability have suffered sexual abuse (Chamberlain et al., 1984), which is well above the rate of one in ten estimated for all children in Britain (Baker and Duncan, 1985). Behavioural disorders, also commonly associated with the physical expression of CP, temper tantrums, challenging behaviours and even psychiatric manifestations, may well arouse relevant suspicion with regard to this aspect victimizing the older CP child or teenager.

All CP children should, therefore, be assessed as comprehensively as possible for more precise evidence of some more or less specific form of learning disability. There would be particular reference to any deviancy in eye-hand coordination. Especially modified techniques will be required in the application of the Ober-2 Eye Movement System with the updated version of the programme. To what extent the Video Eye Position superimposed upon Synthetic Dicholic Sound has relevance in the in-depth study of learning capacity in the CP child, remains to be studied.

Manifestation of mild spastic diplegia and hyperreflexia in a preterm infant surviving with tight heel cords and initial toe-walking may be succeeded by walking attained at 2 years, although no functional impairment by school age. It is important nonetheless to remain aware, however, that they are at high risk for learning disability and behavioural problems, effects that can be far more disruptive of the child's progress than relatively mild motor dysfunction per se.

Other manifestations of the underlying association with "minimal cerebral dysfunction" should include language delay, learning disability, attention deficit, hyperactivity, behaviour problems or emotional lability and minor neuromotor dysfunction. Additions in the case of premature infants could be weaknesses in language acquisition, arithmetical reasoning, mathematical achievement, reading comprehension, and fine and gross motor as well as perceptual skills (Largo et al., 1986).

It is of significance in relation to CP that the application of computed tomography appears to have confirmed that an anatomic variant of the central nervous system may contribute to cognitive disability. In a study of CT scanning in 24 adult subjects of developmental dyslexia (Hier et al., 1978) an unusually high incidence of *reversed cerebral asymmetry* was detectable. The right parieto-occipital region was wider than the left, and their disability was accompanied by verbal defects.

Magnetic resonance imaging can now reveal the location of increased cell activity within the living brain. Described as Blood Oxygen Level Dependent ("BOLD") it can detect increase of blood flow to active areas of the brain by measuring changes in the amount of oxygen bound to haemoglobin. Increased flow is detected in the search for pockets of high oxygen blood. Cortical areas of enhanced neuronal activation can also be identified in this way. Parallel colour changes on the surface of the cortex can reflect this on surgical exposure for treatment of epilepsy, including subpial resection. This can be studied during reading, writing, etc., in connection with the exploration of dyslexia, especially during craniotomy in subjects of CP complicated by seizures. This technique has already been exploited in related studies (Hagland et al., 1992), attempting to unearth pathophysiological changes before and during tongue movements or the *naming* of objects.

## Awareness of the Common Apraxia and Agnosia in CP

In the educational management of the CP child, especially cultivated through the Petö system, it is important to remain fully alert to their high incidence of apraxias and agnosias. Cerebral lesions involving the anterior portions of the frontal lobe may spare the primary motor cortex so that no weakness results, but impairment of voluntary activation of the motor system can nevertheless result. Lesions located more anteriorly on the frontal cortex can produce apraxic impairment of voluntary movement of the eye. The term *apraxia* is applied to this inability to perform certain purposeful movement or movement complexes by will, although still elicitable automatically or reflexly. It might be described as the highest level of motor dysfunction wherein the initiation of complex movements is lost. The child may be aware of the act he is trying to perform but fails to produce the pattern of movement required. This inability cannot be described as apraxic, however, until the subject is well past the praxic age.

The related disorders which have been identified is spastic diplegics comprise:

1. Difficulty in copying shapes, *apraxic* dysfunction rather than *perceptual*.

2. Difficulty in reproducing sequences, visually or audiologically. The order of pictures, or a listing of animals may bring this out.

Other basic difficulties include disturbance of skills in picture completion. A distinctive difficulty arises in the impaired detection of *spatial relations* in pictures, affecting objects in front of, behind or below, or figure-background discrimination.

Matching of shapes or even imitation of actions are specifically affected. But the two main groups of apraxias which can be identified comprise:

1. *Actions involving the use of objects,* such as in the use of toothbrush or comb.

2. *Actions involving movements of the face, trunk and limbs,* as encompassed in closing the eyes, showing teeth or moving tongue, pointing or waving, sitting down on a chair, or kicking a ball. These actions reflect dominant hemispheric function.

Indeed, apraxias for face and limb movements may confuse therapists especially occupational and physiotherapists, who are not aware of its existence.

"Getting lost" in their clothes or the inability to dress in the correct order is accentuated in "dressing apraxia". This and other species of constructional apraxia can be "outgrown" in time given patient and sensitive understanding. Occupational therapists can attempt to circumvent or supersede these anomalies of function, e.g. building of steps with bricks and the copying of block designs, etc. have been exploited.

Constructional praxis also includes drawing with an extension to the use of symbols in writing. Hence a visuomotor defect may contribute an especial element of difficulty in writing (dysgraphia).

*Instead, the agnosias* are disorders of recognition classifiable according to sensory modalities: tactile, visual, or auditory. In *tactile agnosia* there is no identification by touch of the object or of a shape. *Visual agnosia* would relate to failed recognition of objects, pictures, faces, places or symbols (including words). *Auditory agnosia or imperception* more commonly involves recognition of rhythms or words. Thus, *receptive aphasia* is one form thereof. *Finger agnosia* is also a common feature as well as "form constancy" or the ability to reduce many objects to a common factor. By the age of six, the child can be expected to identify nine our of twelve geometrical shapes. Visual agnosias for outline drawing is more common than for objects.

The "gnostic age" of the child must be taken into account, excluding sensory loss of the modality concerned. By the age of two

years, in respect of tactile agnosias, recognition by touch of a pencil or a marble figure or cup can be expected.

When the essential parts of the basic pattern of movement are retained, each segment of a movement runs smoothly into the next. In pursuing the task series as an important component of the Petö system, one realizes that the child is only aware of these segments of movement during the earliest stages of learning a new motor act, whilst these stages are being maintained by vision, or by the "internal language" concept basic to the Petö approach. But in the agnostic CP, *slowness in the initiation of movement* may be a related dysfunction. The *inability to detect spatial relationships* is especially common as is the persistent inability to tell right from left. The movement may even start in the wrong muscle group, perhaps as a result of a restricted or confused choice of motor pattern or possibly reflected in an inappropriate sequence of innervation of muscle groups. A crude and ineffective basic pattern of movement may result, even involving initial contraction of the agonist in a contrary movement. This obviously impairs and slows down the ability to acquire the skills required in the "task series".

*Corporal agnosia* may also be identifiable with underlying disorder of body image, especially for a limb or half of the body. In *hemiplegic CP*, there may nevertheless be bilateral agnostic defects involving the spatial relationships of parts of the body.

# Ocular and Visual Anomalies

This is a highly common association. Indeed Breakey originally claimed in 1955 that a higher proportion than 75% of cerebral palsied children can be expected to develop problems in visual acuity or extraocular muscle movement. Even *optic atrophy* is relatively common in CP. Strabismus is the commonest, being found in 31% of Axel Lademann's series of 64 cerebral palsied children or even in 48.3% of 19 preterm high risk infants developing CP who had been subjected to a systematic video observational study by the Prechtl team (Ferrari, Cioni and Prechtl, 1990). The incidence of oculomotor dysfunctions was highest in serial tretraplegics and diplegia. Routine assessment for phorias and tropias is essential to avert amblyopia ex anopsia. Visual acuity can be tested or rather screened by their ability to follow Stycart's white balls of graded size at 10 feet. Poor visual acuity and myopia appear to be the commonest visual impairment, with restricted fields of vision and failure of upward gaze also included, often in association with strabismus and/or nystagmus.

In the series of Axel Lademann (1968), 37% of 63 of his patients had ocular symptoms which he regarded as sequelae of the brain damage underlying their CP as follows:

| | |
|---|---|
| Divergent strabismus | in 20 |
| Convergent strabismus | in 12 |
| Nystagmus | in 12 |
| Hemianopsia | in 6 |
| Anisocoria | in 15 |
| Optic nerve atrophy | in 8 |
| Severely reduced visual acuity | in 24 |

In several surveys, the relative incidence of blind or partially sighted children has levelled at 14% in Dundee (Douglas, 1961) or 15% in Sheffield (Holt and Reynell, 1967). but in a large survey of 1000 cases, Foley (1977) identified a much lower figure of 4%, although conceding that severe visual defects are to be expected more commonly in association with mental retardation and severe physical handicap, particularly of spastic forms.

The wide range of visuo-developmental anomalies that should receive sensitive attention in relation to the effective management of hypertonic CP was illustrated in the comprehensive study by Yamamoto et al. (1990) of one subject of spastic CP who had suffered frequent apnoeic attacks. These deficits were considered in close correlatotion with the maturation of developmental processes of neuropsychological function. Apart from poor visual acuity there was:

1. disorder of visual directed attention and associative visual agnosia.

2. disorder of visuospatial perception and corporeal awareness.

3. dyspraxia devolution.

Reviewed at 10 years of age, the following neurophysiological deficits remained: (1) visual line agnosia (apperceptive type), and (2) constructive apractognosia.

The MRI localized the basic cerebral pathology to bilateral lesions of the white matter of occipital and parieto-occipital transitional regions and in addition, lesions of the *trunk and splenium of the corpus callosum*.

*Hemianopia*, only usually appreciated when the child begins to read, marks about one third of hemiplegics. Cortical blindness, ostensibly the result of simultaneous damage to both occipital and parietal lobes, is fortunately rare, and linked mainly to severe mental retardation. Foley has also drawn attention to another challenging consequence of bilateral parieto-occipital pathology. This is expressed in "piece-meal vision" wherein only a small portion of the visual field can be attended to at any given moment, so that the whole scene cannot be constructed from the part. Although vision for distant objects may be accurate, the affected CP child can be baffled by nearer objects.

The issue of whether the "associated" ocular disturbances, *including nystagmus*, and sensori-motor difficulties, result primarily from structural lesions, or are secondary to earlier prenatal functional abnormalities of cerebral pathways, remains a problem for future research.

The correlationship of disturbance of visual perception with the lesions in 12 children with spastic diplegia was analysed. Each child was subjected to the Frostig Developmental TIV of visual perception and the Tanaka-Binet Intelligence Test. The Frostig test revealed disturbance of visual perception in two, with Subtest II figure-ground, showing the lowest results. The mean of perceptual quotient proved to be significantly under that of the intelligence quotient ($p < 0.05$ t-test).

Abnormal MRI findings in ten, including six who had disturbance in visual perception, involved lesions of the periventricular white matter extending to semi oral centre and subcortical white matter at parietal and occipital lobes. These corresponded to the superior longitudinal bundle and the vertical occipital bundle, both believed to have vital functions as the major pathways of visual perception, and presumably were interrupted when visual impairment complicated spastic diplegia.

An objective attempt to localize the underlying pathology accounting for the extension to defects in visual perception in spastic diplegics was undertaken by Koeda and colleagues in 1990.

## Visual Impairment

In a review of 55 cases of optic atrophy in Denmark (Petersen, Rosenberg and Ibsen, 1990) perinatal stress factors played a major aetiological role in 58%. The commonest related to prematurity, low birth-weight and perinatal asphyxia. CP was represented as one more additional handicap which also included epilepsy and psychomotor retardation. That it is important to initiate educational stimulation as soon as is possible, reflects the urgent need for early diagnosis. It is also important to stress that many of the obstetrical and other perinatal factors may be preventable.

**Paroxysmal Ocular Downward Deviation**

This abnormality, with paroxysmal ocular downward deviation accompanied by downward movement of the upper  eyelid was recently observed for the first time by Yokochi (1991) predominantly in the preterm. All these infants were subjects of spastic tetraplegia or diplegia, associated with mental retardation, and significantly in most of them, evidence of cortical visual impairment. Fortunately, this phenomenon appears to have resolved spontaneously.

# Hearing Impairment

Hearing loss in the general population of CP has been estimated as approaching one third. But in some estimates (Bowley and Gardner, 1980) a figure of only 15% was tentatively suggested for educationally significant hearing loss requiring the use of a hearing aid. In Dunsdon's series of 1952, however, it reached 60%. In other surveys it has ranged from the 42% (17% severe) in the series of 427 children studied by Fisch (1957) to the 28% (6% severe) of 226 children assessed by Holt and Reynell (1967), both analyses of exceptionally high standard. It was emphasized by Plum (1956) that hearing impairment is commonest by far in the athetoid group, at one time so common a sequel of kernicterus in the West. The decline in kernicterus probably in part accounts for a general reduction in the incidence of hearing impairment in CP. One must bear in mind that a contribution to the hearing impairment in CP may stem from that associated with prematurity per se since hearing loss occurs in 1-5% of infants with a birth-weight below 1500g, and in 5-20% where the birth-weight has been below 800g.

The ex-premature suffers from both high and low frequency hearing loss, that of high frequency having in the past been related to jaundice, atoxic drugs (such as Streptomycin), asphyxia and intraventricular haemorrhage. Equally important to the ex-premature is the incidence of low frequency impairment secondary to conductive loss. This particular problem has commonly been found in very low birth-weight survivors and particularly in infants who have had prolonged naso-tracheal intubation. In the preterm, moreover, there is a lag in the development of expressive speech with respect to receptive speech.

Other aetiological factors are taken into consideration in the hope of facilitating future advances in prevention and/or prenatal therapy. These would include perinatal asphyxia, congenital or acquired cytomegalovirus infections, ototoxic agents, hyperbilirubinaemia of other cause and ambient noise levels.

Great care in the early detection and effective management of hearing loss is crucial in the hope of averting effects upon language development and in maximalizing the potential for treatment. Mainstreaming or integration with their normal peers as early as is practicable (Russell and Shrensky, 1992) is an especially important component, and one particularly vital for the Petö system in which the child is an active participant at all times. The child is expected to respond to the conductor as well as being constantly encouraged to develop speech.

## Cochlear Implantation in Sensorineural Deafness

Some examples of severe sensorineural deafness but intact cochlear nerve who do not respond to conventional amplification techniques may be significantly helped by cochlear implantation (House, 1986) which has already been applied by the UK centre team in Nottingham (Gibbin, 1992) to severe congenital cases. The nature of this multi-channel device, and the indication for its implantation are discussed later.

## Vestibulometry

A large series of over 90 children with spastic diplegia aged 1 to 3 years were studied from this point of view using electronystography (Semenova and Dotsenko, 1988), depending upon computerised definition of the location and severity of the vestibular involvement. The results correlated with the clinical course of the disease, especially relevant to the cases of postnatal meningoencephalitis which were included. One would have appreciated knowledge of the results in examples of ataxic CP. One also records with guarded interest and Western trepidation their rehabilitative claim that

acupuncture could normalize the mesencephalic-cortical control mechanism of the vestibular nystagmus.

On the other hand, a *sensory integration theory* for which Ayres (1985) was mainly responsible, postulates that in sensory disturbance involving the basic vestibular system exercises a significantly adverse effect upon motor development, and especially upon the overall response of the central nervous system to cerebral palsy. Through wide connections of the vestibular nuclei with vital foci in cerebellum, spinal cord, reticular formation, medial longitudinal fascicules, and the cerebral cortex integration is permitted between vestibular impulses and other sensory information concerning gravity, rotation and acceleration which are necessary to maintain normal balance and equilibrium. It is true that lesions of the vestibular structures are the source of a sense of imbalance or dysequilibrium or by vertigo, also a very specific symptom of vestibular dysfunction, and nystagmus.

The relevant hair cell receptors for this system responding to mechanical movement are enclosed within the vestibular portion of the labyrinth in utricle, saccule and the three semicircular canals. Impulses initiated by them are transmitted via the vestibular division of the VIII, the cranial nerve, to vestibular nuclei within medulla and pons. Those within utricle and saccule respond to positional or gravitational change whilst those in the semicircular canals respond to rotational or angular acceleration. In addition, when the head is tilted from a vertical position, gravitational pull is exerted on the otoliths, small calcified particles, which distorts the hair cells and initiate action potentials. In the vestibular nerve, acceleration is any plane is monitored by the three semicircular canals.

The specific list evolved by Ayres (1985) is abbreviated as the Southern Californian PRNT wherein the presence and duration of post-rotatory nystagmus is measured during and after the child is spun in a specialized scooter board or chair.

Simpler processes of testing vestibular function include:

(a) *Caloric stimulation*, with the instillation of a current of warm or cold water into the external meatus. This leads to nystagmus when the vestibular component is intact. The electro-nystography helps to more precisely define the response.

(b) Activation of the oculo-cephalic reflex: rapid turning of the head from side to side, upwards and downwards which in the normal individual evokes eye movement in the opposite direction.

On the basis of such measurements, vestibular stimulation was advocated in cerebral palsy and other motor dysfunction. To achieve this, a programme was evolved in terms of a series of exercise rituals and motor activities exploiting special equipment such as scooter boards, bolster swings and tilt-boards. A systematic programme of proprioceptive and tactile stimuli is added.

It has in consequence been alleged by Clark et al. (1977) that direct vestibular stimulation improves motor performance, even in normal children, as well as in subjects of cerebral palsy, or of Down's syndrome (Offenbacher, 1983). A controlled trial in matched children with cerebral palsy, however, has concluded (Sellick and Over, 1980) that no effects of motor gains could be demonstrated during and after three months of intensive vestibular stimulation of this kind.

## Language Functions

After full audiological analysis, including repeated pure tone audiometry and electrocochleography or mid-brain evoked potentials, each CP child is entitled to a comprehensive analysis of language function. The investigations should encompass the vital components of language comprehension and speech in the hope of a profile of language skills. But sensitive adaptation of appropriate testing for each child by an experienced psycholinguistic consultant is indicated, and an impressively comprehensive set for language assessment, etc., has been ably listed by Lees and Neville (1990) along the following lines:

*For auditory and verbal comprehension*: The test for reception of grammar (Bishop, 1983)

*For confrontational naming*: the word finding vocabulary test
Up to ten years (Renfrew, 1977)
Over 11 years: The graded naming test of Warrington.

For naming by association: Auditory Association Subtests of the Illinois Test of Psycholinguistic Abilities (Kirk et al., 1968).

For short-term auditory and verbal memory and repetition: The Sentence Repetition Test using norms of Gaddes and Crockett (1975) is helpful.

A story-telling technique introduced by Maudler and Johnson in 1977 to elicit a sample of expressive language, is also very useful in an otherwise poorly cooperative child.

## Other Communication Disorders

These have been too often glibly attributed solely to dysfunctions of receptive or expressive language, if not to mental retardation or hearing loss, or permutations thereof. In spite of relatively normal cognitive capacity, moreover, the motor disorder may be sufficiently profound to directly impair motor functions of speech, as in their severe dysarthria co-existing with dyspraxia. But the capacity to communicate is crucial to the cerebral palsied; and is his whole avenue towards creativeness apart from a wealth of human relationships... So that a sensitive awareness is necessary of a far wider range of primary as well as secondary disorders of communication which are so much a burden to the cerebral palsied child. The difficulties accompanying them vary in degree, intensity and characteristic ingredients which may well hinge upon the extent and location of the cerebral damage, and be uniquely specific to it. With increasing refinement of computerized augmentative and other equipment, these difficulties are by no means insurmountable, as alternative means of communication and expression are evolved.

## Non-verbal and Augmentative Communication Aids

There has been growing exploitation in this field of non-verbal and augmentative communication aids. These open up real possibilities for promoting the educational, functional and vocational rehabilitation of even the most severely affected cerebral palsied. Such alternative methods of communication have led to an important breakthrough in the treatment of CP. These devices embody a range of communicative symbols, which the responder can select. These include sign systems, such as those of American sign language, pictographs and ideographs resembling the idea represented such as that of the Bliss system (Bliss, 1965), or other specific letters, words and sentences. The child may indicate his choice by an electronic scanner, or by an encoding system converting coded input into a written display or electronic speech. The appropriate device will depend upon the physical handicap, the language function available, and the child's needs in daily life.

A not infrequent indication for using non-verbal communication is the severe CP complication of *pseudobulbar palsy*, typically accompanying spastic or hypertonic forms. Oral speech production may be rendered difficult if not impossible. Severe dysarthria is another indication. Actual promotion of language is another development, and augmented attempts to use verbal function appears to follow.

The dramatic success of many young CP victims in learning and utilizing such alternative communication, points to a greater underlying cognitive potential than is usually expected. Training in such alternative aids should therefore be offered to all severely affected CP children who still show awareness of the environment, although with evidence of oro-pharyngeal dysfunction expressed in lack of tongue mobility and lip closure, sagging jaw, drooling and swallowing difficulties. In the hope of achieving normal language development, this early stimulation should be begun at an elementary level during the second year of life.

# Speech Disorder

It has been broadly estimated that about 50% of cerebral palsied subjects suffer some form of speech or language deficit or defect. When large numbers of children with CP have been studied at least one half were found to present significant speech defects according to Ingram (1964) in an analysis of their complex speech problems. More precisely, 44% of his children manifested an identifiable speech defect. Most often this was a matter of retarded speech development, especially in the articulation of consonants. Other principal primary deficits include dysphasia, dyspraxia and dysarthria:

## Dysphasia

*Dysphasia* (or disorder of language) reflects disturbance in the acquisition and development of language. This may specifically implicate damage to Broca's cerebro-cortical speech area of the left hemisphere. Functional damage may involve the reception, translation and transmission of information, which can be expected to interfere with the ability to decode language-received via presumably intact sensory channels which are presumably intact but may be encroached upon. A concept of mere difficulties in organizing and selecting speech is simplistic. With input so adversely affected, defects of comprehension characterize the output: "seeing without perceiving, hearing without understanding": either non-fluent telegrammatic speech, or fluency in speech without meaning or content.

## Dyspraxia

In *dyspraxia*, or disorder of voluntary control which may co-exist with dysphasia or dysarthria, the child of appropriate apraxic age is believed to know what he wants to say but cannot execute the movement. He is aware of what he is trying to perform (i.e. he is not agnostic for that particular goal) but cannot achieve the pattern of movement needed. Confusion and mistargetting can follow a simple request to "stick out his tongue". Distinction from supra-bulbar paresis is required in glossal apraxia and may be reinforced by failure to lick his lips in response to a command, although an involuntary response is possible.

**Dysarthria**

As the child acquires language, an ultimately distressing impairment of articulation may become more conspicuous. It reflects a disorder of coordination of voluntary and involuntary movement within speech musculature, particularly of the mouth and tongue. Such sensori-motor disorder appears to involve the smooth synchronous coordination of articulation, phonation and prosody. This must also embrace the coordination control of the respiration needed to attain intelligible speech, with inability to produce a constant but controlled flow of air sometimes loosely attributed to disturbed control of tone and movement in truncal musculature. Difficulties in initiating and sustaining voice may thus be especially recognizable. Gross mistargetting of speech sounds, or incoordination of soft palatal movements leading to nasal escape, linked to inappropriate pauses and short rushes of speech are also notable.

A learning strategy to alleviate this problem includes how to target sounds more accurately, and how to coordinate breathing in a smoother, more synchronous manner. Recourse to palato-pharyngoplasty may be indicated where nasal emission is conspicuously gross. Articulatory drills using a mirror for visual feed-back is usually a helpful technique also useful in improving inspiration and phonation.

It is thus a dynamic disorder sensitive to individual changes in muscle tone, and even of mood. It especially accompanies athetoid or dyskinetic forms of CP which tend to grossly interrupt the fine motor control required for intelligible speech. Drooling is another expression of this loss of control of the speech musculature, which may as a very last resort be radically treated by resection and redirection of the mandibulary salivary ducts.

Prognosis for articulation of speech sounds is limited if there is already poor control of the vegetative functions of chewing, sucking and swallowing, which in itself frequently induces choking and regurgitation. In that context, one should recall that dysarthria may sometimes be a clinical expression of pseudobulbar palsy. Its presence may have already been suggested in early infancy when there is apparent incoordination of the oropharyngeal musculature producing difficulties in swallowing or sucking. Air swallowing may be another manifestation, as is tongue-thrust, with the tongue being pushed against the hole of the nipple. Prolonged drooling may subsequently be the result of such oropharyngeal muscle incoordination.

The conductor in Conductive Education can express her multidisciplinary responsibility in the field of speech therapy by preparing a profile which includes a graphic record of the individual child's speech abilities and disabilities. On the basis of this, a rationale can be outlined and incorporated - when appropriate - into the task series with additional sessions of positive reinforcement built into the programme when necessary. With cheaply-available technology for converting otherwise indecipherable grunts into intelligible speech, the conductor can fulfil her responsibility in respect of speech by enhancing the intelligibility of the exchange, allowing adequate time supported by positive reinforcement. The programme is communication-centred with access to alternative and augmentative means of communication. Counselling, individual or group, should also be exploited, with the therapist as the facilitator in the interaction.

The CP child may in addition manifest other subtle aberrations of communication sometimes encountered in the "normal" child. For example, *phonological*, involving the sound system of language, *phonetic* involving precise targetting and articulation, and disorders of fluency including stuttering. On the other hand, a categorization of three indefinable groups of the reading disabled on the basis of a distinctive pattern of errors has been essayed which may have application to CP. Firstly:

(a) the *dysphonetic* where there is an inability to develop word analysis skills, suggestive of dysfunction of the left cerebral hemisphere; or

(b) the *dyslidotic*, where there is no response to words "as wholes", which points instead to abnormality within the right hemisphere; and

(c) *alexic*, where there is a deficit both in phonetic skills, as well as in the ability to perceive words as "wholes", where bilateral hemispheric involvement is postulated.

One must also keep in mind the possibility, especially in the older CP victim, of related problems associated with acquired secondary cerebral dysfunction consequent upon head or post-concussional trauma or cerebro-vascular accident.

## Left-Handedness in Cerebral Palsy

In Bishop's recent comprehensive exploration of handedness (1992), she has also focused upon relationships between brain function and language development. Particular reference is made to the impairment of language ability and also of right-handed movement following injury to the left side of the brain. In other words, control of precise movement on the right, and of language processing, are both mediated by the left side of the brain whereas visuo-spatial processing is influenced by the right side.

In 57 Japanese children with athetoid CP studied by Yokochi et al. (1990), a left-sided preference was observed in 61%. It was specially common in the more severely affected children. It was hypothesized that the perinatal brain damage underlying athetosis may tend to influence a motor system predominantly involving the right side.

A complex reciprocal relationship is suggested in some individuals in whom left-handedness is associated with the control of speech by the right rather than the left side of the brain. Where there is neurological pathology, as in autism or mental retardation, and/or epilepsy such as is linked to cerebral palsy, there also appears to be a decrease in right-handedness. Ambiguous handedness is also commonly related to spina bifida and hydrocephalus. In premature children, so central to the aetiology of cerebral palsy, this may also be a factor in the decrease in right-handedness

shared with CP. Impaired maturation of or damage to intercommunicating or callosal fibres between both sides of the brain has been postulated. The subtle failures in space perception in cerebral palsy, especially in spastic diplegia, to which we have just alluded, is thus more likely to be a consequence of damage to the right side of the brain responsible for visuospatial processing.

## Emotional and Behavioural Disturbance

Behaviour disorders are especially frequent in postnatally acquired spastic hemiplegia, particularly when complicated by seizures. This does not support the common assumption that disorders of behaviour are predominantly secondary expressions of the frustrations of handicap linked to different environmental stresses including those of the family situation. In the first place, those who work closely with CP children are convinced that they often manifest an underlying lack of so-called "emotional capability", with unduly strong feelings fluctuating freely and difficult to control. Their frustration threshold is clearly low, with violent anger characterizing the frustrations which are usually so much a part of their lives, as is their disturbed self-image and poor self-esteem. Petö certainly recognized this in his emphasis on the necessity for success-orientation in each segment of any task set by the conductor, especially including the basic steps towards daily life-skills so essential in integrating the life of the CP child with that of their family, as well as with their normal peers at school or in their neighbourhood.

Maureen Oswin's study of behavioural problems in a residential hospital school for CP children (1967) also focussed on the element of acute fear afflicting them whenever facing a new situation quite apart from a constantly inherent fear of falling. In such a non-Petö residential situation, a chronically depressive condition is not unexpected, and frequently is expressed in an abrupt withdrawal from routine activities or work. Indeed their capacity to learn is seriously hampered by this general emotional disturbance. Oswin's important conclusion is that the normal phase of emotional instability in early childhood is particularly extended in the CP child. It appears that this aspect of delayed maturation, including delay in the capacity to inhibit strong feelings, may be prolonged for several years. These behavioural phenomena may well be yet another associated product of the limbic, cingulate, diencephalic, or other specific cerebral damage, and therefore a significant part of the "CP dysfunction syndrome". It was largely overlooked before Petö evolved his holistic therapeutic system.

In accord with this view is the study in 1970 of outstanding child psychiatrist, Rutter, and colleagues who revealed that approximately 40% of CP children were rated as psychiatrically disturbed. He preferred to attribute this to an intrinsic component of the brain damage or dysfunction rather than entirely to environmental influences stemming from family and community. A challenging scenario in this context is the occasional denial of the existence of a spastic arm or leg, sometimes demonstrated by the omission of one limb in the child's drawing. Even treatment is sometimes resented for this reason since it serves to constantly thrust the limb into his conscious awareness.

The joyful group atmosphere which is evoked by the conductor-group technique especially enhances the feeling of equal-sharing. It helps to overcome the loneliness of handicap, to lessen or eliminate the intense apprehensiveness, as well as the depression and otherwise characteristic tearfulness. Equal participation means the sharing of frustrations, and with it, the reduction of frustration. The success-orientation helps furthermore to reduce, and eventually erase the fear of failure or of social incompetence. In Petö's holistic approach which the British Hornsey team have so significantly strengthened, it has achieved this not least through the closest integration with both parents and family of the CP child, and within its own home. The cultivation of independence both within the group and school framework is also a vital fundamental theme at all times, and no less in the course of integrative experimentation with his normal peers. The greater the degree of independence, the greater the sense of achievement. Self-confidence and self-esteem will become more and more firmly established... The highest overall priority is given to the value of a stable, consistent and regular routine, minimizing any form of stress, enhancing emotional stability and subduing anything which disturbs and distracts from it. In other words, an accepting supportive setting both in the group and at home, so that our child can consistently enjoy his limited life at home as well as at school.

An international collaborative study of this facet in CP subjects is overdue, and would be worth-while to clarify its meaningfulness in short and long-term management. Its real significance in the Petö-treated groups and in controls would be of considerable relevance.

## Sleep Disorders and Valuable Potential Role of Melatonin

The recent application of Melatonin - the "hormone of darkness" - to control a sleep disorder in the multiply disabled, particularly when associated with brain pathology, has been richly rewarding (Jan, Espezal and Appleton, 1994).

Severe chronic sleep disorders are especially common in multiply disabled children, but are usually sadly neglected. Particularly common are fragmented sleep patterns due to disturbed sleep-wake circadian rhythm (Okawa et al., 1986), and delayed sleep-onset. Nine of 15 children with a sleep disorder which had led to family crises suffered from ocular or cortical visual impairment. Such problems in the blind have been effectively overcome (Sack et al., 1991).

Melatonin orally at night, with a mere 2.5 to 5.0 mg, sufficed to swiftly lead to night-long sleep. What is equally important is the effect upon the daytime aberrations, including self-abusive behaviour and fatigue which hitherto had been the inevitable consequences of the lack of sleep. The chronic tiredness and irritability, age-inappropriate temper outbursts, and bed-wetting, disappeared. The attention span usually improved and so did their general alertness, friendliness and curiosity.

A reassuring feature was how they awakened smiling in the mornings, rather than irritable and abrasive. Often persistent crying during the day subsided and seizure control was greatly improved. The elimination of associated family crises was dramatic, the well-being of the entire family being restored. How critically important

adequate sleep is for the multiply disabled was highlighted by this whole study. At least three of these 15 children suffered from severe spastic tetraplegia, and hyperactivity or severe attention deficit disorder was an alternative problem. Children with delayed-onset are especially responsive and no adverse side effects are recorded.

Melatonin, as a product of the pinealocytes of the Pineal gland plays a crucial role in sleep. The stimulus originates in the retina, then passes via the suprachiasmatic hypothalamic-nucleus, which may be regarded as the central sleep regulator and thence by way of the reticular system spinal cord, cervical ganglia and finally the postganglionic synaptic fibres, to reach the Pineal gland. It is the end product of an endogenous rhythm-generating system in the brain which is synchronised by the light-dark cycle, Melatonin being high in darkness, low in light. Tryptophan is its source, with conversion to serotonin and then N-acetylserotonin before arriving at N-acetyl 5 methoxytryptamine or Melatonin.

## Epileptiform Seizures

To what extent are separate and more specific precentral cortical areas involved in the high percentage of CP children who manifest epileptiform seizures? Emphasized in the earlier findings of Perlstein et al. in 1955, they have been estimated to co-exist in as much as 47% of his 1217 cerebral palsy patients. Likewise, Denhoff and Robinauth (1960), found it a manifestation of more than

half of CP children. In most other cerebral palsy studies, the incidence has ranged between 20 and 40%.

Hemiplegia was particularly conspicuous in the context of the form of CP associated with epilepsy, reaching 46% in one study. In the series of Ingram (1964) there was a sharp and presumably significant differential between right and left hemiplegia, 58.9% being right-sided, and only 29.5% left-sided.

Where intraventricular haemorrhage had been the main source of underlying cerebral damage, seizures are likely to have been its earliest clinical expression whether generalized, focal or of so-called "brain-stem type" marked by apnoea and bradycardia. Blood in the fourth ventricle, or metabolic upset due to respiratory failure, have been invoked as sources. In spite of apparently effective therapy a more subtle convulsive status may smoulder on, however, only to be revealed through 24-hour EEG monitoring. Consequent fluctuations in cerebral blood flow and metabolism may nonetheless influence an extension of haemorrhage, so that continuing anti-convulsant may be justified but only at a level not likely to induce respiratory depression. The prognosis becomes poorer if convulsions persist beyond the first few days. After two to three weeks, their appearance following the initial haemorrhage, or their re-appearance, may herald the onset of progressive hydrocephalus.

The associated porencephaly, as a belated sequel to periventricular leukomalacia, may sometimes be the source of persistent epileptiform reactions. In a personal patient with porencephaly showing increasing tension in the left temporo-parietal lobe, epilepsia partialis continua was linked to left ocular pain and sexual/emotional phantasy pattern typical of temporal lobe epilepsy.

Even acquired aphasia may be associated with such childhood epilepsy (Lees and Neville, 1990). The residual neurological deficit has then been expressed in hemiplegia.

MRI lends itself well to an exposure of focal cortical dysphasia or developmental gyral anomalies as an epileptogenic source. In a recent MRI study of ten epileptic children by Guerrini et al. (1992) two groups were definable. Apart from increased tone, seven subjects with unilateral "macrogyric-like" insulo-opercular changes manifested mental retardation as well as epilepsy. MRI also anatomically characterized the second group of three, in whom a pattern of abnormal gyri and bulging grey matter was associated with ventricular deformation. All had manifested with intractable complex partial seizures, the focal EEG anomalies of the epileptogenic zone corresponding closely with the MRI lesion site. Ablative surgery had thus far proved to be of benefit to one child.

## Infant Onset Progressive Myoclonus Epilepsy
(Hagberg et al., 1991)

This is characterized by a compound of myoclonic seizures, tonic-clonic seizures and progressive neurodevelopmental decline. Although onset may be at any stage in childhood, a number of myoclonic epilepsy syndromes may already emerge in the first year of life. They demonstrate a particular combination of clinical parameters which include previous febrile convulsions, severe myoclonic epilepsy of infancy, or EEG abnormalities such as the "burst suppression pattern" of early myoclonic epileptic encephalopathy. The most likely causation includes non-ketotic hyperglycinaemia, $GM_2$ gangliosidosis, phenylketonuria, the Santavuori variant of neuronal ceroid lipofuscinosis, or a mitochondrial cytopathy demonstrable by 'ragged-red fibres' on muscle biopsy. This latter association is well recognized under the acronym MERRF (Myoclonic epilepsy and ragged-red fibres).

In three of the examples studied by Hagberg et al. (1991) the onset of the myoclonic and generalized tonic-clonic seizures was within the first three days of life. Startle myoclonus also presented in three infants. Either hypotonia or generalized spasticity was associated with severe developmental delay in all their patients. In only two of them was there significant microcephaly. CT scans exposed cerebral atrophy in five of the eight children, with cystic white matter hypodensities in two who had more pronounced atrophy. Cerebellar atrophy occurred in two, with mitochondrial inclusions in cerebellar tissue similar to those in skeletal muscle. Cortical infarction with astrogliosis involving occipital, parietal and frontal lobes was demonstrated histologically in one with prominent cerebral atrophy. MRI in three revealed no significant differences from the previous CT scans. In addition, there was neuronal loss and astrogliosis of dentate nucleus, putamen and thalamus.

Metabolically, a complex 1 respiratory chain defect was identified in three of the eight patients of Hagberg et al. (1991). In one of these, hypotonia was prominent, whilst two manifested spastic quadriplegia. It is probable that tissues other than muscle bore the complex abnormalities, as suggested by the elevated lactate in CSF, as well as serum, and raised lactate to pyruvate ratio in cultured skin fibroblasts.

Other children with complex 1 defects include:

(1) a neonatal group with *hypotonia*, apnoeic episodes, weak feeding and encephalopathy;

(2) a group manifesting Leigh's disease;

(3) another group exhibiting *spastic tetraplegia* from birth; and

(4) a syndrome of mitochondrial myopathy, encephalopathy lactic acidosis and stroke-like episodes. Other epileptic syndromes share onset during the first year of life, with myoclonic seizures, two with specific antecedents:
  (a) preceded by prolonged febrile convulsions in severe myoclonic epilepsy of infancy;
  (b) perinatal hypoxia with non-progressive encephalopathy.

This is diagnostically helpful in differentiating the myoclonic epilepsy syndromes. Generalized spike-wave discharges occur solely in early stages of sleep in the benign form. In juvenile myoclonic epilepsy there is close correlation with a photoparoxysmal response. The infant onset form of Harborg et al. (1991) is characterized by a slow background and multifocal paroxysmal discharges.

# Neonatal Seizures:
## Prognostic Risks for Motor Disability and CP

In an effort to determine the prognostic import of neonatal seizures, a population of 39,000 infants with birth-weight greater than 2500 gm were followed up in a valuable study by Ellenberg and Nelson (1988). Survivors had neither poor Apgar scores (5 minute Apgar scores less than or equal to 5) nor other abnormal signs, a risk for motor disability of only 0.13%, whereas those with low Apgar scores and at least one of five signs compatible with neonatal encephalopathy faced a risk for first year death of 33%, with the survivors of this cluster of events confronted by a risk for motor disability of 55%. Thus amongst the infants with neonatal seizures the risk for CP was 420 times greater if there had been a combination of low 5 minute Apgar score with other abnormal neonatal signs. A tiny subgroup of term newborn was thus identified within the first days of life in whom risk for chronic motor disability of 55%, and for death or disability of 70%.

That some preventive control is attainable is suggested by the Dublin randomized trial involving 13,079 liveborn children reported in 1989 by the Grant, O'Brien, Hennessy and MacDonald team. A special intrapartum care schedule included electronic foetal heart rate monitoring with scalp blood sampling when indicated. This itself was associated with a 55% reduction in the neonatal seizures. Reassessment at the age of 4 years, of children in the intensively monitored group, and 21 in the control group who had survived after neonatal seizures, revealed that three children in each group had CP. Eight other children in the intensively monitored group, and seven in the control group who had not shown neurological signs in the neonatal period, also manifested CP. But the overall results did not support the claim that intensive monitoring has a greater protective effect against CP than intermittent intrapartum monitoring.

# Therapeutic Management
## including Surgical Intervention

The most generally useful drugs are the following:

*Phenytoin*, a hydantoinate which appears to inhibit the spread of seizure discharge rather than prevent their initiation.

*Carbamazepine* (Tegretol) has pharmacologic properties similar to phenytoin. It is the drug of choice for complex partial seizures and temporal lobe epilepsy. It is begun at a low dosage level increasing gradually if indicated over two months. The usual dosage in tablet or syrup form is 100 mg in divided doses rising to 200 mg for a child up to 1 year of age, 200-400 mg up to 5 years of age and 400-600 mg between 5 and 10 years of age, each tablet being 100 mg. In syrup form the carbamazepine is given at the level of 100 mg to 5 ml.

*Sodium valproate* is an inhibitor of enzymes metabolizing the inhibitory transmitter GABA, and has an effective anti-epileptic influence for generalized epilepsy of all types. The usual dosage begins at 20mg/kg/day increasing after 10 days to 30mg/kg/day and thence forward to a maximum of 50mg/kg/day only if necessary.

*Phenobarbitone* is also a safe anticonvulsant for all forms of epilepsy acting as a depressant both for the cortex and the reticular formation.

*Clonazepam*, a benzodiazepine, raises the discharge threshold of the thalamus but not of the cortex. Its broad spectrum of action includes a special value in myoclonic epileptic forms.

Nonetheless at least seizure control is not achieved in 20-30% of childhood cases which leads to profound disruption of their lives (Brorson and Wranne, 1987). The most promising drug now available to bridge this gap is gamma-vinyl GABA or *Vigabatrin* (GVG). It is effective in both partial and generalized epilepsies and can also control symptomatic infantile spasms, a dose of 40-80 mg/kg/day being advised. There is, however, already some evidence that hyperactivity can be a significant side effect.

*Pyridoxine* has also been used empirically in infantile epilepsy, i.e. even in the absence of any specific evidence of pyridoxine dependency. The report from Ohtsuka et al. is a case in point, with 15 examples claimed to have responded successfully out of 118 patients so treated, i.e. a 12.7% efficacy.

**Surgical Intervention in Refractory Epilepsy**

An increasing number of successes are being reported for the use of surgery in intractable epilepsy, although its application to CP is still rare. Limited resections of the pre- and postcentral gyrus has been the principal approach although callosotomy has been used in intractable drop attacks.

If there is a localized lesion or a constant EEG focus associated with SSW, therapeutic investigation should be aimed at identifying an approach which is potentially amenable to surgery. MRI appears to allow better identification of the aetiology of symptomatic PE than CT scanning. In one series, the percentage of abnormal MRI findings reached 38.5% amongst child subjects in whom the CT scan had been normal. The superior definition of lesions included anatomic changes particularly in temporal internal regions, and of cortical modifications making it possible to more precisely specify certain aspects of malformation.

In the light of the improved results, surgery should be considered whenever there is a consistently recurring focus of epileptic spikes in the frontal or temporal lobes, excision of the site of the focus being the objective. The best results have been achieved in temporal lobe seizures in which areas of gliosis or vascular anomalies have been exposed within the temporal lobe. Such temporal lobectomy has been recorded to achieve abolition of attacks in 50%, with convincing improvement in 25%.

The Oxford Group (Oxbury et al., 1993) have recently summed up the results of en bloc temporal lobectomy (16Rt 10L) for chronically drug-resistant epilepsy in 26 children. Thirteen of these revealed brain CT scan evidence of non-atrophic temporal lobe pathology, whilst in eleven others at least one early childhood convulsion was associated with severe depletion of hippocampal neurones. The five-year outcome was impressive in 13 who had not experienced a single post-operative seizure, whilst 7 had suffered only isolated seizures with at least two years freedom from all manifestations of epilepsy.

A more recently advocated neuro-surgical technique for refractory epilepsy has been MST or *Multiple Subpial Transection*. Promising results have been reported in the Landau-Kleffner Syndrome (Robinson et al., 1993). In their challenging account, they cited a previous successful result of a subject with this syndrome in whom the associated *auditory agnosia* was also overcome with restoration of near normal language by six months after surgery.

The propagation of seizure activity from the discharging volume of cortex is interrupted by the transection of horizontal fibres. As far as is practicable, descending fibres responsible for function are preserved, although not infrequently this fails so that hemiatrophy has been a sequel in three of ten cases operated upon by the Morrell team.

In their 10-year-old patient (Robinson et al., 1993) amytal and pentothal suppressive tests applied to the epileptiform discharges represented by bilateral bursts of sharp and slow waves maximal over *both* temporal regions indicated that the bilateral activity was being driven primarily from the left temporal area. The exciting outcome of the MST included elimination of the fits and her near-psychotic behaviour, whilst her intercommunication has reached 50 words and the awake EEG is now entirely normal. Whilst undoubtedly encouraging, the application of such surgical intervention remains to be cautiously exploited.

# Use of SPECT technique to Clarify Haemodynamic Patho-Physiology of the Cerebral Cortex in Epilepsy

The new technique of early single proton emission computed tomography (SPECT) using N-isopropyl-p-[1231] iodo amphetamine was applied to a series of 71 child subjects of epilepsy (Imai et al., 1991). In symptomatic epilepsy especially in the West and Lennox syndromes, SPECT revealed a significant decrease in cerebral cortical blood flow during ACTH therapy. It was suggested that this technique is especially helpful in monitoring the therapeutic effectiveness of ACTH, etc. quite apart from its general usefulness in helping to clarify the haemodynamic patho-physiology of the brain.

# Silent Gastro-oesophageal Reflux in Cerebral Palsy

It has been more recently recognized that gastro-oesophageal reflux, and even prolonged episodes of sleep reflux, are common in the preterm and infant. They have been particularly incriminated in infantile apnoea, pulmonary aspiration and bronchopulmonary dysplasia (Booth 1992). In one subgroup of premature infants with especially severe reflux in the presence of non-obstructive and xanthine-resistant apnoea, treatment with posturing and thickening of feed led to firm *resolution of the apnoeic symptoms*.

The common incidence of feeding difficulties, vomiting and recurrent chest infections in children with central nervous system disorders has been frequently associated with such reflux. An incidence of reflux as high as 75% was revealed by Abrahams and Burkitt (1976) in a small group of children and adolescents with severe spastic CP. Extended *lower oesophageal pH monitoring* has more recently vindicated this extraordinary incidence (Halpern et al., 1991; Staino et al., 1991). An interesting central nervous system association was the *dystonic posturing concurrent with such reflux* in the Sandifer syndrome being cured in the hands of

Puntis and colleagues (1989). Moreover, motor dysfunction of the oesophagus in children with psychomotor retardation and superadded oesophagitis contributes to the oesophageal "dysmobility" as well as leading to severe iron deficiency anaemia.

*Recurrent broncho-pulmonary aspiration* is another risk to be considered in this context. CP children are at any rate already at special risk for broncho-pulmonary aspiration of oral secretions. Use could therefore be justified of a radionuclide "salivagram". A positive test does not necessarily imply that the infant or child is at risk for aspiration after gastro-oesophageal reflux, but as Heyman and Respondek have suggested (1989), sequential images of lung fields after the oral reactivation has cleared could well provide sensitive detection of aspiration following such reflux.

Anti-reflux surgery, especially "Nissanfundoplication" (Rice et al., 1991) plays an important role in these neurologically abnormal infants and children, particularly in those with severe oesophagitis and even profound protein-energy malnutrition as its sequel.

# Swallow and Ventilation Problems: Patho-Physiology

Recent refinements of technique have been applied (Kenny, Casas and McPherson, 1989) to the elucidation of feeding and swallowing problems characterizing CP. The initiation of swallowing is a complex

coordinated sequence of movement of tongue, pharynx and larynx mediated through two cranial nerves - the IXnth or glosso-pharyngeal and the Xnth or vagus. The videotaped output of ultrasound camera and the analogue data derived from physiological measurements of swallowing and ventilation are synchronized. The CP children exhibited much more variability and less control of the liquid bolus than the controls, with impaired control of the posterior part of the tongue in some of the CP children. There was slowing of some segments of the sequence of oral swallow and of the time to reach maximal anterior displacement of the hyoid bone.

A related ventilatory aspect is also worthy of additional exploration. A short-latency apnoea accompanied a saliva swallow, whereas a long latency apnoea attends semi-solid or liquid bolus (alimentary) swallows.

# Hip Subluxation

Apart from referral to a physical therapist to prevent or minimize contractures, hip subluxation should also be excluded as a sequel to the high incidence of adductor spasticity in diplegics or tetraplegics. At least partial subluxation is not uncommon in spastic involvement of the lower extremities. If previously overlooked, it should still be picked up by careful examination and routine x-rays of the hip at 2 years, and at least again at 5. The prevention of hip instability is of greater importance. Since the principal precursor of hip subluxation and dislocation appears to be an adduction deformity of the hip, efforts should be concentrated on this stage, whether or not supported by soft-tissue releases.

A substantial contribution to the study of the implications of hip instability in cerebral palsy, and the prevention of dislocation has stemmed from David Scrutton. Those he considers particularly at risk are those suffering "undue delay in walking, or with very stiff legs". Consequent dislocation may be very gradual, with worsening problems of movement and posture, attended by intensified difficulties of sitting and walking. Pain in the hip is superimposed later...

Another important contribution to the prevention of spastic hip dislocation stems from Heimkes and his colleagues (Heimkes, Stotz and Heid, 1992). Their retrospective analysis of 82 hips of 41 subjects of CP portrays a pathogenic model of such "spastic paralytic dislocation". Reduced activity of the gluteus maximus, medius, minimus and quadriceps femoris muscles, which normally cause a decrease of valgus and anteversion, leads to an increased subluxating coxa valga antetorta with consequent dislocation.

To prevent this trend, it is postulated that these muscle groups must undergo increased activation. And to achieve this activation, this team are emphasizing the essential need for walking as the strongest stimulus for what they define as the dislocation-preventing hip abductors, and hip extensors. It perhaps goes without saying that the erect posture and gait must be encouraged as early as possible. There is still a place, however, for appropriate muscle-relaxing or releasing surgery to overcome antagonistically-effective hip flexors, adductor and inward rotators as well as knee flexors, which can even serve to counteract a dislocation in a severely handicapped child unable to walk.

## Adaptive and Orthotic Devices

Provisional inhibitory casting has gained some popularity in the control of pathological alignment in the ankle and feet. The walking cast is first applied for a 4 to 6 week period. Such sustained stretching contributes to inhibition of hyperactive stretch and tonic reflexes in the foot. Whether this procedure can consistently avert spastic foot deformities and diminish the need for any more radical surgical procedure remains to be confirmed.

The introduction of lightweight *plastic orthoses* in the correction of deformity and improvement of mobility also represent a valuable new trend, especially useful when muscle weakness is a dominant element rather than spasticity. Their corrective effectiveness because of the closeness of fit they permit inside the shoe is another advantage. Most often used for ankle and foot correction, it may be used in combination with metal when knee and hip control is required.

Other adaptive devices are in occasional use, such as the prone standers parapodium, and even crawling devices may be helpful in very special circumstances. There has also been a recent revival of a more scientific interest in seating, mainly to seek optimal head control and hand control. It should be acknowledged first of all that conventional wheelchair models - which are fortunately no part of the Petö armamentarium - rarely meet the requirements for postural support for growing children. The usual soft fling seat adds to trunk instability, asymmetric posture and an internally rotated, adducted position of the hips. A common problem in CP involves increased extensor thrust, tending to make the child slide out of the chair.

The maintenance of the hips, knees and ankles at 90° flexion with a 10-15° posterior tilt of the seat, is recommended to integrate such a tendency. In the floppy hypotonic child, greater stability may be achieved by supporting the lumbar spine in a lordotic alignment.

## Contractures

Contractures, implying a state of shortening of a muscle not due to active contraction, are an insidious and avoidable sequel of spastic disorder. In McArdle's disease, they may be spontaneously reversible, but more often require intervention by repeated stretching, etc. The process has been attributed to a re-arrangement of collagen fibrils within muscle over a longer period. Progressive

85

shortening may arise when muscular action is not opposed by a sufficiently potent antagonist, or one steadily becoming weaker. If neglected, fibrosis makes it increasingly difficult to treat.

Yet another perspective was introduced by the search for an animal model of spasticity in the human being (Wright and Rang, 1990). It was concluded that genetically spastic mice are an homogenous population that embody an abnormally functioning neurotransmitter within the CNS. This model was shown to develop abnormality of muscle growth that ultimately leads to contractures.

Their development, leading to fixed deformity in the CP child, is the most disabling sequel of poor management. Similarly, scoliosis or hip subluxation may well be preventable features of the advanced classical clinical picture which the constantly vigorous active movements and positioning of the child in the Petö system helps us to avoid. Likewise, basic application of the Petö system, even as part of an eclectic approach can help overcome or circumvent the primary disabilities, such as overactive adductors of the lower extremities, which has so frequently invited surgical intervention in the past. Consistent concern

to prevent are nevertheless essential, and passive stretching of the tight soft tissue and ligamentous structures around the joint should be performed on a regular daily basis, The tendo achilles, the knee flexors, hip flexors and the tibial band are the most commonly affected. Contractures at the knee, shoulder, elbow and wrist should never occur once carefully instructed in passive stretching. Parents and even older siblings can help to sustain a regular daily programme of passive stretching, which is effective in preventing deformity, and perhaps also in enhancing mobility.

Where neglect has occurred, lightweight night splints of plaster of Paris can be invaluable in controlling contractures, especially of the tendon achilles and of the wrist flexors. Comfort and the prevention of pressure sores are important considerations.

Although it is our belief that such contractures are avoidable, there is still a disproportionately high incidence, even in excellent centres, for the care of CP. For instance, significant contractures were noted in 45% of 108 CP children admitted to the John F. Kennedy Institute for Handicapped Children in 1977.

## Premature Cervical Spondylosis in Athetoid Cerebral Palsy

The relationship to "overuse" in athetosis has recently been subjected to a somewhat unusual study in the experimental animal. The young rabbit spine was subjected to repetitive extension-

flexion movement through electrical stimulation of the trapezius muscle. It was found that repetitive loads, 200,000 cycles caused more severe delamination of the annulus fibrosus than control at the lower cervical spine. It was also associated with early osteophyte formation at the same disc level.

It was concluded that repetitive movement or overuse served to accelerate the progression of structural abnormalities, such as prematurely generating cervical spondylosis.

## Odontogenesis

Odontogenesis is also frequently disturbed, leading to sufficient abnormality in shape, size or placement of teeth to justify early orthodontic management. In addition, there appears to be a particular vulnerability to tooth decay in the cerebral palsy child population. Defect in enamel formation may in fact be yet another consequence of foetal anoxia, being reflected in a brownish band horizontally crossing the tooth.

## Submandibular Duct Diversion to Overcome Refractory Sialorrhoea in CP

Submandibular duct diversion is now a fairly common procedure for refractory sialorrhoea in CP. A recent report by Hotaling et al. (1992) on six patients with CP (mean age 14.7 years), documented their evaluation by technetium scanning. Successful bilateral function was reported in four of them, with unilateral function adequate in a further two.

## Associated Hypothalamic or Neurovegetative Disturbances including Obesity

Von Howern (1966) drew attention to the common association with obesity, citing 15 examples, although not clearly only in those CP children who are relatively inactive in conjunction with a high caloric intake. In the majority of obese CP children, cranial trauma appears to have been incriminated, possibly extending to bilateral involvement of ventromedial hypothalamic nuclei, and damage to satiety control.

Genetic factors related to the infantile or childhood onset of obesity may be crucial, and dietetic efforts to combat these must be begun early. Otherwise, the obesity can impose a serious additional handicap adversely affecting the functional motor progress, and the incidence of contractures and hip subluxation. To complement a low caloric intake with anorexic agents is not only humane, it is strongly justified in the perspective of an optimal life style for a CP child.

# Growth Deficit

Impaired growth of the affected extremities is characteristic in spastic CP, especially conspicuous in spastic hemiparesis. Almost half of these will show length discrepancies in arm and leg. Such a deficit of 2 to 3 cms in one lower extremity, which peaks by the age of 6-8 years, may have already produced a pelvic tilt and even compensatory scoliosis. Earlier insertion of heel and sole lifts to equalize any such discrepancy in length can prevent this. The routine exclusion and prompt alleviation of scoliosis is also important, again especially in spastic tetraparesis.

General growth is also diminished in children with poor neurodevelopmental functioning of differing sources. Those suffering cerebral palsy are shorter and have a smaller head circumference (Ross, Lipper and Auld, 1985). It is possible that a degree of growth failure during the phase of rapid brain and somatic growth may influence later cognitive function apart from ultimate growth.

The majority of studies whether case control, case series with a population comparison group, or cohort studies have shown a disproportionately high incidence of intra-uterine growth retardation in cerebral palsy. For example, in comparing birth-weight and gestation among cases from a population-based register with those of liveborn controls from the same population, as well as with those of total live births between 1968 and 1975, Stanley (1981) concluded that spastic cases (especially those classified as tetraplegic and hemiplegic) showed increasing proportions of growth retardation in the more recent years. Indeed, a strong statistically significant association was defined by Stanley et al. (1985) between spastic cerebral palsy and poor intra-uterine growth in 134 infants born at more than 33 weeks gestation. Forty-nine cases of spastic diplegia born at term were also compared by Veelken et al. (1983) with 215 term controls. Fourteen per cent were small for gestational age compared with an expected 2.3%. It is apparent that the risk of simple spastic diplegia is directly related to foetal "depletion", foetal immaturity and low birth-weight, as illustrated in figures portraying birth-prevalent rates for the cerebral palsies in other countries. One unproven hypothesis has suggested that there are several avenues through which such factors associated with intra-uterine growth retardation could lead to brain damage. These include intrapartum hypoxia, hypoglycaemia and hypothermia. But by no means yet clarified is whether the intra-uterine growth impact is due to factors specifically underlying prematurity and their effect upon neuronal development at critical stages of maturation, or whether secondary to other risks involved in preterm delivery such as intraventricular haemorrhage and/or periventricular leukomalacia. It has been suggested that the overall effects of foetal growth retardation may serve to make the foetus and infant more vulnerable to the stress of delivery and to postnatal adaptation. "Intra-uterine growth retardation" is by no means a single entity. Of the specific form originally introduced by Russell in 1954, in association with multiple placental infarctions, prenatal bleeding and presumptive "foetal deprivation of supply", cerebral palsy has not manifested in a subsequent series of 42 personal cases. It is better visualized as a final common pathway of differing patho-physiological insults, one of which may produce cerebral palsy. In other words, adverse factors acting during gestation, often in concert with each other, may effect retardation of the foetal growth rate. The practical issue remaining is how medical intervention can minimize the high risk of cerebral palsy among survivors of very low gestational age and birth-weight.

## References

Abrahams P, Burkitt BFE. (1976) Hiatus hernias and gastro-oesophageal reflux in children and adolescents with cerebral palsy. Aust Paediatr J 26: 41-46

Adlard BP et al. (1973) Effect of undernutrition in early life on glutamate decarboxylase activity. Biochem J 130: 12p

Aicardi J. (1991) The argyria-pachygyria complex: a spectrum of cortical malformation. Brain Dev 13: 1-8

al-Rajeh S et al. (1991) Cerebral palsy in Saudi Arabia: a case-control study of risk factors. Dev Med Child Neurol 33: 1048-1052

Alberman ED. (1963) Birth-weight and length of gestation in CP. Dev Med Child Neurol 5: 388-394

Alberman E. (1991) Personal communication.

Amin-Zaki L et al. (1974) Intra-uterine methyl mercury poisoning in Iraq. Pediatrics 54: 587-595.

Andermann E, Palmini A et al. (1992) Familial bilateral congenital perisylvian syndrome: a localized neuronal migration disorder. Neurology 42: suppl 3, 354

Arens LJ, Molteno CD. (1989) A comparative study of postnatally acquired cerebral palsy in Cape Town. Dev Med Child Neurol 31: 246-254

Arens LJ, Molteno CD, Marshall SR, Robertson WI, Rabkin J. (1978) Cerebral palsy in Cape Town - a comparative 12-year retrospective study. S Afr Med J 53: 319-324

Ashkenazi CMV, Russell A, Zadik Z. (1972) Prevalence of cytomegalovirus complement fixing antibodies in Jerusalem and Rechovat Arcas. Proc Israel Paediatr Soc. XVth Nattional Scientific Congress, Beir Harojeh. pp 12-13

Atkinson S, Stanley FJ. (1983) Spastic diplegia among children of low and normal birth-weight. Dev Med Child Neurol 25: 693-708

Ayres AJ. (1985) Sensory Integration and the Child. Western Psychological Services, Los Angeles

Baker AW, Duncan SP. (1985) Child sex abuse: a study of prevalence in Great Britain. Child Abuse Negl 3: 565-575

Baker SP. (1979) Motor vehicle occupant deaths in young children. Pediatrics 64: 860-861

Bishop DVM (1983) The test for reception of grammar. University of Manchester

Blair E, Stanley FJ. (1982) An epidemiological study of cerebral palsy in Western Australia. III: Postnatal aetiology. Dev Med Child Neurol 24: 575-585

Blair E, Stanley F. (1988) Intrapartum asphyxia: a rare cause of cerebral palsy. J Pediat 112: 515-519

Blair E, Stanley F. (1990) Intra-uterine growth and spastic cerebral palsy. I: Association with birth-weight for gestational age. Am J Obstet Gynecol 162: 229-237

Blair E, Stanley F. (1992) Intrauterine growth and spastic cerebral palsy. II. The association with morphology at birth. Early Hum Dev 28: 91-103

Bliss CK (1965) Semantography - Bliss Symbolics. Semantography Publications, Sydney

Boesch C et al. (1989) Magnetic resonance imaging of brain in congenital cytomegalovirus encephalopathy. Pediatr Radiol 19: 91-93

Booth JW. (1992) Silent gastro-oesophageal reflux: how much do we miss? Arch Dis Child Annot 67: 1325-1326

Bowley AH, Gardner L. (1980) The child with hearing loss. In: The Handicapped Child. Churchill Livingstone

Breakey AS. (1955) Ocular findings in cerebral palsy. Arch Ophthalmol 53: 85

Brorson LO, Wranne L. (1987) Long term prognosis in childhood epilepsy: survival and seizure prognosis. Epilepsia 28: 324-330

Campbell S et al. (1986) Qualitative assessment of uteroplacental blood flow: early screening test for high risk pregnancies. Obstet Gynecol 68: 493-506

Carlson DE. (1988) Maternal diseases associated with intrauterine growth retardation. Semin Perinatol 12: 17-22

Chamberlain A et al. (1984) Issues in fertility control for mentally retarded female adolescents. 1. Sexual activity, sexual abuse and contraception. Pediatrics 73: 445-450

Childs B, Evans PR. (1954) Birth-weight of children with CP. Lancet 1: 642-645

Churchill JA. (1958) The relationship of Little's disease to premature birth. Am J Dis Child 96: 779-786

Clark DL et al. (1977) Vestibular stimulation influence on motor development in infants. Science 196: 1228-1229

Cussen GH, Barry JF, Moloney ME, Buckley NM, Crowley M, Daly C. (1978) Cerebral palsy - a regional study. J Irish Med Assoc 71: 568-572

De Long GR. (1993) Effects of nutrition on brain development in humans. Am J Clin Nutr 57: 2865-2905

Denhoff E, Robinauth IP. (1960) Cerebral Palsy and Related Disorders. McGraw-Hill Book Co., New York

Diamond CJ, Jaudes PK. (1983) Child abuse in a CP population. Dev Med Child Neurol 25: 169-174

Dobyns WB. (1989) The neurogenetics of lissencephaly. Neurol Clinics 7: 89-105

Douglas AA. (1961) Ophthalmological aspects. In: JL Henderson (Ed) Cerebral Palsy in Childhood and Adolescence. Edinburgh, Livingstone.

Dowding VM, Barry C. (1988) Cerebral palsy: changing patterns of birthweight and gestational age (1976-81). Br Med J 81: 25-29

Dubowitz LMS, Bydder GM, Muskin J. (1985) Developmental sequence of periventricular leukomalacia correlation of ultrasound, clinical and nuclear magnetic resonance function. Arch Dis Child 60: 349-355

Dunsdon MI. (1952) The educability of cerebral palsied children. Newness, London. 170, 92

Edwards MJ. (1969) Congenital defects in guinea pigs. Prenatal retardation of brain growth of guinea pigs following hyperthermia during gestation. Teratology 2: 239

Ellenberg JH, Nelson KB. (1979) Birth-weight and gestational age in cerebral palsy and seizure disorders. Am J Dis Child 133: 1044

Embil JA et al. (1970) Congenital cytomegalovirus in two siblings. J Pediatr 77: 417-423

Evrard P. (1988) Les troubles du developpment pernatal du cortex cerebral humain. Bull Med Acad R Med Belg 143: 356-368

Evrard P, Lyon G, Gadisseux JF. (1984) Les processus destructifs agissant durant la seconde montré de la grossesse, durant la période de croissance et la differenciation du tissu nerveux. Progrés en Neonatologie, Vol 4, pp 85-106. Basel, New York, Karger

Fernell E, Hagberg B, Hagberg G, Hult G, von Wendt L. (1988) Epidemiology of infantile hydrocephalus in Sweden. Current aspects of the outcome in preterm infants. Neuropediat 19: 143-145

Ferrari F, Cioni G, Prechtl HF. (1990) Qualitative changes of general movement in preterm infants with brain lesions. Early Hum Dev 23: 193-231

Finlay KH. (1958) Postencephalitis manifestation of viral encephalitis. In: WS Fields, RJ Blattner (Eds) Viral Encephalitis. Springfield, Illinois, CC Thomas. pp 69-94

Fisch L. (1957) Hearing impairment and cerebral palsy. Speech 21: 43

Fisher DA, Dussault JH, Sack J, Chopra IJ. (1977) Ontogenesis of hypothalamic-pituitary-thyroid function and metabolism in man, sheep and rat. Rec Prog Norm Res 33: 59-116

Foley J. (1977) Visual defects. In: CM Drillian, MB Drummond (Eds) Neurodevelopmental Problems in Early Childhood. Oxford, Blackwell Scientific Publications

Foley J. (1992) Dyskinetic and dystonic cerebral palsy and birth. Acta Paediat 81: 57-60

Fowler KB et al. (1992) The outcome of congenital cytomegalovirus infections in relation to maternal antibody studies. New Engl J Med 326: 663-667

Freud S. (1968) Infantile cerebral palsies. Translation: LA Russin. University of Miami Press, Miami

Friede RL. (1989) Dysplasias of cerebral cortex. In: Developmental Neuropathology. Springer, Vienna. pp 330-346

Gaddes WH, Crockett DJ. (1975) The Spreen-Benton aphasia tests: normative data as a measure of language development. Brain Language 3: 257-280

Garg BK, Srivastava JR. (1965) Cerebral palsy - a clinical study of 124 cases with a review. Indian Pediat 2: 195-208

Gibbin KP (1992) Paediatric cochlear implantation. Arch Dis Child 67: 669-671

Goldblatt J, Ballo R, Sachs B, Moosa A. (1989) X-linked spastic paraplegia: Evidence for homogeneity with variable phenotype. Clin Genet 35: 116-120

Grant A et al. (1989) Routine formal fetal movement counting and risk of antepartum late death in normally formed singletons. Lancet ii: 345-349

Gross SJ, Oehler JM, Eckerman CO. (1983) Head growth and developmental outcome in very low birth-weight infants. Pediatrics 71: 70-75

Guerrini R et al. (1992) Epilepsy and focal gyral anomalies detected by MRI: electroclinico-morphological correlations. Dev Med Child Neurol 34: 706-718

Guzzetta FF, Shackelford GD, Volpe S, Perlman JM, Volpe JJ. (1986) Periventricular intraparenchymal echodensities in the premature newborn. Critical determinant of neurologic outcome. Pediatrics 78: 995-1006

Hagberg B, Hagberg G, Olow I. (1975) The changing panorama of cerebral palsy in Sweden 1954-1970. Analysis of the general changes. Acta Paediat Scand 64: 187-192

Hagberg B, Hagberg G, Olow I. (1975) The changing panorama of cerebral palsy in Sweden 1954-1970. II. Analysis of the various syndromes. Acta Paediat Scand 64: 193-200

Hall DM et al. (1989) Birth asphyxia. Br Med J 299: 272-282

Halpern IM, Jolly SE, Johnson DG. (1991) Gastrooesophageal reflux: a significant association with central nervous system disease in children. J Pediatr Surg 26: 171-173

Hamano S, Nara T, Nizaki H, Fukushima K, Imai M, Kumagai K, Maekawa K. (1991) Crossed cerebellar diaschisis demonstrable by SPECT in hemiplegic children. No To Hattatsu 23: 58-64

Hansen TWJ, Tydal T, Jorgensen H et al. (1985) Effect of bilirubin on uptake of 5-HT and Dopamine in rat brain synaptosomes. Pediat Res 19: 390A

91

Heimkes S, Stotz S, Heid T. (1992) Pathogenesis and prevention of spastic hip dislocation. Orthop Ihre Grenzgeb 130: 413-418

Heyman S, Respondek M. (1989) Detection of pulmonary aspiration in children by radionuclide "salivagram". J Nucl Med 30: 697-699

Hier DB, LeMay M, Rosenberg PB, Perlo VP. (1978) Developmental dyslexia: evidence for a subgroup with reversal of cerebral asymmetry. Arch Neurol 35: 90-92

Ho M. (1991) Cytomegalovirus Biology and Infection. Plenum Publishing Corporation, New York

Hohenhauer L. (1980) Intrauterine Wachstum skuroen fur den deutchen Sprachrum. Z. Geburtsch Perinatal 184: 167

Holt KS, Reynell JK. (1967) Assessment of Cerebral Palsy. Vol II. London, Lloyd-Luke.

Hotaling AJ et al. (1992) Post operative technetium scanning in patients with submandibular duct divertion. Arch Otolaryngol Head Neck Surg 118: 1331-1333

House WE. (1986) Cochlear implants: present and future. Otolaryngol Clin N Am 19: 217-218

Ikonen RS, Janas MO, Koivikko MJ, Laippala P, Kuusinen EJ. (1992) Hyperbilirubinaemia, hypocarbia and periventricular leukomalacia leukamenia in preterm infants: relationship to cerebral palsy. Acta Paediat 81: 802-807

Illingworth (1985) A paediatrician asks why is it called birth injury. Br J Obstet Gynaecol 92: 122-130

Imai M et al. (1991) Early 1231-IMP Spect in patients with epilepsy. No To Hattatsu 23: 458-464

Ingram TTS. (1964) Paediatric Aspects of Cerebral Palsy. Livingstone, London. 2-14,15,17,18,30

James D. (1990) Diagnosis and management of fetal growth retardation. Arch Dis Child 65: 390-394

Jan JE, Espezel H, Appleton RE. (1994) The treatment of sleep disorders with melatonin. Dev Med Child Neurol 36: 97-107

Jones KL. (1988) Smith's recognizable patterns of human malformation. 4th Edn. Saunders, Philadelphia

Kaiser G. (1988) Sagittal synostosis - its clinical significance and the results of three different methods of craniectomy. Childs Nerv Syst 4: 223

Kalizhnwik ES. (1989) Bilirubin encephalopathy. Zh Neuropatol Psikhiat 89: 45-48

Kenny DJ, Casas MJ, McPherson KA. (1989) Correlation of ultrasound imaging of oral swallow with ventilatory observations in the cerebral palsied. Dysphagia 4: 112-117

Kirk SA, McCarthy JJ, Kirk WD (1968) The Illinois Test of Psycholinguist Abilities. University of Illinois

Kuban KC et al. (1992) Maternal toxaemia associated with reduced incidence of germinal matrix haemorrhage in premature babies. J Child Neurol 7: 70-76

Lademann A. (1978) Postnatally acquired cerebral palsy. Acta Neurol Scand: suppl. 65, 3

Laplaza F, Janvier F, Root L, Tassanawipas A, Cervera P. (1992) Cerebral palsy in twins. Dev Med Child Neurol 34: 1053-1063

Largo RH, Molinari L, Pinto LC, Weber M, Duc G. (1986) Language development of term and preterm children during first 5 years of life. Dev Med Child Neurol 28: 333-350

Largo RH et al. (1990) Neurological outcome in high risk weight appropriate for gestational age in preterm children at early school age. Europ J Pediat 149: 835-844

Lees JA, Neville BGR. (1990) Acquired aphasia in childhood: case studies in five children. Aphasiology 4: 463-478

Little J, Bryan E. (1986) Congenital anomalies in twins. Semin Perinatol 10: 50-64

Longo LD et al. (1973) An anaerobic glycogen-dependent transport of anino acids by the placenta. Nature

Lucas A, Morley R, Cole TJ. (1988) Adverse neurodevelopmental outcome of moderate neonatal hypoglycaemia. Br Med J 297: 1304-1308

Lumley JTA, Wood C. (1967) Influence of hypoxia in glucose transport across the human placenta. Nature 216: 403-404

McCarthy GT et al. (1981) The Physically Handicapped Child: Interdisciplinary Approach to Management. Faber and Faber, London

McIlwaine GM et al. (1979) Scottish perinatal mortality study. Br Med J 8: 1103-1106

Marsal K. (1989) Fetal and placental blood flow. In: F Sharpe, RB Fraser, RDG Milner (Eds) Fetal Growth. Royal College of Obstetricians and Gynaecologists, London. pp 279-308

Martin HB. (1970) Microcephaly and mental retardation. Am J Dis Child 119: 128

Maudler JM, Johnson NS. (1977) Remembrance of things passed: story structure and recall. Cognitive Psychol 8: 111-151

Moll W (1973) Placental function and oxygenation of the fetus. Adv Exp Med Biol 37: 1017

Molteno CD, Arens LJ, Marshall SR, Robertson WI. (1980) Cerebral palsy in Cape Town - a review of 389 coloured children. S Afr Med J 57: 823-826

Morales S. (1989) Use of intrathecal baclofen. Acta Neurochir 46: 39-45

Morales WJ et al. (1989) Efficacy and safety of Indomethacin vs Ritodrine in preterm labor. Obstet Gynec 74: 567-572

Neligan GA. (1976) Born too soon and born too small. Clin Dev Med No. 61

Nelson KB, Ellenberg JH. (1978) Epidemiology of cerebral palsy. In: Advances in Neurology Vol 19, pp 421-435, BS Schoenberg (Ed). Raven Press, New York

Nelson KB, Ellenberg JH. (1981) Apgar scores as predictors of chronic neurologic disability. Pediatrics 68: 36

Nelson KB, Ellenberg JH. (1985) Antecedents of cerebral palsy. I. Univariate analysis of risks. Am J Dis Child 139: 1031-1038

Nelson KB, Ellenberg JH. (1986) Antecedents of CP. II. Multivariant analysis of risks. Neuropaediat 4: 403

Nelson WP. (1988) What proportion of cerebral palsy is related to birth asphyxia. J Pediatr 112: 572-584

Netzar M et al. (1979) Placental transfer of analogues of glucose and amino acids in experimental intrauterine growth retardation. Pediatr Res 13: 100-103

Nicholson A, Alberman E. (1992) Cerebral palsy - an increasing contributor to severe mental retardation. Arch Dis Child 67: 1050-1055

Nicolaides KH et al. (1989) Blood gases, pH and lactate in small for gestational age fetuses. Am J Obstet Gynecol 261: 996-1007

Nicolaides KH et al. (1989) Treatment of fetal growth retardation. In: F Sharpe, RB Fraser, RDG Milner (Eds) Fetal Growth. Royal College of Obstetricians and Gynaecologists, London. pp 333-361

Nigro G, Clerico A, Mondaini C. (1993) Symptomatic congenital cytomegalo-virus infection in two consecutive sisters. Arch Dis Child 69: 527-528

Niswander K, Henson G, Elbourne D, Chalmers L, Redman C, Macfarlane A, Tizard P. (1984) Adverse outcome of pregnancy and quality of obstetrical care. Lancet ii: 827

Norris EH (1916) Morphogenesis of follicles in human thyroid. Am J Anat 20: 411-448

Offenbacher K. (1983) Developmental implications of clinically applied vestibular stimulation. Phys Therapy 63: 338-341

Okawa M, Takahashi K, Sasaki H. (1986) Disturbance of circadian rhythms in severe brain-damaged patients correlated with CT findings. J Neurol 233: 274-282

Ornoy A, Benady S, Kohen-Raz A, Russell A. (1976) Association between maternal bleeding during gestation and congenital anomalies in the offspring. Am J Obstet Gynec 124: 474-478

Oswin M. (1967) Behaviour Problems amongst Children with Cerebral Palsy. Wright, Bristol

Oxbury JM et al. (1993) The condition at follow-up five years after temporal lobectomy in childhood for intractable epilepsy. Abst.

Palmini A et al. (1991) Diffuse cortical dysplasia or the "double cortex" syndrome: the clinical and epileptic spectrum in 10 patients. Neurology 41: 1656-1662

Paneth N, Stark RI. (1983) Cerebral palsy and mental retardation in relation to indicators of perinatal asphyxia. Am J Obstet Gynecol 147: 960-966

Pape KE, Wigglesworth JS. (1979) The clinico-pathological relationships and aetiological aspects of intraventricular haemorrhage. Haemorrhage/ischaemia and the perinatal brain. In: Clinics in Developmental Medicine Nos 69/70. Spastics International Medical Publications, Lippincott, Suffolk. pp 133-148

Peckham CS et al. (1983) Cytomegalovirus infection in pregnancy: preliminary findings from a prospective study. Lancet i: 1352-1355

Perlman JM, McMenamin JB, Volpe JJ. (1983) Fluctuating cerebral blood flow velocity in the respiratory disress syndrome. Relation to the development of IVH. New Engl J Med 309: 204-209

Petersen JR, Rosenberg T, Ibsen KK. (1990) Optic nerve atrophy with particular attention to perinatal damage. Ugeska-Laeger 152: 3865-3867

Pharoah POD, Hornabrook RH. (1974) Endemic cretinism of recent onset in New Guinea. Lancet 2: 1038-1040.

Pharoah POD, Ellis SM, Ekins R, Williams ES. (1976) Maternal thyroid function, iodine deficiency and fetal development. Clin Endocrinol 5: 159-166

Pharoah POD, Cooke T, Rosenbloom L, Cooke RWI. (1987) Effects of birth weight, gestational age and maternal obstetrical history on birth prevalence of cerebral palsy. Arch Dis Child 62: 1035-1040

Pharoah POD, Cooke T, Cooke RWI, Rosenbloom L. (1990) Birth-weight specific trends in cerebral palsy. Arch Dis Child 65: 602-606

Plum P. (1956) Cerebral palsy. A clinical survey of 543 cases. Dan Med Bull 3: 99-108

Powell TG, Pharoah PO, Cooke PW, Rosenbloom L. (1988) Cerebral palsy in low birth-weight infants. 1. Spastic hemiplegia: association with intrapartum stress. Dev Med Child Neurol 30: 11-18

Pryor HB, Thelander H. (1968) Abnormally small head size and intellect in children. J Pediat 73: 593

Puntis JWL, Smith HL, Buick RG, Booth IW. (1989) Effects of dystonic movements on oesophageal peristalsis in Sandifer syndrome. Arch Dis Child 64: 1311-1313

Rakic P. (1988) Defects of neuronal migration and the pathogenesis of cortical malformation. Progress Brain Res 73: 15-37

Rakic P. (1988) Specification of cerebral cortical areas. Science 241: 170-176

Renfrew C. (1977) The Word Finding Vocabulary Test. North Place, Old Headington, Oxford

Rice H, Seashore H, Touloukian RJ. (1991) Evaluation of Nissen fundoplication in neurologically impaired children. J Pediatr Surg 26: 697-701

Riikonen R, Raumavista S, Sinivori E, Seppala T. (1989) Changing pattern of CP in the south-western region of Finland. Acta Paediat Scand 78: 581-587

Robbins TW. (1991) The experimental analysis of sensorimotor "neglect" in animals. 14th Meeting European Neuroscience Association, Cambridge. Eur J Neurosci, Oxford University Press. suppl. 4, p. 303

Robinson RO. (1973) The frequency of other handicaps in children with cerebral palsy. Dev Med Child Neurol 15: 305

Robinson RO, Drew A, Binnie C, Polkey C. (1993) Abst. XIXnth Annual Meeting of British Paediatric Neurology Association, Inst of Child Health, London. p.19

Root L. (1988) Editorial: An orthopaedist's approach to cerebral palsy. Dev Med Child Neurol 30: 569-570

Ross C, Lipper EG, Auld PAM. (1985) Physical growth and developmental outcome in very low birth-weight premature infants at 3 years. J Pediat 107: 284-286

Rudd PT, Peckham C. (1988) Infection of the fetus and newborn. Prevention, treatment and related handicap. Clin Obstet Gynecol 2: 55-72

Russell A. (1954) A syndrome of intra-uterine dwarfism recognizable at birth with craniofacial dysostosis, disproportionately short arms and other anomalies. Proc R Soc Med 47: 1040-1044

Russell A, Shrensky J. (1992) Early Developmental Socio-Educational Integration of Handicapped Infants and Pre-School Children with their Normal Peers. Acorn Scientific Press, London

Russell EM. (1960) Correlation between birthweight and clinical findings in diplegia. Arch Dis Child 35: 548-551

Russell EM. (1961) Cerebral palsied twins. Arch Dis Child 36: 328-336

Ruth V et al. (1988) Prediction of perinatal brain damage by cord plasma, vasopression, erythropoietin and hypoxanthine values. J Pediat 113: 880-885

Rutter M, Graham P, Yule W. (1970) A neuropsychiatric study in childhood. Little Club Clinics in Developmental Medicine, 35/36. Spastic International Medical Publications/Heinemann, London

Sack RL et al. (1991) Melatonin administration to blind people: Phase advances and entrainment. J Biol Rhythm 6: 249-261

Schiff D, Chan G, Poznansky MJ. (1985) Bilirubin toxicity in neural cell lines N115 and NBRIOA. Pediat Res 19: 908-911

Schouman-Claeys L, Picard A, Lalande G, Kalifa G, Lacert P, Brentanos E, Frija G. (1989) Contribution of computed tomography in aetiology and prognosis of cerebral palsy. Br J Radiol 62: 248-252

Scott FP. (1992) Antepartum and intrapartum factors relating to infant retardation. J Obstet Gynecol 12: 385-389

Scoville WB, Milner B. (1957) Loss of recent memory after bilateral hippocampal lesions. J Neurol Neurosurg Psychiat 20: 11-21

Sellick KJ, Over R. (1980) Effects of vestibular stimulation on motor development of cerebral palsied children. Dev Med Child Neurol 22: 476-483

Semenova KA, Dotsenko VJ. (1988) Vestibulometry and its importance in elucidating the pathogenesis and prognosis of the course of nervous system disease in children. Zh Nevropatol Psikhiat 88: 32-37

Shanks DC, Wilson WC. (1988) Lobar holoprosencephaly presenting as spastic diplegia. Dev Med Child Neurol 30: 383-386

Sharav T. (1991) Aging gamete in relation to incidence, gender and twinning in Down syndrome. Am J Med Genet 39: 116-118

Shields JR, Schifrin BS. (1988) Perinatal antecedents of cerebral palsy. Obstet Gynecol 71: 899-905

Sinha SK, D'Souza SW, Rivlin E, Chiswick ML. (1990) Ischaemic brain lesions diagnosed at birth in preterm infants: clinical events and developmental outcome. Arch Dis Child 65: 1017-1020

Srivastava VK, Laisram N, Srivastava RK. (1992) Cerebral palsy. Ind Paediat 29: 993-996

Staino A, Cuechiara SH, Del Giudice E et al. (1991) Disorders of oesophageal motility in children with psychomotor retardation. Eur J Pediatr 150: 638-644

Stanley FJ. (1979) An epidemiological study of CP in Western Australia: changes in total incidence. Dev Med Child Neurol 21: 701-713

Stanley FJ. (1981) Spastic cerebral palsy - changes in birth-weight and gestational age. Early Human Dev 5: 167-178

Stanley F. (1987) The changing face of cerebral palsy. Dev Med Child Neurol 29: 263-265

Stanley F, Blair E. (1984) Postnatal risk factors among the cerebral palsy. In: F Stanley, E Alberman (Eds) The Epidemiology of the Cerebral Palsies. Blackwells, Oxford

Stanley FJ, Blair E. (1991) Why have we failed to reduce the frequency of cerebral palsy. Med J Aust 154: 623-626

Stanley FJ et al. (1985) A Cerebral Palsy Register Methodology: The Western Australian experience. Neuro-epidemiol 4: 146-160

Stanley FJ, English DR. (1986) Prevalence of an risk factors for cerebral palsy in a total population cohort of low-birth-weight (<2000 g) infants. Dev Med Child Neurol 28: 559-568

Stanley FJ, Watson L. (1988) The cerebral palsies in Western Australia trends 1968-1981. Am J Obstet Gynecol 158: 89-93

Steele RJC, Little K. (1983) Effect of seat-belt legislation. Lancet 2: 341

Steinlin M et al. (1991) MRI following severe perinatal asphyxia. Pediat Neurol 7:

Stewart AL, Reynolds EOR. (1974) Improved prognosis for infants of very low birth-weight. Pediatrics 54: 724-735

Sugita K et al. (1991) Magnetic resonance imaging of the brain in congenital rubella virus and cytomegalovirus infections. Neuroradiol 33: 239-242

Suzuki A, Iso A. (1993) Incidence rates of cerebral palsy, mental and motor retardation in Suberkan Tokyo. No To Hattatsu 26: 16

Takahama K et al. (1982) A new type of $\alpha$-amino acid possessing bicuculline-sensitive action in the mammalian brain. Brain Res 239: 294-298

Tanner JM. (1989) In: Foetus into Man: Physical Growth from Conception to Maturity. Chapter 3, pp 47

Tizard JPM (1949) Osteogenesis presenting with delay in walking. Proc R Soc Med 42: 80

Uvebrant P. (1988) Hemiplegic cerebral palsy: aetiology and outcome. Acta Paediat Scand 345: suppl 1-100

van de Bor M, van Zeben-van der Aa TM, Verloove-Vanhorick SP, Brand R, Ruys JH. (1988) Hyperbilirubinemia in preterm infants and neurodevelopmental outcome at 2 years of age: results of a national collaborative survey. Pediatrics 83: 915-920

Vaucher VE et al. (1993) Outcome of 12 months of adjusted age in very low birth weight infants with lung immaturity. J Pediat 122: 126-132

Veelken N, Hagberg B, Hagberg G, Olow I. (1983) Diplegic cerebral palsy in Swedish term and preterm children. Differences in reduced optimality, relations to neurologic and pathogenic factors. Neuropaediat 14: 20-28

Vilensis RA (1985) Effect of maternal oxygen inhalation on the foetus with growth retardation. Pediatr Res 19: 324-327

Villai J, Belizan JM. (1983) Evaluation of the methods used in the diagnosis of fetal growth retardation. Obstet Gynecol Surg 41: 187-199

Volpe JJ. (1992) Brain injury in the premature infant - current concepts of pathogenesis and prevention. Biol Neonate 62: 231-242

Volpe JJ, Herscovitch P, Perlman JM, Raichle MF. (1983) Positron emission tomography in the newborn: extensive impairment of regional cerebral blood flow with IVH and haemorrhagic intracerebral involvement. Pediatrics 72: 589-601

von Howern P. (1966) Obesity as sequel of traumatic injury to hypothalaemia. Dan Med Bull 13: 11-13

Wigglesworth JS. (1989) Current problems in brain pathology in the perinatal period. In: Perinatal Brain Lesions, Eds. KE Pape, JS Wigglesworth. Blackwell Scientific Publications, Boston, Oxford, London.

Wright J, Rang M. (1990) The spastic mouse and the search for an animal model of spasticity in human beings. Clin Orthop 253: 12-19

Yamamoto T, Kudo T, Miyahara N, Miyazaki M. (1990) Disorders of vision in a child with spastic cerebral palsy. No To Hattatsu 22: 253-261

# 2

# DEFINITION AND

# CLASSIFICATION

# OF THE CEREBRAL PALSY

# OR

# CEREBRAL DYSFUNCTION

# ENTITIES

**Introduction**

**Classification**

**Hypertonus or Spasticity**

**Atonic or Persistent Hypotonic Cerebral Palsy, and an Initial Hypotonic Component**

**Dyskinetic**

Athetosis or Choreo-athetosis
Ataxic
Tremor

**Mixed Forms**

**Dystonia and Dyskinesia as a Separate Entity**

**Rigidity**

**Stiffness and The "Stiff Baby" Syndrome**

**References**

# 2

# INTRODUCTION

Essaying a more precise yet comprehensive definition, whilst allowing for the heterogeneity of the *cerebral palsies*, they comprise entities of neuromuscular dysfunction of tone, movement, posture, and balance which are *the long-term clinical expressions of a static non-progressive and irreversible lesion in the pre or postnatal cerebrum and/or cerebellum.* They may arise before, during or after birth, or in hemiplegic forms throughout childhood. Post-neonatal or *acquired* cerebral palsy (CP) as distinct from *congenital* forms, are defined as developing after the fourth week of life. In the subsequent evolution of the growing and maturing CP child, especially during puberty, some clinical changes are inevitable. Nor does the consequent functional disability necessarily remain static. Some functional fluctuations can be anticipated, and variations in the many associated disabilities of vision, hearing and speech, etc. may also be expected. In later life physical deterioration is possible if maintenance is neglected. However, the cerebral palsy entities are rightly regarded as non-progressive disorders in terms of the primary cerebral pathology which remains largely unaltered with time. Although myelin degeneration may very slowly worsen, this appears to have no significant influence upon the axons they enclose which may well have been maximally involved from the time of the initial injury. Scrupulous monitoring will be required to avert potential problems, including those psycho-emotional and behavioural, before

they become irreversible. In so long term a view, withdrawal of services would never be acceptable so that the decline in physical function dependent upon normal aging should be minimized. Apart from transitory initial hypotonia giving way to intensifying hypertonia, choreo-athetosis or ataxia, or adaptations in posture and movement can occur. Especially is this so in spastic diplegia, when the walking pattern may undergo modification or adaptation in later childhood hopefully in response to therapeutic intervention or due to growth of limbs and trunk, as well as weight increments, pre- or post-puberally.

Insufficient is known about the pathogenesis of these entities to use whatever data we possess as a basis for such classifications as proposed by Ford in 1973. The most useful term to describe this composite grouping of entities of CP is still the "Cerebral Dysfunction Syndrome", first coined 30 years ago by Denhoff and Robinauth (1960). I would simply add *plurality*, since one can differentiate syndromes distinctive from those which can be predominantly or solely hypertonic, such as paraplegia or spastic diplegia, whilst spastic hemiplegia is predominantly unilateral. Other major categories or entities are predominantly hypotonic, or choreo-athetoid apart from different entities of ataxia. This serves to emphasize that we are certainly not dealing with one single clinico-pathological entity, but with a coherent spectrum thereof. Each expresses a varying degree of brain damage leading to differing proportions of sensorimotor dysfunction of movement, tone, posture and balance associated with psycho-emotional and specific sensory deficits including agnosias and apraxias as well as organic conduct irregularities, and often interrupted by epileptiform episodes.

A specifically diagnostic classification is also one that should be preferable for epidemiological application. I included a hypotonic group, because the hypotonia can remain as a static or permanent component, although it frequently precedes for a significant but varying period the manifestation of other classical expressions of CP, hypertonicity or spasticity, choreo-athetosis and even ataxia.

With advancing analysis of data derived from correlations of such clinical patterns of dysfunction with those of distinctive neuropathology revealed by brain-scanning and magnetic resonance imaging or exposed at autopsy, a more specific aetiological classification should eventually come within reach.

# CLASSIFICATION

The categorization below (Table 1), based solely upon clinical characteristics, mainly conforms with that proposed by Axel Lademann which takes the qualitative features of the primary motor and movement disability as its basis. The classification is thus a clinical one embodying the number of limbs involved in the spastic forms, although based on the physiological characteristics of the motor dysfunction, with special reference to the associated disorder of tone, movement, posture and balance. The nature of the predominant associated disability or disabilities, whether cognitive, auditory, visual, epileptiform, etc. can be added alongside. Whilst providing an orderly initial descriptive approach to the overall disability, it affords no insight into the aetiology and underlying pathology or pathophysiology of the problem except for a newer concept of a parasagittal cortical infarction and/or ischaemia replacing hypothetical "double hemiplegia". The weakness or lesser degrees of involvement in the milder expressions of the hypertonic or spastic category can be met by using the postfix "-paresis" rather than "-plegia".

The underlying cerebral disease is no longer active, and we categorize the aftermath or consequent form of cerebral palsy which is non-progressive. In essence, there are three main categories of *primary disturbance in tone* which is static or non-progressive: hypotonic, hypertonic, and a mixed evolution of tonal disturbance, with a frequent even characteristic transition from initial hypotonia to hypertonia. The hypotonia itself may be a progressive clinical feature. Alternatively this questions the solely static nature of CP since there can be a gradual "improvement" in tone (to be carefully differentiated from weakness of muscle power) to the extent of an eventual relative normality of tone, such as in the so-called "benign hypotonia" of childhood. This will be discussed in a subsequent

**Table 1**

A.  **Static and Primary Disturbances of Tone**
    Hypotonic
        Atonic or hypotonic diplegia
        Initial hypotonic phase of athetosis or choreo-athetosis, ataxia or hypertonic
            states

    Hypertonic or Spastic
        Spastic monoplegia
        Spastic hemiplegia
        Spastic paraplegia
        Spastic diplegia
        Spastic triplegia
        Spastic tetraplegia (or Quadriplegia)
        Spastic double hemiplegia (Parasagittal cortical syndrome)

B.  **Dyskinetic: Primary Disorders of Movement, Coordination and Balance**
    Athetosis
    Choreo-athetosis
    Ataxic syndromes: Ataxic CP
    Dysequilibrium
    Tremor

C.  **Mixed Forms: Consistent and non-progressive disturbance of tone combined with
        disorder of movement and coordination**
    Hypertonus plus athetosis
    Hypertonus plus ataxia
    Hypotonia plus athetosis
    Hypotonia plus ataxia
    Hypotonia and intermittent extensor hypertonicity

chapter with particular reference to certain metabolic disorders with progressive clinical manifestation, or with the preliminary inclusion of specific syndromes showing initial transitory diminution of tone, such as Downs or Prader-Willi. Another chapter will be devoted to both the neurophysiological detail and a compound of clinical diagnostic data highlighting each of the entities simulating different components or categories of CP.

In respect of *spastic* dysfunction, it is also split topographically for clinical purposes. The so-called mixed forms should be more specifically delineated, rather than leaving them as a confusing heterogenous assortment.

# HYPERTONUS OR SPASTICITY

The hypertonic forms comprise over 60% of all forms of CP. Not typically evident at birth but becomes identifiable after a few months.

The fully fledged spastic form presents the following clinical features: increased muscle tone or increased velocity-dependent resistance to passive movement of "clasp knife" character, reflecting "give-way" after a build-up of resistance, accompanied by a positive stretch reflex. It is also attended by:

(a) Hyperactive deep-tendon reflexes, although typically initially diminished in infancy

(b) Possibly elicitable clonus at ankle and other joints

(c) Positive Babinski reflex

(d) Depressed or absent *superficial* reflexes
   - abdominal
   - cremasteric

(e) Loss of control and of differentiation of finer voluntary movements

(f) Suppression of associated movements.

Delayed postural development is typically associated, including prolongation or perpetuation of postural reflexes such as the tonic neck and neck righting reflexes. The extent of such disability varies, so that a topographical clinical grouping is justifiable under this heading:

1 **Spastic Monoplegia** (Brachial or crural)
Solely involving one limb. Whilst there has been convincing documentation of its occurrence (Crothers and Paine, 1959; Wood, 1975) i.e. not turning out to be a spastic hemiplegia, it is rare for some degree of hypertonus not to eventually emerge in the other extremity *on the same side*. However, two examples of monoplegia with one leg solely involved, were identified amongst 19 infants developing CP in the series of preterm infants observed through sequential one-hour video recordings by the team of Prechtl, the great Dutch neuro-developmental scientist (Ferrari, Cioni, Prechtl, 1990).

2 **Spastic Hemiplegia**
Unilateral involvement of the extremities, with relative sparing of the contralateral limbs. It is especially characterized by asymmetric responses. Perhaps the earliest of these could be a unilateral Moro reflex, or later, the lack of a parachute response *on one side only...*

Within this category, there is still clinical room for use of the term *"plegia"* to represent complete paralysis, whilst "paresis" indicates a partial dysfunction. This is especially relevant in describing gradations of hemiparesis, ranging from almost complete lack of function to the mildest degree of functional impairment which is far commoner than is generally recognized.

Under the heading of "Neonatal and Infantile Hemiplegia", their clinical definition, aetiology and epidemiology has been more fully dealt with in Chapter 4.

3 **Spastic Tetraplegia**
Total body involvement, with a significant and considerable *involvement of all four limbs*, whether or not it is relatively

greater in upper or lower extremities, although usually the latter are more severely affected. Since the term "quadriplegia" can be designated as an etymological bastard of *both* Greek and Latin origin, a preference should lean towards "tetraplegia". Muscle tone tends to increase rapidly and uniformly in all four limbs. Righting responses are severely impaired, as is later sitting posture. The characteristic disability of the upper limbs is soon complete: adduction of shoulders, flexion of elbows, pronation of forearms, flexion of wrists and fingers; and in the *lower extremities*: flexion and adduction of hips, scissoring of legs and right heel cords. The constant or predominant extension is the most conspicuous characteristic especially if the ankles are closely apposed or scissored over one another. Involvement of the supranuclear connections of the lower cranial nerves bilaterally influences muscles of the lower part of the face leading to poor feeding, swallowing difficulties, drooling, lack of facial expression and interference with speech and its maturation are other sequelae. *Quadriplegia* is therefore a superfluous term unnecessarily superadded to connote acceptably *equal* involvement of all four limbs: tetraplegia being the preference as above. But the following familiar clinical subgroups are included:

## 4   Spastic Diplegia

Where upper extremities are affected less than the lower, although there is involvement of arms and legs on both sides, albeit of lesser degree. Rather than a separate clinical entity it is probably better envisaged as a less intense or unequal variant of tetraplegia, wherein equally significant involvement of all four limbs can be differentiated.

Likewise, the older term "paraplegia" or spastic paraplegia referring to involvement confined to the legs, should be discarded and replaced by "spastic diplegia" since there is always some associated involvement of the upper extremities however slight.

## 6   Spastic Bilateral or "Double Hemiplegia" or Parasagittal Cortical Lesion

"Double hemiplegia" has always been an hypothetical concept. I postulate that it should be replaced by a "parasagittal cortical lesion", infarctive or ischaemic, to which fuller reference is made in reference to its newly established MRI localization in Chapter 6. Its clinical expression equates to that hitherto described as tetraplegia of "double hemiplegic" type with bilateral involvement of all limbs, the *upper extremities being affected to a greater degree than the lower*. Severe brain damage is usually apparent from birth, with repetitive seizures and particularly intense feeding difficulties stemming from a bulbar component. Relative lack of movement gives way to increasing hypertonicity in all four limbs.

## 7   Spastic Triplegia

A rare involvement of three limbs. But perhaps not so uncommon as has been believed, with the topography somewhat loosely delineated as "diplegic involvement of the lower limbs linked to hemiplegic involvement of one arm".

## Dystonia vs Transient Hypertonus of Infancy

Intermittent or remittently progressive and possibly mixed forms of dystonia and dyskinesia especially with a torsional component, should not be categorized as conforming with the consistently static non-progressive character of CP. They constitute a separate entity of movement and postural disorder which nonetheless earns a place in this text, to be defined and described separately in a chapter on "The Dystonias" (Chapter 5), which I regard as a separate manifestation lending itself to precise clinical definition. The progressivity of dystonic syndromes in any case transfers them from CP to a number of neurometabolic degenerative entities. This should serve to clarify the differential diagnosis, and perhaps finally overcome some semantic - and clinical - confusion which still prevails. One rational consequence of this would be my plea to substitute "transient hypertonus of infancy"

for what has already tended to assume the time-hallowed term "transient dystonia" of which my friends Drillien, and Nelson and Ellenberg became so fond of describing in the course of otherwise meticulous observation.

In the description of individual cases, the co-existence of a predominantly associated primary problem such as visual, audiological, speech/language impairment could be added. Relevant clinico-pathological knowledge is not yet ready to justify the addition of other attributes which could complete a more comprehensive classification such as:

(a) a degree of intellectual or cognitive deficit;

(b) a more precise classification of functional capacity;

(c) identifiable aetiological risk factor(s);

(d) a genetically-determined basis.

# ATONIC OR PERSISTENT HYPOTONIC CEREBRAL PALSY AND AN INITIAL HYPOTONIC COMPONENT

*A relatively rare* type of CP is manifested by *persisting hypotonia* disproportionate to the degree of microcephaly and mental retardation usually associated. Extreme forms, including atonic diplegia, as well as athetoid and ataxic types were first emphasized by Yannet and Horton (1952). The superimposition of *flexion contractures* and *positional deformities* in later childhood may impart an impression of muscle

tightness and an erroneous diagnosis of spastic CP. Athetoid children may exhibit different degrees of muscular tension, apparently sensitive to position and anxiety. Indeed it is often difficult to say whether there is "pure" athetosis or whether there is accompanying rigidity or spasticity. Choreic movement, with rapid irregularly-repetitive or discrete involuntary jerks may accompany. There may also be a static tremor. Ataxic CP may also be preceded by an infantile phase of hypotonia. A fuller presentation of the early diagnostic identification of the neonatal and infantile hypotonic element appears in Chapter 4.

# DYSKINETIC

## Athetosis or Choreo-athetosis

The major category expressed in disturbance of movement and/or of co-ordination is *Dyskinetic*: Athetosis. This constitutes approximately 10% of the incidence of CP. Athetosis represents an impairment of motion. Characterized by fluctuating muscle tension, in which attempted activity precipitates a succession of slow smooth, writhing, involuntary movements or even spontaneously are marked by frequent involuntary writhing or torsion sometimes dominated by choreiform irregular twitch. Quick, jerky, spasmodic staccato and more proximal movements of individual muscles and small muscle groups of the extremities or of the face or of all muscle groups (*choreic* element) are then superimposed upon voluntary effort, especially during mental stress. This element is especially accompanied by general muscle weakness and ineffectuality in attempted action. These may mask as well as interfere with normal movement of limbs, face and tongue, so that the child is often first referred because of delay in motor skills. The involuntary movements may either be continuous, or are precipitated by voluntary active movement. The accompanying disorderly changes in tone may extend to the bulbar musculature as well as face, trunk and all four extremities. An instability of opposing postures whether flexion and extension, or pronation and supination, is also an intrinsic component, mainly involving the distal musculature. It is subdued during sleep if the child is secure posturally.

Whilst at one time often preceded by a history of kernicterus, this dyskinetic form of CP may still follow hyperbilirubinaemia and feeding difficulties. At least initial *hypotonia* is still characteristic and the deep tendon reflexes are normal or slightly increased. The early hypotonia, however, eventually gives way to hypertonicity, which may nevertheless diminish when the child is posturally secure. Tonic neck and neck-righting reflexes persist, with a classical diagnostic suggestion that a persistent tonic neck reflex in a 1-year-old with motor delay, or of axial hypertonus, points to the probability of this form of CP.

The pathognomonic movements emerge very gradually, often not until 3 years of age, with tremor and choreiform jerks appearing first in fingers or toes. Abnormality of movement may first be observed as the child is playing with toys, drinking from a cup or later in walking. With involvement of supranuclear connections of the lower cranial nerves, grimacing, drooling and dysarthria become manifest. The dysarthria per se depends upon an inability to curb involuntary movements of the mouth and tongue as well as inability to sustain a constant flow of air because of truncal dyskinesia. Severe hearing impairment is another common association.

The dyskinetic child is eventually outstanding because of the combination of involuntary athetoid or choreo-athetoid movements of the trunk and limbs with grimacing, drooling, dysarthria and dysphagia. Underlying the speech defect, *the inability to emit a uniform flow of air to the larynx* because of disturbed or increased axial tone is a second major element. Since the source of cerebral damage is mainly in the basal ganglia motor system, with relative sparing of the cortical mantle, intelligence is usually normal, but the dyskinetic child is usually especially in need of specific specialist help from speech and language pathologist, as well as otolaryngologist and audiologist.

## Ataxia

Constitutes another 10% of CP incidence. Dysharmonic, imprecise muscle movements and poor body balance, with lack of a sense of position in space, incoordination of movements, and instability of gait predominating. The hypotonia may already be noticeable in infancy, along with normal or slightly reduced deep tendon reflexes, and absent stretch reflexes. Walking is on a wide base, with trunk weaving and arms held akimbo to maintain balance, sometimes showing intention tremor of limbs, or axial tremor. Especial difficulty in eye-hand coordination and control, even on finger-nose testing, may with care and patience be already identifiable towards the end of the first year, or beginning of the second. The motor handicap or imbalance will become apparent as soon as the child begins to sit upright, and certainly when he stands. Nystagmus and/or esotropia may be associated anomalies. Accentuation of the instability in standing or attempted walking on closure of the eyes characterizes the sensory ataxia in which there is impairment of responsiveness to proprioceptive stimuli. Also, in association with hypotonia, it appears in so-called "mixed" forms. Pathology in this context is mainly centred on the cerebellum, and in particular the vermis.

The more fundamental differentiation of these ataxic cerebral palsies will be dealt with subsequently in relation to metabolic and other disorders simulating CP. Meanwhile a simplified subdivision would be as follows:

(a) *Cerebellar forms* characterized by hypotonia, disturbed balance and incoordination of voluntary movement.

(b) *Sensory ataxias,* as already mentioned.

(c) *Motor or ataxic diplegia,* wherein spasticity of diplegic distribution is superimposed on other ataxia variants. The majority are associated with pre- or perinatal factors. Those of very low birth weight may be survivors of neonatal or immediately prenatal intraventricular haemorrhage. Likewise postnatally acquired or congenital hydrocephalus are characteristically followed by ataxic diplegia (Hagberg et al., 1975).

(d) *The dysequilibrium syndrome.*

As well as hypotonia, there is especially defective postural function with disproportionately severe difficulty in sustaining an upright body posture and the positional sense of the body in space. Motor delay is

prominent, whilst relatively marked language delay and mental retardation were emphasized by the outstanding Swedish team led by Hagberg (1974).

(e) *Congenital ataxias.*

Ataxias also arise occasionally in association with hydrocephalus and more frequently as one component of progressive metabolic disorders, particularly of pyruvate metabolism, which will be outlined in the subsequent chapter of progressive disorders simulating CP.

## Tremor

This rhythmic disorder of movement may be added here, although dealt with more comprehensively in Chapter 4. It manifests involuntary rhythmic alternating movements of varying strength but individually constant frequency. At rest, it is uncommon in children, but may be noticeable only when the child attempts to use the limb (i.e. an intention tremor).

When occurring as a major motor manifestation, such as in only two of the series of Crothers and Paine (1988), they have supported the tenuous view that it represents a rare entity of CP. One of these cases was postencephalitic and it may suffice to regard tremor as either a significant feature of extrapyramidal CP possibly of encephalopathic source, or as an associated component, often of a predominant athetotic category.

## "MIXED" FORMS

Motor dysfunction incorporating two or more of the above states. Involvement is manifest of pyramidal and/or extrapyramidal components of the "motor ganglia" circuitry of the motor control system. Hence *initial* or *persistent* hypotonia may be demonstrable, but predominantly there is evolution into a combination of

*Spasticity*, mainly reflecting pyramidal dysfunction with marked hyperreflexia and a marked tendency to contracture in the usual spastic distribution, and *extrapyramidal* or motor ganglia dysfunction reflected in incontrovertible Dyskinesia with a choreic or choreo-athetoid component, or with parallel cerebellar involvement, reflected in *Ataxia*.

Hypotonia may thus exist in the early stages of spastic CP with hypertonicity eventually taking over... It also accompanies the predominantly ataxic form of CP, although many forms of CP (spastic, dyskinetic and hypotonic) may have an ataxic component. Because of the more extensive pathology likely to underlie these mixed forms, the clinical expression is also more likely to be tetraplegic as opposed to diplegic. Some degree of ataxia may be superadded but the different entities of predominant ataxia are outlined in Chapter 19. An element of tremor may occasionally co-exist.

The so-called "mixed" forms should therefore be more specifically delineated, rather than leaving them as a confusing heterogeneous assortment. Dystonia I regard as a separate clinical manifestation, and one which lends itself to precise clinical definition. The progressivity of dystonic syndromes, in any case, transfers them from cerebral palsy to a number of neurometabolic and degenerative disorders. Hence it seemed justifiable to devote a separate chapter to dystonia, with a plea that meticulous diagnostic differentiation could be of significant benefit to patient and physician alike. One rational consequence of this, is my substitution of "transient hypertonia of infancy" for the now time-hallowed term, "transient dystonia", of which my respected colleagues, Drillien and then Nelson and Ellenberg became so fond.

# DYSTONIA AND DYSKINESIA AS A SEPARATE ENTITY

Other types of disordered movements, sometimes loosely attributed to extrapyramidal CP, include dystonia and ballismus. To reiterate a previous comment, and that elaborated in subsequent Chapter 5, dystonia is not classifiable as an underlying category of CP, but reflects a separate entity of disordered tone and movement such as is exemplified by intermittent or remittent hypertonus *initially precipitated by intention*. An apt description would therefore be "intention dystonia", or when writhing is superimposed, characterized as "*torsion dystonia*". One of its underlying entities is a genetically determining enzyme disorder first described by Russell and Yatziv in 1985. This was explained by an underlying permutation of deficit in arylsulfatase A and its iso-enzymes B and C, accounting for a failure of breakdown of sulfatides within the myelin sheath, and thus a newly-defined variant of metachromatic leukodystrophy, uniquely marked by relatively normal intellectual capacity.

Peripheral nerve involvement is the dominant feature in this, as in the classical forms of metachromatic leukodystrophy or sulfatide lipidosis of the infantile form of which it is an early feature. In both the new entity and the established forms, there is a marked slowing of nerve conduction velocities, with confirmation of an histochemical and electronmicroscopic diagnosis following sural nerve biopsy, and lysosomal enzyme assay.

An auxiliary form of dysfunction of tone may be superadded here: rigidity.

# RIGIDITY

Elevated muscular tension and resistance on passive movement, in both flexion and extension, is constant giving rise to the *lead-pipe* or *cogwheel* phenomena. It represents an extreme form of hypertonicity, and is classically associated with Parkinsonism and Wilson's hepato-lenticular degeneration. In the rapidly evolving Wilsonian form, it assumes the guise of facio-linguo-pharyngeal "rigidity", also producing facial masking together with dysarthria and dysphagia as well as rigidity of the limbs as the earliest motor manifestation. As the disease progresses beyond 7 to 10 years, the rigidity tends to become generalized and accentuated.

The "clasp-knife" phenomenon produced during flexion against resistance in hypertonic forms of CP is not reproducible in rigidity. Instead, the "lead-pipe" or "cogwheel" phenomena are associated features, when rapid flexion and extension of the arm is attempted with several hindrances or hold-ups to the movement, communicating a slow moulding or a jerky and staccato feeling. Apart from this distinction, it may nevertheless be hard to differentiate "spastic tetraplegia" when the degree of hypertonus is so severe, and it also becomes difficult to decide whether the tendon reflexes are truly exaggerated. Is it a matter of degree of hypertonicity? Conversion of tetraplegia into complete decerebrate rigidity may depend upon total de-afferentation of the reticular formation (Ward, 1945). Furthermore, the EMG of the two conditions, tetraplegia and rigidity, are almost identical (Denny-Brown, 1949).

In terms of infancy, Ringel et al. (1978) recorded a sporadic example of severe muscular rigidity dating from birth. The intense involvement of muscle tissue was also reflected in an extremely high serum CK (indeed 45 times the normal). The muscle biopsy revealed an unusual trilaminar structure. Muscle rigidity and weakness have been an uncommon clinical expression of congenital hypothyroidism, in the Debre-Semelaigne syndrome. A degree of rigidity equalling that in tetanus may even reflect "reducing body myopathy" as well as that of amyopathy to which reference has already been made in relation to trilaminar fibres (Ringel et al., 1978).

Rigidity is also a particularly striking feature of Trisomy 18. Its characteristic "fisting" is a compound of fingers rigidly flexed across the palms, with the index finger overlapping the middle finger. Indeed, rather than a CNS source, the rigidity appears to stem from joint and ligamentous fixation. The many anomalies found in association include the microcephaly receding chin, low-set and receding ears, pointed beaky nose, cryptorchidism and herniation whether inguinal, lumbar or umbilical. The feet with prominent heels are characteristically "rockerbottom".

109

# STIFFNESS AND THE "STIFF BABY" SYNDROME (HYPERREFLEXIA)

A somewhat different impediment to movement is also marked in an autosomal recessive disorder of generalized hypertonia in flexion from birth. Later the acute diffuse hypertonia can make them fall like a log. Exaggerated startle reactions follow truncal stimuli. The hypertonia diminishes over the first two years although startle responses persist (Kok and Bruyn, 1962).

The hypotonia associated with cerebellar lesions is well known, but in the *decerebellate* animal, *rigidity* is profound and thought due to what is postulated as "alpha rigidity". In the *decerebrate* animal, however, the rigidity due to stretch reflex hyperactivity, is attributed to "gamma rigidity". In contrast, it has been hypothesized that the cerebellum inactivates the stretch reflex at the same time as it increases the drive to the motor neurones.

## References

Carlson DE. (1988) Maternal diseases associated with intrauterine growth retardation. Semin Perinatol 12: 17-22

Crothers B, Paine RS. (1959) Disorders of the nervous system in childhood. In: The Natural History of Cerebral Palsy. Cambridge Press, London. p 299

Crothers B, Paine RS. (1988) Effects of growth retardation and aswphyxia on brain electrolytes. Paediat Res 7: 494-499

Denny-Brown DE. (1949) Interpretation of the electromyogram. Arch Neurol Psychiat 61: 99-128

Denhoff E, Robinauth IP. (1960) Cerebral Palsy and Related Disorders. McGraw-Hill Book Co., New York

Ferrari F, Cioni G, Prechtl HF. (1990) Qualitative changes of general movement in preterm infants with brain lesions. Early Hum Dev 23: 193-231

Ford FR. (1973) Diseases of the Nervous System in Infancy, Childhood and Adolescence. CC Thomas, Springfield. 3,6,37,41,49,53,60

Hagberg BA. (1972) The Dysequilibrium syndrome in cerebral palsy. Acta Paediat Scand: suppl 226

Hagberg B, Sanner B, Stern M. (1974) The dysequilibrium syndrome in cerebral palsy. Acta Paediat Scand, suppl. 226

Hagberg B, Hagberg G, Glow I. (1975) The changing panorama of cerebral palsy in Sweden 1954-1970. Analysis of the general changes. Acta Paediat Scand 64: 187-192

Hagberg B, Hagberg G, Olow I. (1975) The changing panorama of cerebral palsy in Sweden 1954-1970. II. Analysis of the various syndromes. Acta Paediat Scand 64: 193-200

Kok O, Bruyn GW. (1962) An unidentified hereditary disease. Lancet 1: 1359

Lademann A. (1978) Postnatally acquired cerebral palsy. Acta Neurol Scand: suppl. 65, 3

Ringel SP, Neville HF, Ousler MC, Carroll JE. (1978) A new congenital neuromuscular disease with trilaminar muscle fibres. Neurol (Minneapolis) 28: 282-289

Russell A, Yatziv S. (1985) A metabolic basis for idiopathic torsion dystonia: a new variant of metachromatic leukodystrophy. World Pediat Child Care 1: 25-29

Ward AA Jr. (1945) Decerebrate rigidity. J Neurophysiol 10: 89-103

Wood GE. (1975) Cerebral palsy in childhood. Etiology and clinical assessment with particular reference to Bristol. In: The Handicapped Child: Assessment and Management. Blackwell Scientific Publications, Oxford

Yannet H, Horton F. (1952) Hypotonic cerebral palsy in mental defectives. Pediatrics 9: 204-211.

# 3

# DIAGNOSTIC NEURODEVELOPMENTAL AND OTHER CRITERIA IN EARLY DETECTION

**Early General Manifestations in the Preterm, Full-Term Neonate and Infant**

**Early Deviant Neurodevelopmental and Clinical Criteria**

**The Usual Timing of Diagnostic Detection**

**Neurodevelopmental Reflexes**

> Traction Test and "Pulling Up to Sit"
> Head Balance
> Grasp Reflex
> Other Reflexes at Spinal Cord Level

## Brain Stem Reflexes

Asymmetric Tonic Neck Reflex
Symmetric Tonic Neck Reflex
Positive Supporting Reactions and Placing
Negative Supporting Reaction
Tonic Labyrinth Reflex

## Automatic Movement Reactions

Persistently Abnormal Movement Pattern in Diagnosis
Moro Reflex
Suspension in Space
Neck-righting Response
Equilibrium Reactions
Sitting
Prone Kneeling
Standing

## Cerebral Cortical Reflexes

Simple Test of Balancing Ability
Parachute Reactions
Babinski Reflex Response and Rossolino Version

## Assessment of Motor Disability

Gradation of Motor Disability

## References

# 3

# EARLY GENERAL MANIFESTATIONS IN THE PRETERM, FULL-TERM NEONATE AND INFANT

Alertness to the concurrence of unfavourable circumstances, and its prenatal clinical manifestation such as foetal distress in the preterm, early neonate, or infant, should contribute to the subsequent diagnostic process. This may have thus been preceded, especially in the preterm earlier than 34 weeks, by what may have been recognizable foetal symptomatology consequent upon subependymal or germinal matrix bleeding, or upon other preceding, parallel or ensuing hypoxic/ischaemic lesions in periventricular zones. In both, there is sparing of direct damage to the cortical mantle. Characteristically, its overall clinical expression is therefore either *prenatal*, mainly in some form of foetal distress or aberration of foetal heart rate or rhythm, or *perinatally* in a non-specific and generalized upset beyond that expected in the typical normal infant. The neonate is hypotonic and often unresponsive in the first few hours. Increasing irritability follows, and unilateral or multifocal seizures may be frequent. The ensuing pattern on the second or third day could include persistent apathy or undue restlessness, feeding resistance, tense fontanelle, apnoeic or cyanotic bouts and other respiratory irregularities, with or without earlier intense respiratory distress. Prolonged hypotonia and prolonged need for tube feeding would have ominous prognostic implications for future severe handicap or death, especially

when accompanied by hypothermia, a high-pitched or "cerebral" cry and vomiting. It is nevertheless reassuring to know that even severe neurological signs may subsequently resolve. *In the preterm*, prolongation of the apnoeic spells not responding to stimulation would be especially sinister. *In the full-term*, when involution of the germinal matrix is apparently complete, the cerebral damage would tend to be more peripheral, probably stemming from choroid plexus haemorrhage predominantly involving the cerebral cortex (Fig. 3) and underlying hemispherical white matter.

Before Rh immunization prevailed in the prevention of "Rhesus incompatibility", its kernicteric sequel, was one of the commonest universal sources of cerebral palsy. Initial signs of the neuropathy usually followed within two to three days of the onset of jaundice marking the first day of life. Clinical manifestations are comparable to those of the anoxic-hypotensive syndrome, shock or even intraventricular haemorrhage, with apathy, hypotonia, lethargy and poor suck reflex interspersed later with episodes of opisthotonos, muscle spasms and seizures. Still later sequelae, perhaps not evident in surviving infants even before the second or third year, comprise a classical triad of severe choreo-athetosis, difficulties with vertical gaze and degrees of deafness,

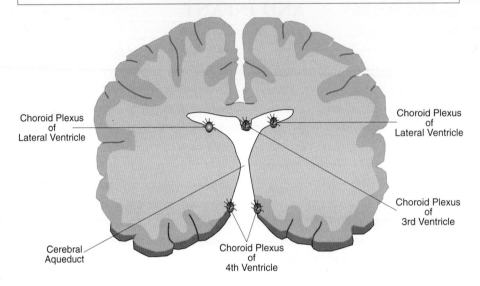

**Diagrammatic Localization of Choroid Plexus Bleeding Mainly at Term**

Choroid Plexus of Lateral Ventricle

Choroid Plexus of Lateral Ventricle

Choroid Plexus of 3rd Ventricle

Cerebral Aqueduct

Choroid Plexus of 4th Ventricle

including the high-tone form, linked to mental retardation. Commoner causes of severe hyperbilirubinaemia in developed countries would now include ABO incompatibility and various hereditary disorders, such as G6PD deficiency.

It was repeatedly demonstrated clinically that the brain tissue of *preterm* infants was highly vulnerable to less severe degrees of hyperbilirubinaemia. This was particularly expressed in the yellow staining of brain nuclei despite the absence of overt neuropathic signs in those who died of hyaline membrane disease, intraventricular haemorrhage or other factors related to extreme prematurity. Although the unconjugated bilirubin believed to be the

toxic substrate could interfere with many intracellular enzyme systems within the neurone, the precise nature of its toxicity at cellular level has not yet been clearly defined. Studying hippocampal slices in culture, Hansen et al. (1985) demonstrated interference with electrical activity. Suppressive effects upon DNA synthesis and mitochondrial function of the neural type cell were invoked by Schiff et al. (1985).

Whilst albumin binding of the toxic bilirubin within the intravascular compartment can be sustained at bilirubin/albumen molar ratios of less than one, the brain is considered to be protected, although the degree of protection is inversely related to the degree of prematurity. On the other hand, Levine and colleagues (1982) have indicated that even such levels of albumen-bound bilirubin could become potentially toxic should there be disruption of the blood-brain barrier. Such *bilirubin encephalopathy* constitutes a more generalized cerebral syndrome in the neonate resulting from widespread yet specifically focussed infiltration of unconjugated bilirubin into brain cells, especially those of major nuclei, such as the globus pallidus and subthalamic nuclei as well as the hippocampus (Karp, 1979). Neuronal loss follows, attended by fibrillary gliosis and varying degrees of demyelination. That such pathogenesis of encephalopathy is restricted to the newborn period was long ago contradicted in the documentation by Blashke and colleagues (1974) of its appearance even as a consequence of the Crigler-Najjar syndrome in an adolescent.

More specific neuropathic features either manifest or elicitable in the preterm or full-term neonate, which are indicative or predictive of possible underlying brain damage or defect that may ultimately express itself in cerebral palsy, will be discussed in the subsequent outline of early deviance of neurodevelopmental parameters (Chapter 3).

Almost any form of the cerebral damage characterizing the neonatal period may develop *in utero*. However, the pathological outcomes vary. Thus where there has been a subependymal or massive intraventricular haemorrhage in utero, for example, presentation at birth may be with hydrocephalus suggestive of a diagnosis ranging from congenital malformation to infection. Likewise, anoxic/ischaemic damage months before birth producing damage to medulla and spinal cord could in due course result in an infant with skeletal deformity and hypoplastic lungs. In any event, the infant who had sustained prenatal episodes of anoxic/ischaemic damage might subsequently on delivery appear to be the victim of asphyxial birth injury. Objective initial assessment of cerebral status in such ostensibly asphyxiated neonates, in particular including initial and serial comprehensive neuroimaging, is now almost mandatory.

## EARLY DEVIANT NEURODEVELOPMENTAL AND CLINICAL CRITERIA

Deviations in the manifestation and timing of early infantile automatisms and postures, including those assumed in suspension, may provide valid diagnostic clues to disturbed or delayed development of motor function in a child under 18 months. These infantile responses may be asymmetrical or qualitatively abnormal, and an abnormal basis may in fact be conveyed by their failure to appear at the normal age, or conversely by their persistence beyond the age at which they are normally expected to disappear. Such signs are best interpreted in conjunction with various other findings, apart from known perinatal and postnatal history.

The maturing of an inherently abnormal nervous system poses differing physical or neurological problems at different stages of development. Assessment should therefore be an ongoing or serial process.

Early infantile extremity and axial *hypotonia* is more weakly associated with cerebral palsy in general. Nevertheless a strong association was eventually to emerge with:

(a)  Minor Neuromotor dysfunction (MND), or

(b)  Mild motor delay and relatively mild neuromotor abnormality.

The search continues, however, for simple and effective screening tools for the identification of cerebral palsy as early as in pre-term infants who are so vulnerable to this disorder. As Marilee et al. indicated, the most predictive components of the developmental examination at this age [age corrected for degree of prematurity = Term Age Equivalent (TAE)] are likely to be threefold, meanwhile overlooking prediction of ultimate cerebral palsy by the technique of neuroimaging at birth not yet available when the clinical criteria below were first cited:

1  Abnormal cranial nerve and oromotor function;

2  Hyper-irritability;

3  Neck extensor hypertonia, frequently associated with later diagnosis of cerebral palsy.

Indeed, extensor hypertonus affecting trunk as well as neck muscles have long been accepted as important signs of impending spasticity.

In the management of such a neonate demonstrating the three signs above, or merely neck extensor hypertonia, the infant is better placed in a side position so as to avoid too frequent or too intensive head lifts. Marilee's team also concluded that their form of neonatal examination enhanced the predictability of perinatal risk factors in respect of motor outcome.

Further physical signs gradually becoming conspicuous during the second half of the first year encompass three main groups:

1  *Abnormalities of tone;*

2  *Delayed emergence of normal postural reactions;*

3  *Persistence or perpetuation of abnormal patterns of movement.*

Postural tone is often low early in infancy following brain injury, but eventually spasticity takes over. A sequence or parallelism of mechanisms may include:

-  Depression of inhibitory mechanisms normally curbing excitability of motor neurones;

-  Augmented excitability especially of gamma stretch-receptor system

-  Interference with reciprocal innervation leading to impeded control of fine and complex movements - and apparent weakness.

There are more subtle clinical features that require careful surveillance during the first months following premature birth, or suspected perinatal injury. The issue of *paucity of spontaneous movement* as a token of cerebral pathology in early infancy is again worthy of emphasis, and such movement patterns as are present would be limited and stereotyped. In addition, there is often poor visual following with relatively suppressed facial expression, and reduced

"turn-taking" behaviour in response to social stimuli.

# THE USUAL TIMING OF DIAGNOSTIC DETECTION

Serial monitoring of the head circumference may more promptly reveal deceleration or even arrest of cranial growth accompanying premature closure of fontanelles and sutures as in craniostenosis. Such secondary microcephaly would reflect declining growth of the brain, damaged under the impact of anoxia, haemorrhagic infarction or progressive metabolic upset.

In the full-term, because the *primary* site of the cerebral lesion mainly *involves the upper limb girdle*, an accurate diagnosis of motor dysfunction is often practicable by 3 to 6 months in severe spastic tetraplegia. But since the major focus of injury may manifest later in the lower limbs, particularly in the parasagittal category, accurate diagnosis is frequently deferred until immature albeit independent walking is otherwise expected, i.e. between 12 and 18 months. In general, however, the more severe and extensive the lesion, the earlier the diagnosis. In the preterm infant, all evaluations should be made from the

corrected age. In general, the likely times for detection of hypertonic neurodevelopmental sequelae can be predicted as early as 3 to 6 months for severe tetraplegia, whilst accurate diagnosis of spastic forms of moderate degree may be deferred until 6-12 months. The hemiplegic with moderate disability can also be identified by 6-12 months, whereas most diplegics are mild and are not firmly detectable until 9-18 months. If of moderate degree, signs are likely to be obvious earlier, say by 6-12 months, whereas when of severe degree, experienced identification or prediction may be reached by 3-6 months.

In ataxic forms, incoordination of hand movements may be recognizable before the end of the first year, with the recognition of general imbalance or dysequilibrium possible in the second year. Likewise, dyskinetic phenomena are not likely to be superimposed or recognized until well into the second year.

# NEURODEVELOPMENTAL REFLEXES

Evolving from the caudal towards the cephalic level of control, these protective and maturing reflexes of the first two years

of life carry the normal child through to the characteristically *mature* human form of bipedal walking. For instance, the various body-righting and balancing reflexes are essential to maintain balance in walking. The spinal cord is the mediating source of some of these reflexes, whilst the brain stem is operative for some, others are mediated at midbrain, and others at cortical levels.

The relevant reflexes thus mark a phase which all normal children traverse. Motor behaviour in the neonate is indeed dominated by these so-called *primitive reflexes* which include the spinal cord and brain stem reflexes, and serve to protect his or her early survival whilst establishing the foundation for ongoing motor as well as cognitive development.

As *postural* and *behavioural* responses to *sensory stimuli*, tactile, proprioceptive, and vestibular, *the most relevant* are: rooting, sucking, grasp, Moro, asymmetrical tonic neck and tonic labyrinthine reflexes.

*Primary spinal cord reflexes* such as flexor withdrawal, extensor thrust and crossed extensor are elicitable from birth to their disappearance between one and two weeks. These reflexes result in limb movement mediated by flexor muscle contraction away from the source of stimulation. Both ontogenetically and phylogenetically, the flexion reflex is one of the most primitive reflexes of the central nervous system. It is already present by the seventh to eighth week of gestation. *Its initial absence or impairment would have pathological significance.* But of more practical relevance, *abnormal persistence* beyond this period would signify serious underlying cerebral damage, ultimately to be manifest as cerebral palsy in particular.

During activation of flexor reflexes, ipsilateral flexor motor neurone excitation together with extensor inhibition (*reciprocal innervation*), flexor motor neurone inhibition and extensor excitation follow contralateral to the side of stimulation (double reciprocal innervation). Under normal conditions, this crossed extension reflex stabilizes the body as the ipsilateral limb is flexed.

The most significant of the secondary or *brain stem reflex group* are those which can directly influence or modify development. They start appearing *at about the second week of life*, and such as the asymmetrical tonic neck reflex, is normally most evident or most easily elicitable at 2 to 3 months when it appears to prepare the way for *the integration of head turning, visual fixation* and *reaching-out*. It may indeed be fundamental to the establishment of visually directed reaching-out along with eye-hand coordination, *but should disappear after six months*. Persistence beyond this is considered indicative of brain damage having occurred in utero or early life. Other "brain stem reactions" include the symmetric tonic neck, the positive and negative supporting reflexes and the tonic labyrinthine. Midbrain reflexes, such as neck, labyrinthine and optical correcting, both begin to appear at the fourth month, being finally suppressed after two years of age by assertion of cortical control.

In essence, *the postural reflexes* do not appear at the normal time, *or persist* beyond the normal timing. Marked head lag may therefore persist beyond the usual time, and there is delay in rolling over or sitting and the parachute defensive reaction is delayed beyond one year. However, in severe impending manifestations of CP, this may never be more than fragmentary.

Abnormalities of other specific cutaneous or superficial reflexes diagnostic of central nervous system lesions, are dealt with later. For instance, the more primitive form of flexion reflex, the Babinski sign, represents a modification of the local cord reflexes in the presence of corticospinal tract disease. Likewise, other forms of flexion reflex, *abdominal and cremasteric*, are no longer elicitable after lesions of the corticospinal tract (direct activation pathway).

Gradually progressive lessening of hypotonia on serial examination without oncoming hypertonicity or dyskinesia during the second or third year of life, should be recorded as indicating so-called congenital benign hypotonia or the hypotonic component of Down's or Prader-Willi syndromes. Nonetheless, it may also be a feature of otherwise progressing and slowly worsening multifocal syndromes such as the developmental regression of the Rett disorder, so often mistaken for CP during two or more of its developmental phases. To these a subsequent section is being devoted because it should be more widely appreciated that the associated progressive component diagnostically excludes the true entities of cerebral palsy.

## Traction Test and "Pulling Up to Sit"

Holding the wrists, the infant is gently pulled up 15 to 20cm from supine whilst observing for head lag and ability to overcome the force of gravity. Continuing observation is also worthwhile - with continuing readiness to protect the head - when returning the baby to a supine position, noting the degree of spontaneous contraction of back, shoulder or neck musculature and of overall head control, or conversely, the persistence of hyperextension of neck and back, which is also evident in the prone position in the hypertonic infant.

## Head Balance

This measure modified from Bayley (1969) could be added as an additional parameter of nuchal and head control. The child is placed prone on a firm surface, and ability to lift the head and shoulders from the surface (continuing later with the use of hands or elbows) and to hold the head up for more than 30 seconds.

# Grasp Reflex

Stimulus contact by gentle stroking of the palm, or pressing of a finger transversely across the palm, elicits this firm grasping response. Stretching of the finger flexors constitutes another stimulus. Even in terms of this familiar primitive reflex, attention should be paid to the strength and "tonicity" of the reflex, including its "traction reinforcement phase" with progressive contraction of forearm muscles. But when not elicited the hands should remain freely open, whereas *persisting "fisting"* is abnormal. Distinction should be made on the basis of an array of other criteria reflecting those chromosomal anomalies *without cerebral palsy* which are characterized by "fisting", such as Trisomy 18.

It is so consistently elicitable in the neonate that it is an especially useful diagnostic index. Any variation from the fully normal reaction is a reliable indication of probable abnormality. Its diagnostic value is illustrated in several ways. In determination of maturity, for example, it is less evident in the less mature neonate. In detection of abnormality, its absence, weakness, extensor strength, or persistent asymmetry, may each indicate relevant abnormality. It normally fades after a few months, usually by 4 to 5 months, so that early diagnosis of motor cortical damage is likely to be reflected in its *persistence* beyond 4 to 5 months.

In terms of the feet, the contact stimulus becomes a supporting surface, on contact with which there is flexion or "crumpling"... Until this particular reaction fades, *usually between 7 and 8 months*, walking is in any case impossible whereas after 8 months, the feet become essential for anti-gravity support and balance. Meanwhile, other sensory responses include *tactile avoiding reactions*, the stimulus being light contact with the back of the hand or forearms.

The infantile *"tactile placing reactions"* are yet another emerging sensory response - when contact is with the forearm, of the shin or dorsum of the foot, i.e. when the infant is suspended but brought briskly forward so that the limb or dorsum of the foot strikes the edge of the table, or when either foot or hand is briskly "placed on the surface (Fig 4). This reaction is commonly absent or limited in the mentally subnormal. Likewise in the athetoid, it is often absent in the arms which are folded away, whilst the so-called "athetoid dance" sometimes expresses responsiveness of the legs.

# Other Reflexes at Spinal Cord Level

### Flexor Withdrawal

With the child supine, legs in extension, and head in a neutral position, the sole of the foot is pinched. A positive reaction until two months of age is a *slow flexion response* with uncontrolled flexion at the knee, whereas a brisk avoidance response is negative. Persistence or reappearance of the slow flexion response *beyond 2 months* also becomes abnormal.

# PLACING

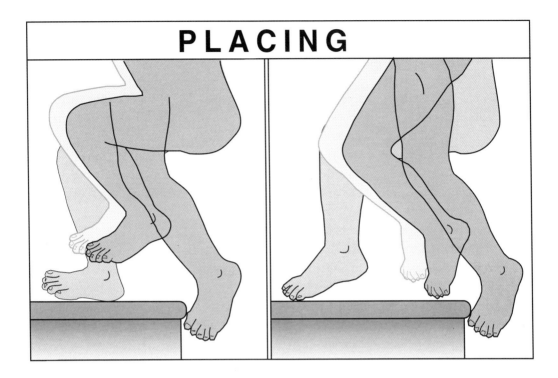

**Extensor Thrust**

With the child supine, the sole of the flexed leg is pinched. Slow extension, without kicking the stimulus away, is a positive reaction up to two months of age. Persistence after 2 months is abnormal.

**Crossed Extensor**

(a) With the child supine, and both legs in extension, tap the medial aspect of one thigh just above the patella. Stiffening, adduction and internal rotation of the opposite leg is normal until about 2 months, whilst relatively protracted persistence beyond 6 months would be distinctly abnormal.

(b) In another version of this test, which appears to be a more readily applicable and specific response, the leg is kept extended at the knee whilst the sole of the foot is repeatedly stimulated by firm strokes (with finger or other firm object). The opposite leg flexes and then extends. As the extension phase is linked to some adduction at the hip, the impression is that the moving leg is crossing the stimulating hand.

This reflex is present in both premature and full-term infants, gradually fading during the first year, although it is difficult to ascertain the precise time of its disappearance. If still present at one year of age, it may be the only clue to a predictive diagnosis in some babies who eventually demonstrate cerebral palsy.

# BRAIN STEM REFLEXES

## Asymmetric Tonic Neck Reflex (ATNR)

This is a reflex derived from proprioceptive receptors in the neck. With the child supine, rotation of the head first to one side and then subsequently to the other, extensor hypertonus is increased on the side to which the head is turned. The arm and leg *extend* on that side, with *flexion* of the arm and leg of the opposite (occipital) side. This is normally most readily elicitable at 2 to 3 months, persisting up to 4 to 6 months. Such postural automatism may develop immediately the head is turned, or be delayed for 20 to 30 seconds. Whether even this delay bears any pathogenic significance is not yet fully understood. It may be more conspicuous when done with the child sitting or even standing supported. At 3 or 4 months, the reflex reaction may remain in the tonic neck pattern for minutes, even though 30 seconds is the more usual duration. In CP, the ATNR is commonly *obligate*, i.e. he cannot escape from the pattern. An obligate tonic neck pattern is abnormal at any age. It persists longer, and is stronger in Dyskinetic forms of CP. Perpetuation of the reflex reaction as long as the stimulus continues is an hypertonic effect.

Persistence of this neck reflex beyond 6 to 7 months is characteristic of cerebral palsy, although its undiminishing intensity may make underlying cerebral palsy already apparent after only 4 to 5 months.

Whatever degree of reflex is elicited, it is typically more striking in the supine position, although sometimes even more so when sitting or standing. Such strong reflex reactions are incompatible with rolling, or with balance in independent standing or walking.

## Symmetric Tonic Neck Reflex

Again, this is a proprioceptive reflex derived from neck receptors. Supported prone across the thighs of the examiner, the neck is passively *flexed*, when the arms flex and legs extend. When the neck is *extended*, arms extend and legs flex. This reaction is normal until 4 to 6 months, but abnormal if persisting beyond 6 months.

## Positive Supporting Reactions and Placing

Lifting the child by the axillae, he is bounced several times so that his feet gently touch the floor. Incidentally, the infant "slipping through the hands" in this manoeuvre would be characteristic of hypotonia. When his feet are in contact with the floor, continue to hold the child in a vertical position whilst checking for increased extensor tone in the legs, and ability to bear weight. A sustained position in plantar flexion and adduction is then expected. This positive supporting reaction to bearing weight is present at birth, and should disappear by 2 to 3 months. It is important to realize that it makes a *reappearance once more at about 6 months* in preparation for supported walking beginning 2 or 3 months or more later. An abnormal reaction is sustained plantar flexion and increased tone of adduction beyond 4 months. The most likely abnormalities would be absence of the normal response, its general disorganisation, or its exaggeration, in unvarying fashion.

In the most severe encephalopathies likely to be expressed as CP, the positive supporting reaction is pathologically intense. It is elicited as soon as the infant is held in vertical suspension or when the feet first touch the surface. In the infant with predominant spasticity, some evidence of a normal supporting reaction is seen by 12 to 15 months, with flexion at the hips and knees, equinus at the ankles, and scissoring, although the "placing" reaction is not easily demonstrable.

It is believed that in the infant destined for dyskinetic forms of CP, the *supporting reactions are deferred* until later, i.e. even from 18 to 26 months. The extrapyramidal source leads to general disorganisation of this reflex, which is more poorly developed than the *placing* reaction. In spasticity, the reverse is true.

When there is little or no equinus or scissoring, the child is more likely to be hypotonic.

Curiously enough, extensor hypertonus during vertical suspension is an *asset in supporting although a liability in placing* which tends to be effected with both feet at once irrespective of only the dorsum of one foot being rubbed against the underside of the table top in a mechanical fashion.

## Negative Supporting Reaction

Again, lifting the child by the axillae, and bouncing him up and down several times, suddenly hold him in space. A positive response until 4 months of age is considered to be increased flexor tone in the legs, with thighs and knees flexing. Persistence beyond 4 months, however, is regarded as abnormal.

## Tonic Labyrinthine Reflex

With the infant both in prone and supine positions, and head in midline, the tone of the flexors and extensors of arms and legs are tested. When prone, flexor tone dominates; when supine, extensor tone predominates. Normality of this is acceptable until 4 months of age, with persistence beyond 4 months considered abnormal.

# AUTOMATIC MOVEMENT REACTIONS

## Persistently Abnormal Movement Pattern
## in Diagnosis

Considered one of the more important diagnostic tests. It exploits the inability of the CP child to achieve an isolated discrete movement. A single movement is expected to set off a complete stereotyped total body pattern. The retention of a primitive reflex is not implied. They are patterns never seen in movement.

## Moro Reflex

In the full-term infant this reflex, attributed to a response of the stretch receptors of the neck, should have disappeared by 6 months. Although its retention beyond 6 months may be seen in cerebral palsy, that is a relatively infrequent finding but is an example of abnormal persistence of a primary reflex impeding and delaying development. Manipulative skill is one of man's greatest assets, and this becomes attainable only as this reflex wanes.

Hip flexion may be the last element to go, and may still be identifiable for months through gentle contact by the examiner's hand against the child's knees. From the outset there should be no confusion with the startle response which is a mass myoclonic movement, and may emerge in sleep following a sudden noise, or some movement, or some event evoking sudden anxiety or fright.

## Suspension in Space

(a) **HORIZONTAL**: Landau reflex

With *horizontal suspension* of the child in space in a prone position through support of the thorax, muscle tone is assessed. Absence of elevation of the head and of the lower extremities is less specific, although mainly indicating hypotonia of neck and trunk.

In the normal response, the neck spontaneously extends with some stiffening or extension of the back and raising of lower extremities. The full Landau reaction is considered present when there is elevation of the head above the horizontal, and arching of the spine so that it becomes concave. This degree of spinal extension does not normally appear until about one year, but normality of this response would be accepted between 6 months and 2½ years. A reaction labelled as Landau 2 by Touwen (1976) is the loss of extensor tone when the head is flexed, unless an hypertonus state prevails. Overall failure of this reflex to develop by 10 to 12 months is also abnormal. Maintenance of the "rag-doll" or inverted "U" position, with both hands and feet hanging down loosely, implies muscle weakness such as in the congenital myopathies, or in the basic generalized hypotonia of a tonic or hypotonic CP. In the hypertonic child, excessive reflex contraction of musculature is mostly evidenced by the ability to sustain arching in this hypertonic postural response, although usually associated with other clear signs of hypertonicity.

Such reflexes appear at a slower pace in cerebral palsy, and the automatic movement reactions such as the Landau in particular may only emerge by the age of 2 years.

## (b) VERTICAL

While the infant is in vertical suspension, lifted until the toes are about 10-15 cm from the table top, note any tendency for the legs to scissor, and for arms to flex in early manifestation of spastic diplegia. The weight should be evenly distributed and without extensor thrust. Adduction, extension, or scissoring of the lower extremities, are also classically typical of spastic tetraplegic cerebral palsy, and the scissoring in vertical suspension may appear months before other manifestations of hypertonicity. Such hypertonus of limbs is linked to hypotonia of the trunk and its axial musculature in such an infant. In the infant destined to develop dyskinetic cerebral palsy or choreo-athetosis, however, the hypertonic trunk becomes a constant feature once the neonatal *rigidity* - such as may stem from kernicterus or anoxic insult - wears off.

## Neck-Righting Response

Righting responses are poor in the neurologically disadvantaged infant, as is subsequently in the spastic tetraplegic. On turning the head, look for the emergence or not of the neck righting reflex. In cerebral palsy, the normal response after turning the neck to one side, of rotation of the body as a whole in the same direction, is *absent between 1 and 6 months*. Thus the positive response will emerge only after 6 months or more.

*Righting reactions* serve the function of maintaining normal alignment of the body parts to one another, as well as the normal orientation of the head within space. These brainstem and midbrain reactions emerge initially in prone and supine positions, and become fully mature in these positions by 6 months of age. As well as neck-righting, they include head-righting on the body, body-righting on the head, body-righting on the body, and optical-righting. Head-righting upon the body may be the result of kinaesthetic stimuli from the neck, or from optic or labyrinthine stimulation. Each may predominate at different stages of development. The righting responses advance to equilibrium reactions.

As these reactions develop or mature, the child can roll over, move to sitting, four-point kneeling, half-kneeling, standing, and thence ambulate with rotation around the body axis, and with increasing extension against gravity.

As already mentioned, the physiological basis for initiating orienting movements of eyes, head and body appears to derive from complex interconnections arising from deep cerebellar neurons (Westby et al., 1991). Excitatory activity therefrom is mediated via the cerebellar-tectal projections to cells in the region of the superior colliculus, in turn under basal ganglia influence via a Nigro-tectal pathway.

The primary reflexes fade after serving their purpose, or as they are superseded by more mature responses. Elements of secondary reflexes, such as the righting reactions, persist throughout life, for example in the continued maintenance of posture, whilst movement against gravity is only possible as a result of the continued interaction of reflex postural mechanisms.

## Equilibrium Reactions

A group of automatic reactions which are more complex than righting reactions are specific to man. Their purpose is thus to maintain the erect or upright position. The body is thereby adapted to shifts in its centre of gravity, and to modifications of extremity positions relative to the trunk. The five basic reactions in prone  supine,

prone kneeling with  elbows extended, sitting and standing are elicited by labyrinthine stimulation. Reactions in prone and supine are tested on a tilt board. In both, the normal reaction pattern is of side flexion of head and trunk together with abduction of arm and leg on the raised side.

## Sitting

Using a static supporting surface with feet unsupported:
*Sideways*: tilting to the right evokes side flexion of head and trunk to the right with extension of arm and leg.

*Backward* tilting produces forward flexion of head, trunk and arms.
*Forward displacement*: pushing the trunk forward produces extension of head and trunk.

## Prone Kneeling

Also tested on a tilt board. On the raised side, slight flexion of limbs with slight drop in supporting tone. On the

lowered side, there is bracing of the limbs in extension and slight abduction.

## Standing

Testing is by passive movement at the hips...  To the right, is followed by slight

side flexion of head and trunk, to the left with abduction of left arm and leg.

# CEREBRAL CORTICAL REFLEXES

These are used to test balancing ability under the influence of cerebral cortex and cerebellum.

## Simple Test of Balancing Ability

*With the child sitting*, edge him gently to one side. The arm on the falling side extends and fingers open up, whilst the neck corrects so that it is brought to a neutral position. The positive response should appear normally by 10 to 12 months *when the child is already able to stand.*

*When standing*, tilt to one side. Flexion of the knee ensues on the side to which falling is threatened, whereas the opposite knee extends and tries to cross over towards the direction of momentum and before he takes a forward step to catch up with gravity.

*Pressed back*, the neck flexes and he takes a backward step.

*Pressed forward*, the neck extends to bring the head to neutral, and forward steps are taken to catch up with gravity.

Such positive standing responses should appear in the sitting position by 10 to 12 months, and in the standing position by 15 to 18 months. Asymmetric responses are abnormal. The absence of balancing reflexes for sitting after 12 months is abnormal, as is their absence for standing after 18 months.

Consistent *unilateral* failure is associated with hemiparetic cerebral palsy, although of course brachial palsy, injuries, or other painful lesions of one upper extremity or clavicle may lead to comparable asymmetry of response.

On the other hand, bilateral suppression or distortion of this reaction marks both spastic and dyskinetic forms of cerebral palsy. As well as hyperextension of the limbs as a whole, there is spreading and slight hyperextension of fingers so that both proximal and distal functions are tested. Especially when combined with a "fisted hand", the eventual manifestation of spasticity is confirmed.

## Parachute Reactions

In testing for the beginning of this response after one year is reached, hold the child by the waist and tilt forwards or lower the face gently towards the table top. Arms then extend and first abduct, with extension of the fingers as if to break a fall.

Any asymmetry or bilateral impairment of this typical "defensive" reaction, is abnormal. In *hemiplegia*, in addition to the asymmetry of the parachute response, asymmetry of limb movements may be obvious. In the supine position, a sensitive sign of hemiparesis would be for one lower limb to fall into external rotation at the hip with the foot pointing laterally. Failure of one arm to swing normally in pendular fashion is also a sensitive clue to hemiparesis, with asymmetrically "associated" swinging especially helpful in detecting mild degrees of hemiparesis.

Rolling the infant over a large beach ball will help to smoothly elicit a parachute response if present, since opening up the palm with extension of the fingers is part of the response. It also helps open up the spastic adducted thumb. This "defensive" response normally begins to emerge at about 7 months, being present in most normal infants after 10 months of age. Although absence is not to be regarded in itself as abnormal before one year, suspicion of abnormality remains if there is *total* absence of any such response after 8 months. Failure to elicit may serve not only to demonstrate malfunction of the upper limbs, but also to confirm that paraparesis in the upper limbs objectively completes a tetraparesis. And this may be demonstrable long before hyperreflexia is elicited in the arms. It is basically considered to be more a vestibular reaction than an ocular one.

*A poor or absent parachute response*, or one which is more abnormal distally than proximally, and with delay in thumb-forefinger-grasp for small objects (normal at 9 to 12 months), points rather to future athetosis.

## Babinski Reflex Response and Rossolino Version

On stroking the lateral plantar surface from heel to toe, a positive response is marked by dorsiflex extension - or dorsiflexion - of the great toe accompanied by spreading or fanning of other toes. This Babinski response is typically positive in normal infants and does not become clinically significant until the end of the second year, when myelogenesis of the pyramidal tract has presumably been completed. Beyond the second year of life, this positive response would be indicative of pyramidal tract damage. In its slight modification comprising the Rossolino version, reflex flexion of the toes and extension of the great toe is induced by stroking its plantar surface. The same response may be elicited by applying a stimulus at a distance from the big toe as in the following modifications which could be especially exploited if the Babinski is equivocal. *The Chaddock sign*, extension of the big toe may be induced by stroking along the lateral malleolus or dorsolateral aspect of the foot. Downward stroking along the medial aspect of the tibia is used in the *Oppenheim sign*, whilst the calf is squeezed in *Gordon's sign*.

It can be regarded as a fractionated *withdrawal reflex* mediated by local spinal cord mechanisms akin to a nociceptive withdrawal response. Normally, the corticospinal tracts exercise suppression of such withdrawal responses, and the toes remain immobile or curl down. In infancy, no such suppressive influence is apparent, so that the extensor plantar response is normal. Possibly lack of "suppression" at this stage may be consequent upon immature and incomplete myelogenesis of the corticospinal pathways. Once complete, early in the second year of life, persistence or return of this extensor response will become abnormal.

It is thus supportive evidence of pyramidal damage, especially of an underlying component of cerebral palsy of the hypertonic form, particularly when complemented by hyperactive deep tendon reflexes and ankle clonus. These responses more strictly reflect the bi-pyramidal syndrome: of abnormally brisk reflexes, hypertonus and diminished muscular power, being consequent upon upper motor neurone lesions involving the corticospinal tracts, relatively frequent in all types of central nervous disease. It is even a common manifestation of the encephalopathy of metabolic disorder which is distinctively *progressive* or intermittent as in the hyperammonaemia of Reye's syndrome or in Tay Sachs or the demyelinating encephalopathies in contrast to the non-progressive pathology of cerebral palsy, or of relevant anatomical malformation such as platybasia compression by a medulloblastoma or other cerebellar neoplasm.

In this early age period as already suggested, interpretation of this sign is usually more uncertain. Flaccidity rather than spasticity may well be prominent in the initial phases of cerebral palsy. This may well be due either to the fact that the facilitative reticular spinal mechanisms from which spasticity derives, have not yet developed, or to immaturity of myelinization. Ultimately, in damage involving the internal capsule, one must recall that fibres of the direct activational or pyramidal pathways are intermingled with those of the indirect activational or extrapyramidal system. So that the result of such combined damage to these systems adds increased tone and spasticity to the list of findings. A clinical pattern of flaccid paralysis linked to a positive Babinski is unusual, occurring only after small lesions localized to the medullary pyramidal motor cortex. The rare associated monoplegia of a leg (or arm) is the more likely result of limited pathology of the motor cortex.

In association with hyperreflexia, an important sign of pyramidal tract lesions is also relative, i.e. the *depression of superficial abdominal reflexes*.

Hypoactive or reduced plantar responses are more typically associated with the hypotonic and cerebellar ataxic categories of cerebral palsy. It also characterizes many of the metabolic and other disorders simulating CP in part of their course, including the torsion dystonia linked to a permutation of arylsulfatase deficiency (Russell and Yatziv, 1985) together with other peripheral neuropathic disorder.

*Prognostic predictability* has been laid at the door of the presence or absence of these reflexes by clinicals with long-term experience in cerebral palsy, whether they be present, intensified, weak or absent. They have especially suggested that a poor prognosis for walking to have been associated with an unduly strong and persistent asymmetric tonic neck reflex, crossed extensor and Moro, together with the absence of a parachute response.

# ASSESSMENT OF MOTOR DISABILITY

No adequate objective measurement of the magnitude of the underlying motor disability has been evolved as yet. Strength in the arms is solely one indirect criterion, and this can be gauged through measure of the hand-grip using the hand-held dynamometer as described by Fleishman (1964). Another parameter that is testable is that of manual coordination. For this assessment, the Pardue pegboard test has long been exploited (Costa et al., 1964). In one example, the hemiplegic group, abnormal slowness is a characteristic response, even when allowed to use the best hand or both hands together. It may prove a very useful screening test for the minor degrees of hemiplegia to which I have already referred as possibly a separate entity.

In estimating motor disability in the lower limbs in the older CP child, Bruininks (1978) has proposed a modified Oberetsky test of running, speed and agility.

## Gradation of Motor Disability

Nevertheless, some form of "severity index" would be helpful or a system for classifying the extent of the disability in relation to what could be considered "normal" functional activities linked to lifestyle for a particular age. Such *gradation or degree of motor handicap* could then be embodied descriptively within this clinical classification, perhaps along the lines proposed by Perlstein (1952), as follows:

### Grade I        Slight or mild
The affected child manages everyday functions without difficulty. Walks and talks although physical movements are somewhat clumsy.

### Grade II        Moderate
Manages everyday motor functions with difficulty and necessitating some assistance. Clinically, speech is indistinct, and there is some difficulty in hand control. Gait is unsteady.

### Grade III        Severe
Fails to manage everyday motor functions at all, or only succeeds with considerable assistance. Is reflected in little control of arms, hands and legs, whilst independence is severely limited.

# References

Bayley N. (1969) Manual for the Bayley Scale of Infant Development. Psychological Corporation, New York

Blashke TF, Birk PD et al. (1974) Crigler-Naggar syndrome: an unusual course with neurological damage at age eighteen. Pediat Res 8: 573-590

Bruininks RH. (1978) Bruininks-Oberetsky Test. Examiners Manual, Circle Pines, American Guidance Service

Costa LD, Scarola LM, Rapin I. (1964) Purdue pegboard scores for normal grammar school children. Perceptual Motor Skills 18: 748

Fleishman FA. (1964) Basic Fitness Tests. Examiners Manual. New York, Prentice-Hall.

Hansen TWJ, Tydal T, Jorgensen H et al. (1985) Effect of bilirubin on uptake of 5-HT and Dopamine in rat brain synaptosomes. Pediat Res 19: 390A

Karp WB. (1979) Biochemical alterations in neonatal hyperbilirubinaemia and encephalopathy: a review. Pediatrics 64: 361-368

Levine RL, Ferericks AB, Rappaport SL. (1982) Entry of bilirubin into the brain due to opening of the blood-brain barrier. Pediatrics 69: 255-259

Perlstein MA. (1952) Infantile cerebral palsy. Classification and clinical correlations. J Am Med Ass 149: 30-34

Russell A, Yatziv S. (1985) A metabolic basis for idiopathic torsion dystonia: a new variant of metachromatic leukodystrophy. World Pediat Child Care 1: 25-29

Schiff D, Chan G, Poznansky MJ. (1985) Bilirubin toxicity in neural cell lines N115 and NBRIOA. Pediat Res 19: 908-911

Touwen B. (1976) Neurological development in infancy. Clinics in Developmental Medicine, No. 58. London S.I.M.P. with Heinemann Medical. Philadelphia, Lippincott

Westby O, Collinson C, Redgrave D, Dean P. (1991) Deep cerebellar neurons provide tonic excitatory drive for cells in intermediate white layers of contralateral superior Colliculus. 14th Meeting European Neuroscience Association. Eur J Neurosci, Oxford University Press, suppl. 4, p. 302

# 4

# EARLY DIAGNOSTIC

# IDENTIFICATION OF

# CEREBRAL PALSY

# COMPONENTS

# AND THEIR

# NEUROPHYSIOLOGY

## Hypotonia

## Hypertonicity or Spasticity: Early Diagnostic Identification and Neurophysiology

Patho-Physiology

## Chorea, or Choreiform Movements

## Athetosis

Further Neurophysiological and Other Aspects of Athetoid Manifestation

Role of GABA, etc., in Basal Ganglia Function especially of Caudate, Putamen and Subthalamic Nuclei

## Early Diagnostic Identification of Ataxia and the Dysequilibrium Syndrome

The Ataxic Pattern characterizing the Dysequilibrium Syndrome

Patho-Physiology of Ataxia

## Congenital Hemiplegia

Associated Movements and Postural Changes
Additional Early Diagnostic Criteria
Aetiology
Acquired Hemiplegia
"Double" Hemiplegia or Parasagittal Cortex Syndrome
Atypical Hemiplegical and Multifunctional Patterns of Hemiplegia
Management

## Tremor

## Possible Activation of Fundamental Cerebral Protective Mechanisms Against Neuronal Death: The Role of Glutamate Receptors

## The Role of Superoxide Radicals, Effects of Hypoxia and Hyperoxaemia Evaluated in Cultured Neurones

## References

136

# 4

# HYPOTONIA

## Initial Hypotonia: in Neonate or Early Infancy during which there appears to have been a Subtle Diminution of Tone from Birth

The premature infant is relatively hypotonic, and in the initial relatively hypotonic pattern of the first 6 to 9 months of life, the muscles remain flaccid with reduced tone presumably because of the absence of excitatory input to the gamma motor neurone. These are small and more diffusely arrayed than the alpha motor neurone. Whatever the cerebral source of the hypotonia may be, flexion and extension movements of the legs are infrequent or absent, as well as the limbs being flaccid and lacking in tone. A very gradual increase of tone, however, marks later childhood.

A transitory hypotonic phenomenon, which is not relevant in terms of the sustained short term hypotonia under discussion, is the so-called "silent period" which follows transient although continuous phasic contraction of a muscle such as may be produced as a tendon-jerk reflex. A transient reduction of activity of the motor units may be induced by several reflex mechanisms:

1. Reduction or cessation of muscle spindle discharge.
2. The inhibitory discharge of the tendon organs or receptors.

3. Recurring inhibition of the alpha motor neurone.

The muscle spindle discharge is regarded as the *gamma bias* of the spindle ascribed to gamma motor neurone activation of the intrafusal fibres. A low gamma bias may be envisaged as underlying the absence or prolongation of this silent period and hypotonic state.

Flexor tone, with resistance to extension of all limbs, is prominent in the full-term neonate. Furthermore, when lifted forward from the supine, the head does not fall back more than 45°. Hypotonia would be considered significant if head lag is much in excess of this, and if there is floppiness when the limb is gently shaken without flexor recoil. If accompanied by *alertness* of the baby, this may reflect muscle or anteriorhorn disease, *whereas associated apathy* and *diminution of consciousness* would instead suggest either the influence of maternal drugs, sedatives or analgesics if there is no underlying sepsis or severe intracranial damage.

Other manoeuvres may be used in testing hypotonia in the neonate or infant:

in *horizontal suspension*, hypotonia of neck and trunk is illustrated by an abnormal posture not only without elevation of head and lower extremities but with conspicuous *drooping of both* as the infant slumps limply into the so-called inverted "U" position. In spastic babies, the trunk is often hypotonic despite apparent hypertonicity of the limbs. Nevertheless, the head is elevated above the horizontal. Upward arching of the spine so that it becomes concave is more typical as the infant approaches one year of age. In the future, choreo-athetotic child, hypotonus of the trunk is typical during infancy once any initial neonatal rigidity stemming from kernicterus or anoxic insult has subsided. Hypotonia is also characteristic of cerebellar ataxia, when it is commonly associated with hyperreflexia as well as nystagmus and subsequent dysarthria.

The *scarf sign* can be a useful criterion of hypotonia in the infant and child. The arm is drawn gently across the chest and the elbow normally fails to quite reach the mid-sternal line. In the hypotonic, the elbow extends beyond the midline with ease.

The *popliteal angle* is another useful parameter of tone in the legs of the newborn and infant. The leg is flexed on the abdomen and the knee is extended. Extension beyond 80° is allowed in the normal full-term.

## Traction Test or "Pulling up to Sit"

Head lag is especially clarified in this test in which the infant is gently pulled up to 15-20 cm from the supine whilst observing for head-lag, shoulder bracing and ability to overcome the force of gravity.

Clinically, the profound hypotonia from birth in the "floppy infant" of "rag-doll" posture encompasses syndromes of multiple aetiology, as vividly portrayed in the Dubowitz monograph (1980), including the congenital myopathies. The growing group of known *metabolic* myopathies still require confirmatory diagnostic biopsy and electron microscopic cytochemistry in addition to initial metabolic and electromyographic investigation. These ultrastructural analyses are being increasingly exploited to pinpoint the location of chemical elements by *electron probe microanalysis*, as well as by assay of enzymes and other proteins, e.g. by the especially important technique of electronmicroscopic *immunolabelling*.

# Early Diagnostic Identification of Hypotonia

Early diagnosis of hypotonic states, relevant from the newborn and early infantile phase, warrants special consideration. Indeed, diminished tone to an abnormal degree is the commonest disturbance of tone in the "neurologically compromised" neonate, and may express pathology of cerebral hemispheres or of cerebellum and spinal cord, as well as of peripheral nerves, or of myoneural functions. In the neonate, and in early infancy, it first implies identification of relative lack of tone and the diagnostic differentiation of "the floppy infant" in various forms which nonetheless present a common clinical picture. Presentation in the infant, however, may be because of relative immobility, although this is typically associated with three more specific features particularly well enunciated by Dubowitz (1980), slightly rephrased as follows:

1. *Deviations of Posture and Movement* which are unusual or even bizarre.
2. *Significantly reduced resistance to passive movement.*
3. *Joint mobility* excessive in range. (Analysis and correlationship at the end of this section).

Although the degree and extent of hypotonia is especially clear in the supine position, it can be clinically accentuated - as already emphasized - by pulling up the infant from supine, whilst assessing head control or lag. Particularly when reaching prone suspension, the posture of head, trunk and limbs is observed. Initial "floppiness" in the baby is also the characteristic response in congenital myopathic and other disorders to be subsequently discussed in Chapter 18. Movement of the limb should initially be slow and then rapid. The response in a child with normal muscle tone is consistent regardless of speed. In general, a slow smooth passive movement should produce less resistance than fast movement. The *clasp-knife response* to fast movement, characterized by initial resistance followed by sudden release, is typical of spastic diplegia. Other descriptive labels include the *lead-pipe* or *cog-wheel* reactions expressing rigidity in

response to slow or fast movement, as well as "waxy" to both slow and fast movement. In the athetoid CP, there is classically fluctuating tone, varying from moment to moment. Whilst hypotonicity is the typical response to lesions of the basal ganglia, hypertonus of rigid type may also be associated.

It is important to assess whether any significant *degree of weakness*, including *facial* weakness, is associated with the hypotonia. This helps determine whether there is a basic neuromuscular disorder or myopathy, or whether it is derived from a disorder of the central nervous system. Simple manoeuvres help in this regard: the degree of ability to raise a limb against gravity, and the withdrawal response of a limb to a painful stimulus. Further assessment will be required to determine whether the underlying condition is suprasegmental or involves lower motor neurones and muscles.

If diagnostic decision is in the direction of a neuromuscular disorder, principal causes could be spinal muscular atrophy, such as also outlined in the section of Disorders Simulating Hypotonic CP in Chapter 18, principal causes could be spinal *muscular atrophy, a congenital myopathy, or congenital muscular atrophy, etc. A more specific CNS basis, for example, would include early and severe spinal muscular atrophy of the Werdnig-Hoffman form*, or its later infant manifestation of Kugelberg-Welander, demonstrating paralysis and immobility of legs linked to lesser paralysis of the arms. The face is spared therein, whereas facial weakness is typical of the congenital myopathies and of myotonic dystrophy. But sucking and swallowing difficulties may *present* in both. *The superimposed finding of contractures and/or skeletal anomalies* would in particular point to congenital muscular dystrophy or congenital myotonic dystrophy, with the addition in the latter of a prenatal history of hydramnios as a possible source of the limitation of joint extension at elbows and knees. Muscle tone is also strikingly diminished if there is interruption of the afferent proprioceptive input to the cord or of the afferent arc of the stretch reflex.

*The posture* adopted whilst supine may reveal asymmetry in muscle bulk, power and movement. The excessively relaxed "pithed frog" posture is often found in spinal muscular atrophies and myopathies, but is also characteristic of ascorbic acid deficiency and many metabolic disorders from *idiopathic hypercalcaemia, renal tubular acidosis, nephrogenic diabetes insipidus* and *hypoaldosteronism,* as well as to the neurometabolic encephalopathies such as in *hyperglycinaemia,* or the neonatal *organic acidaemias* including maple syrup disease.

Severely incapacitated infant subjects of Werdnig-Hoffman disease exhibit a disproportionate alertness. An overall developmental delay of motor, social and language skills would instead point to mental retardation, also indicated if the head circumference was found to be below the third percentile. Presentation with infantile hypotonia will be accompanied by other pathognomonic features in familial dysautonomia, when even *taste* will already be impaired etc., (Russell and Perlman, 1992), or in the Downs and Prader-Willi syndromes.

*Myasthenia gravis* is another rare source of hypotonia and weakness in infancy, presenting with muscle weakness and progressive fatiguability stemming from defect of neuromuscular transmission in the presynaptic area. A transient neonatal form may derive from a mother suffering from the disorder or about to develop symptoms. In the congenital form, anomalies of jaw growth (Russell and Shapiro, 1994) may be the conspicuous postnatal clue to prenatal defect of oro-masticatory muscle function.

## Basic Muscle Tone and its Clinical Assessment

Before appraisal of such reflex responses and automatisms, a preliminary assessment of muscle tone is a routine requirement. During flexion and extension of arm or leg, muscles are stretched and a mild *resistance to passive movement* is elicited which is referred to as muscle tone. In part, "tone" is due to the intrinsic elasticity of the tissues, but in practice is mainly the result of the activation of motor units by stretching of the muscle spindles, or is subjectively appraised on the basis of degree of resistance on passive movement of an individual joint.

Such resistance to passive movement is therefore gauged, as is the subjective appreciation of tone on passively *palpating and manipulating the musculature.* An increase in the input to *alpha* or *gamma* motor neurones would effect an increase in muscle tone. A reduction in either the afferent input from the muscle spindle, or of the efferent activity of these lower motor neurones would bring about a lowering of muscle tone. Such loss of muscle tone identified in response to passive movement is usually described as flaccidity.

Conversely, a significant increase in the resistance to passive movement could indicate the hypertonus of spastic cerebral palsy which may later come to be convincingly supported by extensor hypertonicity of the legs held in extension; still later in a scissoring posture, etc.

While sitting-up the child, note the presence or absence of resistance. If marked hip flexion accompanies this, it may imply spasticity of the hamstrings, and indicate a retesting of knee and ankle jerks to confirm their hyperactivity, or even the eliciting of ankle clonus, both characterizing hypertonic CP. Whilst *checking the hips for dislocation*, even at such early stages, abnormal limitation of abduction and other so-called expressions of hypertonus are sought. Even at three months, one should exclude an *asymmetrical* response which could also point to *unilaterally* increased muscle tone. Indeed, whenever passively flexing or extending arms and legs, there should be routine evaluation of joint mobility as well as of muscle tone, since not uncommonly an associated hyperflexibility of joints, often genetically determined, introduces a confusing element in both the assessment of tone and of developmental status. The role of Golgi tendon receptors in this connection has not yet been adequately clarified. This likewise applies to the contribution of mechano-receptors in the muscle spindle itself, or the adaptation of tonic receptors therein, or elsewhere in muscle, in continuing to initiate or sustain impulses in adjacent axons as long as the stimulus remains. They must serve to maintain tone whilst keeping the central nervous system constantly appraised of the postural and equilibrium status of the body.

Conversely, head-lag and its tendency to fall back during the traction test would point to hypotonia. Also the head should be turned looking for the emergence or not of the *neck righting reflex*. The clinical elicitation of hypertonia in vertical suspension, or of hypotonia in horizontal suspension, should be clearly expressed, as outlined subsequently under "suspension in space".

**Locus caeruleus in the "control" of tone**

Significant results are emerging from the study of potential sources of pathophysiology involved in "damage" to the immature brain underlying disorders of muscle tone. The *Locus caeruleus*, a group of melanin-pigmented cells rich in norepinephrine located in the lateral portion of the tegmentum of the upper pons and lower midbrain, and other midbrain structures adjacent to it, appear to have an important physiological role in the control of muscle tone. Electrical stimulation of structures rostral and ventral to the locus caeruleus (the caudal pontine, reticular, and cuneiform nuclei and ventral parts of the inferior colliculus) evoked remarkable enhancement of muscle tone in the biceps as well as tonic vibration and tonic stretch reflexes (Jüch et al., 1991). It appears that activation was thereby involved of descending pathways derived from the mesencephalic loeoniotes region. Possibly this is the outcome of excitatory action upon alpha motor neurones on the one hand, and to augmented fusimotor drive on the other hand. Note the revelation of involvement of the *inferior colliculus*, whilst it is of interest that the neurones of the other corpora quadrigemina of the tectum, the *superior colliculis*, is also implicated (Westby et al., 1991). This is the target of tonic excitatory drive from deep cerebellar nuclei involved in the initiation of orienting movements of eyes, head and body, presumably via cerebellar-*tectal* pathways. The *posterior lobe of the cerebellum, in particular the large lateral hemispheres*, also appear to be specifically concerned with maintenance of limb tone. Lesions thereof are especially associated with hypotonia as well as *dyssynergia* or limb ataxia.

## Significance of Hypotonia in the Preterm Infant

In appraising hypotonia in the premature infant, one must keep in mind that premature infants are primarily hypotonic. Greater flexor tone is demonstrated immediately after birth in temporary perpetuation of the flexed posture *in utero*, although a more hypotonic posture is assumed within 12-72 hours after delivery. The development of tone and reflexes prior to term is guided by two patterns - caudocephalad and centripetal (distal to proximal). Premature infants less than 28-30 weeks are generally hypotonic, mild flexor tone being detected in the lower extremities by 31 weeks, and in the upper extremity by 34 weeks (Allen and Caputo, 1990). Flexor tone then becomes stronger, peaking at term (with flexor hypertonia in both upper and lower limbs, as well as fisting) to be lost or become more balanced with extensor tone after term.

By 3 to 4 months, tone has typically become equal in all extremities, with the hand unfisted most of the time.

With respect to axial tone, mild hip adductor tone is identifiable by 31-33 weeks becoming stronger by 35-37 weeks, and strong enough to overcome gravity by 36-37 weeks, so that the normal prone posture of a full-term infant incorporates flexion of all extremities, with the buttocks up in the air due to strong hip adductor and flexor tone (Saint Anne Dargassies, 1977).

Truncal hypotonia can be appraised in the premature infant by holding them in ventral suspension and measuring the curve of the back. With progressive improvement, a horizontal position is briefly attainable by term, or 40 weeks PMA.

Whilst *neck flexor tone* may emerge by 33 weeks (Allen and Capute, 1990) it takes longer to mature than any other aspect of tone. Measured by the manoeuvre of pulling the infant to a sitting position from supine, whilst observing the position of the head with respect to the body, he should first be able to modulate forward movement so that it no longer slams forward by 37 weeks, and can then actively flex forward even against gravity.

The pull-to-sit manoeuvre may be stressful in hypotonic infants or where there is an increasing risk of atlanto-occipital instability as in Down's syndrome. One may instead gently rock the infant back and forth in the sitting position.

Neck flexor tone is balanced against the development of neck extensor tone. Predominance of the latter signifies abnormal development. Neck extensor hypertonia is indicated by increased space behind the shoulders or in the pull-to-sit manoeuvre or when rocking in sitting. These children also show head lag on pull to sit, or the head remains extended on rocking in sitting, even against gravity. Most term infants have a head lag on pull to sit from supine but by 2-3 months the infant can actively flex the neck so that the head remains in line with the body on pull to sit.

## Hypermobility: Ligamentous, Tendinous and Other Causes of Joint Mobility and Apparent Hypotonia

To clinically differentiate ligamentous laxity and joint hypermobility from muscle hypotonia in early infancy is especially difficult, albeit a day-to-day diagnostic problem during the first few years of life. Neurodevelopmental delay and the contribution or otherwise of hypotonia are the common differential factors. To begin with, they may co-exist. Later undue mobility of joints but otherwise normal muscle tone becomes clearer.

Joint hypermobility in infancy is a relatively common trait with a prevalence of about 17%, but especially high amongst Africans and Orientals, the latter which may be mirrored by the "lotus position" of Buddha with the soles of his feet facing upwards. Such hypermobility of the joints of fingers and hands is exploited by Thai dancers. In European terms, this feature in reflexion of joint laxity could be labelled the "benign hypermobility syndrome". It is postulated that the range of movement of a given joint in different individuals is distributed in a Gaussian manner, although it occurs twice as commonly in females. Hypermobile individuals are simply at one extreme of this normal distribution, although occasionally there may be an underlying pathological situation.

Congenital disorders of connective tissue may thus be attended by sufficient delay or defect in postural control to suggest hypotonia. Joint laxity is also especially seen in the Marfanoid syndrome described by Walker et al. (1969). Of the eight types of Ehlers Danlos syndrome now recognized, for example, Types 3 and 7 especially demonstrate joint laxity and recurrent dislocation of joints, whereas the characteristic elasticity of skin and bruising, etc., are more prominent in the remaining types (Byers et al., 1983). Ligamentous laxity is also a cardinal feature of the autosomal dominant form of osteogenesis imperfecta alongside hypotonia (Tizard, 1949) linked to delay in walking.

In the presence of moderate to severe mental retardation with an IQ in the range 40-60, hyperextensibility of joints should be remembered as a feature of *the fragile X syndrome* with a "fragile" site near the tip of the long arm of the X chromosome at band Xq27.3. This is now recognized as the commonest inherited cause of mental handicap. It has an incidence of 1:1,100 in males and 1:700 in females. Characteristically, there is epilepsy, elongation of the face with large and everted ears, prognathism and repetitive jocular speech patterns with evidence of perseveration. However, in addition the hyperextensibility in this syndrome is also envisaged as one manifestation of a more generalized connective tissue dysplasia, linking aortic dilatation, mitral valve prolapse and pectus excavatum.

Muscle tone or the joint structure help to determine joint mobility. Lack of tone may be associated with varying abnormality, including that of the CNS such as cerebral palsy or mental retardation. An excellent objective study by Tirosh et al. (1991) was applied to 60 children between 54 and 60 months. The principal objective was firstly to assess the gross and fine motor proficiency of such children either with or without associated motor delay and secondly to assess any residual association between joint hypermobility and gross motor dysfunction at the age of 5 years. The prevalence of the latter association was significantly higher than in the children without abnormal motor development. But of particular importance in reference to the whole subject was that children with such hypermobility and motor delay were significantly likely to present the same association when they reached the age of 5 years. Fine motor problems also persisted into later childhood whereas previous reports have claimed complete resolution of both fine and gross motor defects.

In relation to a possible contribution from the central nervous system the cerebellum has an important function. As long ago as the First World War, Gordon Holmes (1917) showed that in unilateral destructive lesions of the cerebellum, there is very rapid development of abnormal hyperextensibility of the fingers without any resistance being felt, quite apart from the characteristic hypotonia. Protective reflexes must be concurrently diminished, or are in abeyance.

Joint movement is restrained partly by the muscles and partly by the capsular tissue and the ligaments of the joints, although this braking effect may be less pronounced. In terms of muscle, the resistance to stretching of a complete muscle depends not only upon tone but also if the motion is moderate partly upon the intrinsic properties of muscle fibres and partly upon its constituent fibrous tissue (endomysium and perimysium). It remains to be clarified whether a relative lack of the muscle's meshwork of connective tissue contributes to hypermobility.

Reduction of such hypermobility with age is part of the natural history of man and this may be compatible with the above hypothesis. Certainly the hypermobility is naturally greatest in infancy. Note the beautiful Shakespearean reference to this in Hamlet (III ii 71) "Be soft as the sinews of the newborn babe...". so that diagnostic and prognostic confusion is also greatest in those first two to four years of life, not only with the mild to moderate hypotonia of cerebral palsy, but also with "benign congenital hypotonia". At the very least it is inescapably responsible on conventional testing or observation for what is called "neurodevelopmental" delay in motor milestones. If overlooked, temporary errors in prognosis as well as diagnosis leads to much unnecessary parental anxiety.

In simple testing of the child for multiple joint mobility rather than selective joint involvement such as is often confined to hyperextension at the wrists. the fingers of either hand may be hyperextensible, or the thumbs can be pressed back into the forearm. Can he also press the palms of his hands upon the floor? Hyperextension of knees, and

even of hips, can lead to much provisional disability, apart from diagnostic misjudgment.

It is possible, however, that a basic mutational anomaly of collagenous proteins is responsible for the later severity of "hypermobility", akin perhaps to that found in Ehlers-Danlos syndrome.

Consideration should be given at this point to the hyperextensibility associated with osteogenesis imperfecta such as we have already mentioned as reported by Tizard (1949). Their undue laxity may be limited to the extremities. But in some examples, it also involves knees and hip joints (as well as elbows and shoulders) of a degree already emphasized. Sometimes in my experience at the Hornsey Centre for Cerebral Palsied Children, it may on occasions actually co-exist with spastic diplegia although by no means so frequently as with hypotonia. One example of the latter was the Cohen syndrome, its early hypotonia "flabbiness" and hyperextensibility of joints coexisting with shortness of stature, adiposity and mental retardation. Minor dysmorphic features include anti-mongoloid slanting of eyes, broad prominent nasal root, microcephaly, large ears and maxillary protrusion. In that perspective, the genetic defect identified in the case of Sippola and Prockop, where the joint hyperextensibility was considerable, is especially challenging. They found a short deletion from the product of one of the $\alpha2(1)$ alleles, and it is reasonable to presume that the deletion leading to poor alignment of the cleavage domains of the three chains serves to alter the rate of conversion of procollagen to collagen, the fibrous framework of bone, skin and tendon. Further exploration of this facet is certainly called for, as well as possible genetically-determined structural or functional anomalies of tension receptors I would like to postulate within the Golgi tendons or related tissue. These appear to act as a sensitive feedback to individual motor units and the tension they are generating. The tendon organs embody receptors located within the fascia of muscle tendons. They are considered to be physically discharged by stretch of the muscle tendon. Because they are in series with the muscle fibres, muscle contraction with resultant phasic stretch of the tendon results in tendon organ discharge. The tendon organ afferents just project centrally through fibres (Group 16) only slightly smaller than the primary spindle fibres and then enter the dorsomedial portion of the dorsal horn.

Occasional association with a specific metabolic defect may yet prove to have similar or other significant implications. For instance, adenic phosphoribosyl transferase deficiency leading to urinary calculi is known to underlie marked *hyperlaxity of joints linked to muscular hypotonia*. The urinary tract calculi is made up of 2,8-dihydroxy adenine and are responsible for frequent renal colic from about 9 months of age. Its excretion is reduced by a combination of a low purine diet with allopurinol (20 mg/kg/day). Even without such therapy, the hypotonia per se gradually lessens the conventional developmental delay - particularly of motor milestones - and

unsupported walking is achieved by 2½ to 3 years of age.

Conversely, a greater depth of study of infantile syndromes characterized by the opposite phenomenon of progressive stiffening and immobility of joints may provide information relevant to the aetiology of hypermobility of joints. For instance, in the Moore-Federman syndrome of familial dwarfism with stiff joints, both sexes are affected equally in this disorder of autosomal inheritance emerging between the ages of 3 and 5 years of age. The stiffness progresses slowly until there is complete inability to clench the hand. Concurrently, there is a decline in the height of the vertebrae confirmed radiologically, whilst there has been a steady widening of the phalangeal metaphyses. Hepatomegaly is associated but no mucopolysaccharidosis or other metabolic basis comparable to the Hunter/Hurley syndromes.

The *Leri-Johnson syndrome* is an autosomal dominant syndrome pre-eminently of progressive impairment of the articulation of joints. There is also evidence of premature ossification of bone. The limited motion of joints attended by stiffness also affects the spine. Localized intensifications comparable to the carpal tunnel syndrome or metatarsalgia may prevail as well as flexion contractures of interphalangeal joints, together with semi-flexed internal rotation of the upper limbs and external rotation of the legs. Radiologically, bone shafts show long irregular streaking assuming the so-called "candle-wax" formation subperiosteally.

# HYPERTONICITY OR SPASTICITY: EARLY DIAGNOSTIC IDENTIFICATION AND NEUROPHYSIOLOGY

Characteristically, there is resistance to passive movement at an individual joint which is followed by the sudden release defined as the "clasp knife" phenomenon. It is predominantly felt in the arm flexors and the leg extensor muscles. Rigidity constitutes a constant resistance to passive movement of both extensor and flexor muscles. There is a consistent association with exaggerated or brisk deep reflex responses, an extensor or Babinski response, diminished active movements, clonus, and eventually disuse atrophy with the knee partially flexed, abrupt but guarded dorsiflexion of the foot. Sustained clonus invariably reflects hypertonicity and a lesion of the upper motor neurone tract. [In the newborn, it is regarded as sustained when it exceeds 5-10 beats.]

When crawling, the infant with spastic lower extremities will drag them, but later walks on tip-toes when there is rigidity, or marked spasticity, the head retracts into opisthotonos, and both head and heels are bent backwards.

In *vertical suspension* in space, adduction, extension or scissoring reflects spasticity. This may amount to an initial phase of rigidity of the lower extremities, with passive resistance to both extension and flexion, whilst adductor spasm of the hips sustains them in a scissored position. A spastic phase then takes over with flexion of hips, knees and to a lesser extent of the elbows. In less pronounced diplegia, impaired dorsiflexion of the feet may be solely in evidence with heightened tone at the ankles leading to walking in equines ("toe walking"). In still lesser degrees of diplegia, the leg spasticity is accompanied by impaired coordination of fine and rapid finger movements linked to weakness of wrist extensors.

In horizontal suspension, there is excessive reflex contraction of muscles so that head retraction may be accentuated, and the head is in any case held above the horizontal, the legs are raised with upward arching of the spine so that it becomes concave.

The Landau reaction or Landau 2 (Touwen, 1976) is valid at that point, so that when the head is passively flexed, extensor tone is lost.

In vertical suspension in space, adduction, extension or scissoring reflect spasticity.

## Parachute reaction
This is tested by suspending the child by the waist or thrusting him gently face down, or rotating him forwards on a large ball. In most normal infants, the reaction is elicited by 9 months, and its absence is not considered abnormal before 1 year. It is less demonstrable normally after 2 years. It comprises extension of the limbs as a whole, and particularly of the upper

limbs with spreading and slight hyperextension of the fingers.

Testing both proximal and distal function, it should invariably be compared with the child's ability to grasp small objects. One can demonstrate *suppression* or if not distortion of the parachute reaction in both spasticity and choreo-athetosis. A poor or absent response, or more abnormal distally than proximally, with delayed thumb-to-forefinger grasp for small objects (normal range 9-12 months). This negative response would especially suggest spasticity when combined with a fisted hand. A unilateral or asymmetric reaction would indicate an hemiparesis. My experience concurs with the claim of Baird and Gordon (1983) that it may help to identify a cerebral paraparesis apparently solely involving lower limbs as a tetraplegia long before either a stretch reflex or even hyperreflexia are elicitable in the arms.

# Patho-Physiology

## A. Hypertonicity

Several studies have claimed that disturbed coordination of muscle activity accounts for or significantly contributes to the summation of impairment of motor function in the spastic child (Nashner et al., 1983). Mycklebust and colleagues (1986) stressed that this functional incoordination is marked particularly by lack of relaxation of antagonist muscles. *Alpha* motor neurones are somatotropically arranged in the ventral horn, those innervating the axial musculature being medial to those supplying muscles of the extremities. Within the latter, *extensor motor neurones* supply extensor muscles, while groups of *flexor motor neurones* innervate flexor muscles. Muscles in functional support of one another, such as the gastrocnemius and soleus, are *synergistically* responsible for plantar flexion of the foot, whilst those acting in functional opposition to them are antagonists, such as the anterior tibialis responsible for dorsiflexion thereof. Electromyo-graphic exploration (Paneth and Kiely, 1984) has indeed confirmed that reciprocal excitation of antagonists is particularly characteristic of the clinical grouping of such spastic states. And in 1988, Harrison also indicated a possible role for functional abnormalities of the *spinal interneuronal* networks accounting for the motor dysfunction of spastic CP, that is in addition to the more *direct* primary corticospinal and related effects of brain damage.

Mainly in terms of *reflex excitability* Lance (1980) offers an interesting explanation:

"In both cerebral and spinal spasticity, the stretch reflex responses obtainable from extensor and flexor muscle groups of the upper and lower limbs increase linearly with increase in the velocity of stretch. The reflex component of the increased tone may therefore be measured in terms of the threshold velocity required to evoke reflex activity, and the slope of the EMG-velocity relationship. The implication is that the velocity threshold of stretch necessary to elicit a reflex is reduced, and the amplitude of a reflex response to a given velocity of stretch is increased in spasticity".

*Stretch Reflex*

The response initiated by afferent discharge from the muscle spindle is a stretch reflex. This is not clearly functional until the 17th week of gestation. Thereafter it continuously activates extensor and axial muscles towards *stabilisation of trunk and limbs*. Ultimately this serves to counteract the downward force of gravity central in the maintenance of the upright posture.

This basic automatism - a monosynaptic or myotatic reflex - is thus a fundamental element of anti-gravity postural adjustment, adaptation and stabilization. Tapping on a tendon to produce a sudden stretch of muscle initiates an efferent discharge from the muscle spindle, or rather a phasic synchronous discharge of primary muscle afferents which triggers the monosynaptic stretch reflex. The increased resistance to passive movement which is evoked by increased tonic stretch reflexes is termed *spasticity*. When a spastic muscle is stretched beyond a given length, the increased tone - or resistance to stretch - suddenly gives way to an abrupt loss of the resistance to stretch. This *clasp-knife* response is due to the activation of Group II spindle afferents which produce a length-dependent inhibition of the stretch reflex.

The spindle may be described as a group of specialized intrafusal (or encapsulated) muscle fibres, the spindle being built around 3 to 12 intrafusal fibres. Within the centre of these are at least two types of sensory receptors, primary or secondary endings which are sensitive to measurement of length and velocity of stretch in a muscle. Other equivalent sensory organs include the Golgi tendon organs and bare nerve endings or intrafusal fibres activated by gamma motor neurones.

The reflex is of two types: phasic and ionic. The phasic monosynaptic type is triggered by synchronous discharge of primary spindle afferents. In other words, a phasic response is thereby excited by neurones innervating motor units of that muscle and its synergists, with concurrent inhibition of antagonists: a pattern of so-called *reciprocal innervation*. This thus serves to activate extensor and axial muscles sustaining stabilization of the trunk and limbs whilst counteracting the force of gravity to sustain the upright posture. The spindles are especially numerous in muscles exercising fine control, e.g. the intrinsic muscles of the hand.

Contributing to this function is the *static* or *tonic stretch reflex* initiated by change in the length of muscle, activity which is involved in clinical tone. When muscle is *passively* stretched, intrafusal fibres are also stretched and the spindle sensory discharge is enhanced. When a spastic muscle is stretched beyond a specific length, the enhanced tone abruptly gives way: the "clasp-knife" response. This is ascribed to Group II spindle efferents evoking a length dependent inhibition of the stretch reflex. Section of the dorsal root is designed to interrupt both the afferent limb of the tonic stretch reflex and the phasic stretch reflex to effect a dramatic reduction in muscle tone.

But the generation of *active muscle power* is a phasic component, comprising more than a continuous synchronous discharge of gamma motor neurones. 1a afferents appear to have an increased rate of discharge even when muscle shortens during contraction. A clear implication is that in the synchronous activation of gamma and alpha neurones during voluntary movement, spindle firing is maintained by alpha-gamma co-activation. It has recently been confirmed by Murphy and Martin (1993) that the nervous system must modulate the independent contraction of intrafusal and extrafusal fibres. This is attained by adaptational adjustments of the balance between activation of static and dynamic gamma motor neurones.

Muscle tone has two connotations: firstly clinical and secondly, physiological. The first goes back a century to the definition of Foster emphasizing the examiner's *feeling* of resistance when passively moving segments of limbs or trunk in a resting state. *Passive muscle power* and *muscle tone* are used interchangeably in assessing the degree of passive resistance to movement.

Evidence for its physiological basis swings between *myogenic* or *neurogenic* sources. The former begins with the acceptance of a slight but sustained

contracture especially within anti-gravity muscles. A continuous *input* of efferent impulses is matched by a constant return of afferent impulses from the stretch receptors of the muscle spindles. This enhanced muscle tone would be due primarily to increased gamma activation, basically to increased sensitivity of muscle spindles to the stretch of anti-gravity muscles. In turn, the gamma neurones are susceptible to regulation by the supraspinal systems already referred to, reticulo, vestibulo and cerebello-spinal, operating ultimately via interneurones, excitatory and inhibitory. So that the cerebellar facilitation of extensor tone is mediated through communication between the spino-cerebellar and lateral vestibular tract as well as with the reticular nuclei of the brainstem.

*The active component of muscle power* as distinct from passive muscle power or tone is evaluated in the infant in two ways, first gauging *activity* or spontaneous movement, secondly *reactivity* or the infantile reactions. Firstly, the degree of vigour expressed in spontaneous arm and leg movement, fluently alternating between flexion and extension. A sick preterm is characterized by a frog-like position and paucity of movement. As well as being weakly expressed, there is a lack of variation in speech and amplitude subsequently becoming more rigid with the limbs held mainly in extension. The second approach is to gauge the reaction to a particular test demanding and measuring an ability to adjust in posture and movement. The traction test is a good example, with the initial reaction being flexion of the arms at the elbow.

This is typically absent in the sick or preterm infant whilst being pulled to a sitting position. Arms remain fully extended without co-contraction of the shoulder girdle.

*Hyperactive Stretch Reflexes and Clonus*

Upper motor neurone damage leads to hyperactive tonic stretch reflexes, which in turn leads to an increase in the resistance to passive movement which is termed spasticity. Underlying this is a highly sensitive state of the alpha-motor neurones to synchronous afferent volley. If constant stretch is first applied, a sudden additional stretch or tendon tap may then elicit the repetitive jerking of *clonus*. This classically reflects a lesion of the upper motor neurone, typically alongside hyperactive stretch reflexes and bilaterally positive Babinski. In contrast, however, both flexion reflexes leading to abdominal wall or cremasteric contractions elicited by cutaneous stimulation are eliminated by the same level of lesion.

In spastic diplegia, a crossed adductor response is often spontaneous when the knee jerk is elicited, the opposite thigh adducting reflexly.

*Clonus* is apparently the result of hyperactive stretch reflexes re-exciting themselves. Whether sustained or unsustained (only one or two beats), it is most likely to be elicitable when ankle jerks are tested. Although a known product of an upper motor neurone lesion, it may arise spontaneously, or metabolically in response to hyperammonaemia, or be elicitable even when the tendon jerk is unobtainable during anaesthesia, general or spinal. Likewise, it may appear spontaneously in hepatic failure, then in association with hyperactive reflexes and extensor hypertonus, with the underlying metabolic impact of hyperammonaemia probably a common factor shared with similar findings I have observed in congenital hyperammonaemia, or Reye's syndrome.

*Reversal or Reduction of Hypertonicity by Vibration*

It was claimed by Walsh (1992) that the application to the forearms of a vibrator run at twice the mains frequency in order to treat stiffness or relieve muscle pains, quickly reduced muscle tone measured at the wrist. Lower frequencies proved to be even more effective.

In addition to direct effects upon the contractile properties of muscle and upon spinal excitation, presynaptic inhibition may be decreased possibly as a significant source of tone and spasticity. Such vibration can also inhibit the H-reflex as well as selectively reducing tendon jerks (i.e. except for the jaw jerks), so that the overall response appears to depend upon the balance between these processes (Whitlock, 1990).

According to Burke (1988), however, an underlying imbalance between excitation and inhibition of the *alpha* motor neurone stems directly from *a loss of inhibitory input*, possibly through neuronal changes subsequent to an upper motor neurone lesion. Descending tracts from suprasegmentary sources, reticulo, vestibulo and rubrospinal, coordinate *alpha* cell activity and inhibit *gamma* anterior horn cells. Vital complementary control is also exercised by what is sometimes known as the first control circuit, the cerebellum, and by the second control circuit, the basal ganglia, the functions of which are more fully discussed elsewhere (Chapter 4). It is believed to be concerned primarily with *learned* automatic behaviour and with the preparation and maintenance of *background support or posture* for motor activity. The afferent neurone from the muscle spindle influences segments above and below its spinal cord segment to maintain a precise agonist-antagonist balance *reflected in optimal tone and posture.* In cerebral palsy, it is believed that inhibition is reduced because of damage to descending tracts with excessive x-activity evoking spasticity. Decreasing facilitation or increasing inhibition could then relieve the spasticity. When spasticity is the major factor interfering with independent function or daily care of the child, it is the post-operative experience of Peacock and Arens (Arens et al., 1989; Peacock and Standt, 1991) that neuro-surgical section of the afferents or posterior nerve rootlets bilaterally from L2 to S1 which have shown an abnormal response to stimulation (tetanic muscle contracting at 50 stimuli per second and diffusion of contractor muscle groups) has produced dramatic reduction of the hypertonus. Although these results have excited controversy, Peacock and Standt (1991) has convincingly postulated that by confining division of the sensory nerve rootlets to those demonstratively related to the hyperactive muscle responses, the facilitatory input to the alpha motor neurone is reduced. The functional improvement thereby accomplished is also conceived to be dependent upon the degree of strength and motor control innately possessed by the child.

Basic "release" from gamma inhibition, even though mediated through *release from inhibition* of a *facilitatory integration in the reticular system,* has become perhaps a more precise hypothesis. Indeed, acknowledging the *dual system* of innervation of muscle via alpha and gamma systems, spasticity may be visualized as a response to release of the gamma system from higher inhibitory control. This may stem mainly from the *basal ganglia motor system,* and its loop circuitry with the sensorimotor cortex. Alternatively, it may be visualized as a *'withdrawal' of inhibitory control of the facilitatory integration* within the *reticular substance* of the brain stem acting upon the gamma system. The Bobaths went on to postulate that this evoked the "release" of, or as expressed differently in *an abnormal persistence of,* a number of abnormal postural reflexes (tonic or static reflexes), with variable interaction underlying varying patterns of spasticity.

The more recent consensus of evidence agrees that the major suprasegmental or supraspinal reinforcement of the motor neurones controlling *posture,* and indirectly of *tone,* stems from the projection systems originating in the *reticular formation* but in communication with *vestibular nuclei.* These Group A descending pathways effect coordination of extensor/flexor "balance" via consistent but contrasting motor events: on the one hand activating extensor muscular responses, and on the other inhibiting flexor activity. Indeed this function has been *more specifically attributed to the excitatory dorsolateral reticular formation* extending from the midbrain through the rostral medulla. Its activity evokes excitation of extensor motor neurones but inhibition of flexor motor neurones which are expressed as postural tone, with terminals mainly focused on the gamma motor neurone. Conversely, *loss of excitatory input to the gamma motor neurones* which innervate the muscle spindles leads to *reduction in muscle tone* and flaccidity, or distinctive hypotonia.

It is postulated furthermore that these systems are normally in balanced control via cortico-reticular pathways, as expressed through inhibition of extensor muscle contraction and facilitation of flexor activation. Cerebral damage could thus interfere with such cortical controls so that unchecked pontine-medullary pathways would induce hyperexcitability of the extensor motor neurones to make spasticity or hypertonicity clinically manifest.

The coordinated contraction of many muscles or their automatic activities involved in normal motor function, for instance in the maintenance of the erect posture in sitting or standing, is mediated through indirect pathways. In addition to the major extrapyramidal pathways already touched upon, the cerebellum also plays a major role in the coordination and correction of movement errors. In particular, this is influenced by the paravermal cortex of the cerebellum

which mediates facilitation of *extensor tone*, whilst its vermal cortex subserves the same facilitatory function in respect of *flexor muscle tone*. More recent evidence (Holstege, 1991) invokes *monoaminergic innervation from the lateral Limbic motor system* as a significant factor in the modulation of behavioural or motivational states.

The supraspinal control of both active and passive muscle power is exercised through medial and lateral brainstem pathways. Medial pathways end on interneurones and proprioneurones in the ventromedial part of the intermediate zone of the cord which innervate axial and *proximal* muscles and subserve the maintenance of posture necessary for differentiated movements under the control of motor cortex. The reticulospinal tracts (medial and lateral) with both *excitatory* and *inhibitory* connections with spinal interneurones and motor neurones are vital for the maintenance of muscle tone in the anti-gravity muscles. Similarly, medial and lateral vestibulospinal tracts deriving from vestibular nuclei maintain *control of balance and posture*, influenced by signals from the vestibular labyrinth. The *tectospinal tract*, originating in the superior colliculus has an important role in the coordination of head and eye movements.

But the main lateral descending pathway remains the corticospinal tract. Via arcuate fibres it reaches the internal capsule, thence to the ventral pons and medulla, to form the medullary pyramids. After pyramidal decussation in the medulla, the fibres cross the midline to descend in the dorsolateral column as *lateral* corticospinal tracts. This is especially concerned with *fine finger movements* required for manipulation. The *ventral* corticospinal tract transmits projections to motor neurones in the ventromedial column innervating axial and proximal muscles.

Distal muscles required for movements of reaching out and manipulation are in the mammal under the control of the rubrospinal tracts. But in man, these functions appear to have been assumed by the phylogenetically newer corticospinal tract.

So that the passive component of muscle power or muscle tone is sustained by *facilitating influences* via reticulospinal and vestibulospinal pathways whilst active muscle power reflects the maturation of cortical control. Damage to the corticospinal tract particularly where it fans out into the internal capsule can lead to intensifying passive muscle power, and hence spasticity. This is apparently the result of lost cortical connections with inhibitory interneurones that normally suppress the excitatory input of the 1a affarents to the motor neurones.

Active and passive muscle power should be in optimal balance. When the active component affecting axial and proximal muscles exceeds the passive, as may occur in the preterm, the posture and mobility of the infant is modified inducing hyperextension of the neck and back muscles, forcing the infant to lie on one side with persistence of infantile motor asymmetrics and interference with the maturation of sitting. This is probably the basis of the more or less transient disturbance of tone first described by Drillien (1972).

## B. A Biochemical/Metabolic Basis of Muscle Activity

Discovery of the vital role of the Calcium ion in the contractile system of vertebrate striated muscle has led to the finding of a third factor in addition to *actin* and *myosin*, the so-called "regulatory proteins" comprising tropomyosin and a new protein, troponin. Intracellular dependence of the calcium was later traced from phosphorylase to kinase and phosphodiesterase and thence to definition of the modulator protein: "calmodulin" by Kachiochi. The principal function of the troponin appears to be to repress the fundamental process of *actin-myosin-ATP* interaction by influencing the actine filament through tropomyosin. The concept has since evolved that the troponin-tropomyosin system is responsible solely for regulatory function.

Other regulatory proteins, leiotonin A and C, a new calcium-binding protein, are involved in the activation of the myosin-actin-ATP interaction in the presence of Ca ion - in contrast with troponin which represses this interaction in the absence of Ca ion. It can moreover fully activate this contractile system in which it is incorporated together with myosin, actin and tropomyosin, at a molar ratio of about one-hundredth of actin.

An even more fundamental role of the filaments themselves - so basic to muscle function - is also crucially influenced by enzymatic processes. So that minute proportions of ß-actinin, a factor inhibiting the network formation of actin filaments, can swiftly abolish the structural viscosity of actin filaments. And gelsolin, a new factor isolated from macrophages is maximally effective in inhibiting the gelation of actin filaments at a ratio of less than one hundredth to actin. The intimate correlationship of these intracellular metabolic processes, linked to extracellular influences of potassium as well as calcium ion, on the fundamental contractile system of muscle on the one hand, and upon the cerebro-spinal complex of neurogenic control on the other hand, remains a challenging field of future research in

respect of the patho-physiology of anomalies of muscle tone, movement and overall postural balance.

In explaining the phenomenon of *passive muscle "power" or tone* the neurophysiological mechanisms already mentioned are not necessarily the whole story. For instance, a complex interaction between the *visco-elastic properties* of skeletal muscle and their reactions to stress. Likewise, as emphasized in Chapter 4, on "Hypermobility as a component of so-called hypotonia", phenomena peculiar to connective tissue and ligaments also condition resistance against stretch and movement.

# CHOREA, OR CHOREIFORM MOVEMENTS

This refers to the random, almost continuous, occurrence of rapid irregularly jerky involuntary movements of major joints, trunk and face, which are abrupt, and purposeless, and typically brief and unsustained, without significant change in tone. The movements appear spontaneously and whenever the arms are extended. When held above the head, they move into pronation.

These fragments of purposive movement succeeding one another in disorderly fashion are associated with "*motor impersistence*", contraction being unsustained as classically demonstrated by the inability to keep the irregularly fluctuating tongue protruded without being gripped firmly between the teeth, or by an unsustained and fluctuant "milk-

maid" grip. The involuntary movements render voluntary movement ataxic. Another manifestation of a choreiform character may be an expression of endocrine or neuro-endocrine disorder as in childhood hyperthyroidism or the hypoadrenocorticism of Addison's disease. In terms of newer concepts of neurotransmitter control, chorea is basically ascribed to overactivity of dopaminergic neurones.

Particularly large amplitude movements of a flinging or flailing character are known as ballistic. Such movements may be partially suppressed or "concealed" by incorporating them into semi-purposeful movements known as parakinesia. Ballistic movements are often unilateral, and have been attributed to a

155

lesion of the contralateral subthalamic nucleus (Corpus Luysii), or to multiple small infarcts in the contralateral striatum.

The character and distribution of the movements differ according to their source. When congenital they often merge with athetosis. In the persistent chorea of Huntington, they remain predominantly distal for many years, even assuming a resemblance to a coarse static tremor.

A transitory or acquired subacute choreiform disorder characterizes Sydenham's Chorea associated with rheumatic fever, is not infrequently complicated by true rheumatic carditis. It is thus part of a post-streptococcal immunological syndrome wherein antibodies of protein structure to streptococcal antigens are akin to proteins within the membranes of striatal and other basal ganglia neurones. So that antibodies to these antigens are believed to evoke choreiform movements by also attacking basal ganglia neurones, especially of caudate and subthalamic nuclei.

# ATHETOSIS

These are also irregular continuous involuntary movements which are slower, coarser and more writhing and "snake-like", recurring around the long axis of a limb. Although most often appendicular, it may also affect the axial musculature including the neck, apart from the face and tongue and have been attributed to release of alternating grasp and avoidance reactions resulting from cortico-striatal fibre degeneration. In terms of tone, a "lead-pipe" type of increase in tone may be associated in later childhood. Choreo-athetosis has sometimes been regarded as a form of chorea which may even be responsive to anti-choreic therapy. It is better nonetheless to distinguish chorea and athetosis as two forms of movement which are nevertheless sometimes conjoined or interwoven.

## Further Neurophysiological and Other Aspects of Athetoid Manifestation

Although this CP entity is dominated by the positive symptom of involuntary irregular and arrhythmic movement, there is a tendency for most voluntary movements to be destroyed in advance by contrary movement. Indeed, the normal shadowing of a voluntary act by its opposite voluntary act, in the nature of balancing a controlling function, is grossly disturbed and "out of phase" in the athetoid. Any defect of postural reaction is shared with some impairment of postural fixation of the trunk and with some general movement and early attempts at locomotion especially directed at such defects of postural fixation lacking fixity of the trunk. Despite the profusion of such movement there is relative immobility, with protracted delay in locomotion except perhaps by wriggling and rolling.

The dyskinesia affects almost all muscles including respiratory, but is mostly evident in face, tongue, neck and arms. Absent in early infancy when hypotonia and defective postural reactions predominate, the arrhythmic movement tend to be confined to toes and fingers.

The movements may be absent in repose or when attention is deeply held, but are provoked or accentuated by a sense of insecurity, by emotion, startle response, or wish to perform a voluntary act such as feeding. Violent throwing, even ballistic-type movements of the body, may prevent voluntary action. Attempts to bring the child to a standing position is often characteristically interrupted by a sudden collapse of the trunk or hips ("jack-knife"). Holding the legs firmly in extension, avoiding flexion, may avert this response.

Overactivity of the tonic neck and labyrinthine reflexes may be associated. *Visual* avoiding reactions are also typical elements of their pattern of movement, the head and eyes being often averted from the desired object. Similar *tactile avoiding reactions* affecting the feet are also characteristic - and when exaggerated have been labelled the "athetoid dance".

Although the most severe form may be attended by the absence of speech, the "sparing" of the cortex by the predominant localization of pathology to the motor ganglia or striatum in particular, cognitive development may be normal even high.

Conventional patho-physiological explanation has glibly referred to disinhibition of fairly primitive reflexes linked to a failure of cortical or higher entities to gain control of, or to assimilate, the "basic movement pattern". These have been termed release phenomena, which in this instance have been confined to dyskinesia and overactivity of primitive brain stem reflexes. Their gradual emergence during the second half of the second year is in part explained by the completion by then of myelinogenetic development of these pathways, and / or the maturation and uninhibited activation of striatal-related basal ganglia (caudate and putamen).

On the other hand, there have been great advances in our understanding of the vital potential of neurotransmitter balance in dyskinetic disorders. Certainly the concept of chemical neuro-transmission, involving the synaptic release of a transmitter from axonal terminals, has long been firmly accepted, and major transmitters identified. The concept of neurotransmission at axo-neuronal junctions also encompasses the synthesis and storage of a transmitter within presynaptic elements. Release is through a calcium-dependent process initiated by depolarization, and thence by interaction with postsynaptic receptors or recognition sites - so triggering a transient alteration in the permeability of the membrane to certain ions. Modification in membrane excitability, important in modulating neuronal excitability, may possibly involve the participation of cyclic nucleotides as second messengers.

Changes in neuronal excitability may depend rather upon diffuse release of particular neurotransmitters with influence upon intracellular metabolic processes. These may be especially relevant to specific CNS changes induced in various progressive metabolic disorders to be subsequently outlined rather than the control of membraneous ionophores. Hence the term *neuro-modulator* may be more apt than neurotransmitter (Kupferman, 1979).

The activating role of acetylcholine, and its elimination by cholinesterase, is well established as central to the physiological balance within the motor unit which is the physiological core of reflex and voluntary contraction. We have also witnessed the dramatic benefits of l-dopa in Parkinsonism which have followed identification of dopamine (3-hydroxy tyramine) and its conversion properties, as a *nigro-striatal* transmitter. But GABA - gamma aminobutyric acid - appears to be the most important *central inhibitory transmitter* since *gabergic interneurones* occur at all levels of the

brain and cord. It has been shown that *gabergic synaptic inhibition* is blocked by Bicuculline and Picrotoxinin.

One of the most important advances in this field has been the exploration of immunohistochemical methods in the localization within nerve terminals of glutamic acid decarboxylase, the enzyme responsible for the synthesis of GABA from glutamate. The decarboxylic acids, *aspartic* and *glutamic*, excite all central neurones. It s possible that since the prime function of the brain is information transfer, processing and storage, the metabolism of these excitatory amino acids is concerned predominantly with their functions as excitatory transmitters. It is likely moreover, that the major excitatory pathways including long, ascending and descending tracts are glutamergic or aspartergic.

But the application of direct studies of GAD and its GABA neurotransmitter product after imposing prolonged neuroleptic damage upon basal ganglia with consequent dyskinesia, has produced the most exciting clues to their possible role in movement disorder possibly akin to that in cerebral palsy.

## Role of GABA, etc., in Basal Ganglia Function
### especially of
### Caudate, Putamen and Subthalamic Nuclei

Pathology of the striatum, comprising the integration of Caudate nucleus and Putamen can be considered as a recurrent theme in several long-term movement disorders. In Huntington's Chorea, for

example, atrophic changes in the head of the Caudate nucleus has been well demonstrated by nuclear magnetic resonance imaging (Byddel and Steiner, 1982). Atrophy is recognizable against a detailed anatomical background, both medial and lateral margins of the head of this nucleus being clearly definable. Pathological changes connected to excessive organelle accumulation of copper are instead concentrated within the lenticular nucleus and thalamus in Wilson's disease. These have been pinpointed more accurately by NMR imaging than with CT. Likewise, there has been a recent important MRI exposure of localization of basal ganglia pathology by Yokochi et al. (1991). In 6 of 22 children with athetotic CP, symmetrical high intensity areas were found in both the thalamus and putamen. In another 5, they were defined only in the thalamus, and in 1 solely in the putamen. More discrete MRI localization to the putamen was attained by the Lily Dubowitz team (Rutherford et al., 1992) of symmetrical bilateral cystic lesions in the posterior putamen in all three cases of athetoid CP following upon hypoxic-ischaemic encephalopathy. Their athetosis was already manifest within the first year of life.

It is a challenging thought that the ingenious demonstration in adult *tardive dyskinesia* (TD) through actual brain tissue "punchings" of basal ganglia, (Fig. 5) of significant enzymatic as distinct from histological changes within the caudate nucleus or the medial segment of the globus pallidus, subthalamic nucleus and substantia nigra and other basal ganglia components following neuroleptic therapy (de Long et al., 1985), may not be so far removed from the pathogenesis of dyskinetic CP in infancy and childhood. Clinically, the main involuntary

movement is in the oro-facial region, although there is also choreoathetoid movement. In CP of prenatal origin, there appears to be a closely analogous localization of cerebral pathology; for example the involvement of the head of the caudate nucleus, and/or the Putamen, in subependymal/germinal matrix bleeds.

The *Dopamine supersensitivity hypothesis* in tardive dyskinesia (TD) postulates that the neuroleptic impact is upon dopamine receptors of the basal ganglia. An enzyme significantly influenced would be *glutamate decarboxylase* (GAD), the GABA synthesizing enzyme, which would be thereby reduced. Studies in the Caudate nucleus of the cebus apella monkey including autopsy assays after chronic neuroleptic dosage (Anderson et al., 1989), have in fact confirmed a *marked decrease in GAD* after neuroleptic therapy. An alternative theory therefore involves changes in the GABA system, with TD as the outcome of neuroleptically-induced destruction of subsections of GABA-containing neurones in the basal ganglia. Whichever theory is relevant, it is significant in relation to the foetal or infantile situation that factors closely relevant to CP such as *anoxia* and *reduced cerebral blood flow in particular, adversely* influence this same enzyme (GAD) which is responsible for the synthesis of GABA from glutamate. One of the most important advances in this area has been the development of immunohistochemical methods for the localization of GAD within nerve terminals. Because of direct connections with both the substantia nigra and globus pallidus, the subthalamic nucleus has also been considered of

# Distribution of basal ganglia punchings in typical horizontal section of human brain

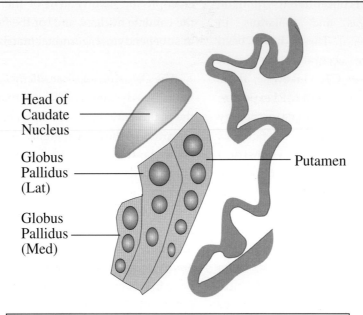

Head of Caudate Nucleus

Globus Pallidus (Lat)

Globus Pallidus (Med)

Putamen

**Gaba Sources in Dyskinesia Tardive**

especial import in regulating the neurotransmitter output of these areas. The depressed GAD-levels may of course be more closely related to the dyskinesia than the long term neuroleptic treatment per se. Therefore *reduced GABA function stemming from reduced GAD activity in* the subthalamic nucleus - as well as striatum - may also be a significant factor underlying the dyskinesia of CP.

Lesions of the caudate nucleus in primates, including man, have been shown to induce *ballistic movements* of the extremities. And even in autopsies of the brain in Huntington's chorea, there was a significant loss of neurones and volume within the subthalamic nucleus (Crossman et al., 1984), as distinct from the atrophic changes in the head of the caudate nucleus already mentioned (Byddel and Steiner, 1982). Conversely, microinfusions of GABA antagonists into the subthalamic nucleus of monkeys produced dyskinetic ballistic movements comparable to those following upon the lesions studied. It appears, therefore, that GABA innervation of the subthalamic nucleus appears to be critical (Lange et al., 1976). In this context, one should keep in mind the frequent sites of cerebral haemorrhage in the preterm. Arising from the subependymal/germinal matrix, it frequently involves the region of the head of the caudate nucleus, or caudothalamic notch, which is also associated with the recently recognized entity of thalamic haemorrhage (Trounce et al., 1985).

Experimental studies in the ape, say of the effects of restoring GABA to striatum or subthalamic nucleus by *microinfusion* or otherwise may provide promising therapeutic leads in overcoming the CP forms of choreo-athetosis (Fig. 5)

Another promising, albeit delicate, avenue for allied experimental study is the development of *microelectrophoretic methods* - using fine glass micro-electrodes for insertion into single neurones - also lends itself to the direct exploration of mechanisms of synaptic excitation and inhibition at a cellular level.

In infants and children, the neuropathology has been linked in bilirubin encephalopathy (or kernicterus) and post-asphyxial encephalopathy (Volpe, 1987) to the chronic scarring of the basal ganglia known as status marmoratus. Like hemi-ballismus, hemi-athetosis may occur, and in the adult post-hemiplegic hemi-athetosis, it has been specifically identified with lesions of the putamen segment of the striatum (Dooling and Adams, 1975). The pathology in choreo-athetosis is certainly predominantly localized to the basal ganglia rather than cerebral cortex so that intelligence may be preserved. Athetosis is therefore often a pure disorder of motility, with the intellect spared, although speech defects, especially dysarthria, may be associated.

# EARLY DIAGNOSTIC IDENTIFICATION OF ATAXIA AND THE DYSEQUILIBRIUM SYNDROME

Ataxia refers to both incoordination of movement and disturbance of balance which may be primarily truncal or limited to the limbs.

In addition to the more generalized manifestations of incoordination in hand movements and reaching out we shall discuss later, the infant's posture is especially studied, noting the position or attitude of the body when standing (i.e. his "station"), or when recumbent forwards or backwards. Truncal ataxia is

characterized by unsteadiness on sitting or standing, being attributed primarily to involvement of the cerebellar vermis (Fig 6). Whilst ease of performance, and the presence of abnormal associated movements are essential detail in testing, indications of undoubted clumsiness or unequivocal unsteadiness are of primary importance. The child is persuaded to straighten up, extend his arms palms down and place his feet together. Beyond 18 months or so, the ataxic child will separate his feet to achieve the wide base

# CEREBELLUM
## as viewed from its dorsal surface

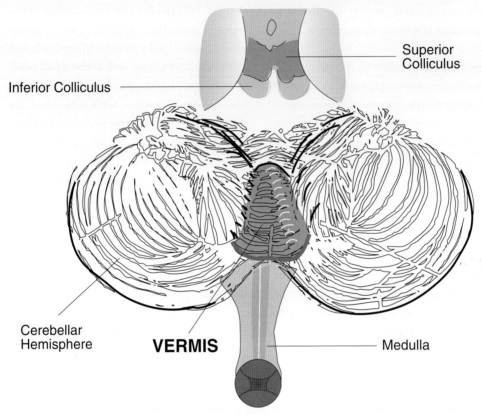

Superior Colliculus

Inferior Colliculus

Cerebellar Hemisphere

**VERMIS**

Medulla

he needs to balance. Whilst counting to 10 in the older child, look for a tendency to sway or fall in a consistent direction. Repeat with his eyes closed, which mildly accentuates swaying in cerebellar ataxia, or much more so in sensory ataxia. Vestibular ataxia, ascribed to bilateral labyrinthine disease, is also augmented when the eyes are closed.

The child may also be persuaded to stand on one foot, then the other, for 10 seconds on each... Then, if ataxia is mild or subtle, it may be justifiable to encourage the child to walk along a line marked on the floor for at least 2.5 metres putting the heel of one foot in front of the toes of the other, and then to even walk backwards along the same line. Next, to hop a short distance forward on one foot, and to hop back on the other.

Ongoing observation of the child's spontaneous activity is always worthwhile, especially when reaching out towards and playing with a toy, or retrieving a ball. Incoordination may then be clearly exposed, often in association with intention tremor. His ability to stand with his feet together thus becomes important. Likewise, whether he can walk in tandem fashion, or turn quickly?

Coordination and balance is furthermore tested in the older child by the classical tests: heel to shin or knee or toe, or upraised finger to nose or his father's nose. Self facilitation in fixing the position of one hand on one side of his body to attain stability will tend to make his basic ataxia less conspicuous. Once walking is achieved in sensory or cerebellar ataxia, the child tends to keep his eyes fixed on the floor. Later, the heel would be brought down to the floor first and then a slapping contact of toes. In the presence of an unilateral lesion, say of the cerebellum, forward progress on the affected side takes longer and there is a tendency to sway towards that side. When, for example, a cerebellar tumour is in the right cerebellar hemisphere, a few steps alternately forward and backward leads to a slow drift to the right. Where the cerebellar lesion is midline, especially a medulloblastoma, the child tends to fall.

An *ataxic gait* embodies jerky unsteadiness, staggering irregularly to either side or swaying forwards or backwards, and the wide base adopted to improve the imbalance and often vainly to overcome it. *Truncal tremor* may be associated.

Ataxia may occur in isolation, although all forms of CP, spastic, dyskinetic or hypotonic, may have an ataxic component. It may be, however, an ominous harbinger of an insidiously progressive disorder such as Friedreich's ataxia, if not of a much more acutely progressive metabolic disorder.

Ataxia therefore comprises an irregular unsteadiness involving incoordination of all movement, and eventually of gait. The unsteadiness prevails despite the wide base adopted to improve balance. When confined to standing posture, its instability is defined as not attributable to muscular weakness. In this context it can be aptly described as a disorder or decomposition of movement stemming from a breakdown of the normal coordinated implementation of a voluntary movement. *Motor ataxia* is summed up as a failure to produce normally smooth coordinated motor acts, including interference with fine finger manipulation. In the absence or interruption of tactile or proprioceptive stimuli, the term *Sensory Ataxia* is applied, and is accentuated by closing the eyes, cutting off visual control, when proprioceptive input is sufficient for stability to be sustained. This is reflected in the Romberg sign, when the standing child is unsteady with eyes closed but not when open. Even in cerebellar ataxia this may produce slight accentuation. In other words, unless the patient can effectively monitor movement of his limbs and voluntarily correct their errors, he will stagger, stumble and fall.

# The Ataxic Pattern Characterizing the Dysequilibrium Syndrome

This is often claimed to be a distinguishable variant (Hagberg et al., 1974), with less involuntary movement of the limbs but more unsteadiness than is usually found in ataxic CP. Not only is there a failure to develop postural control, and an inability to maintain equilibrium when standing, falling fails to excite compensatory mechanisms. This ataxic pattern is also encountered in the Marinesco-Sjogren syndrome where allowance should be made for more or less severe visual impairment derived from the associated cataracts.

Such exaggerated imbalance implies a lack of awareness of the body's relationships, and of a tendency to fall, especially from the standing position, with a lack of compensatory or defensive reaction, especially involving the flocculonodular lobe, and its important connections with the vestibular nuclei. In terms of cerebellar signs, there is a chronology which is related to the archicerebellum developing early prenatally, and in connection with vestibular structures.

There are transitional forms between dysequilibrium and ataxia in which classical symptoms of ataxia are present and are probably due to involvement of structures developing later (oreocerebellar structures). In the typical form of dysequilibrium, "titubation" or gross tremor of the trunk is very common. Clinically it is identical with the jerky truncal tremor/ataxia/apraxia of Rett syndrome. In some instances of dysequilibrium, delay in language development and perceptual disorders are prominent.

# Patho-Physiology of Ataxia

Throughout child development, a special feature of cerebellar function is the capacity to produce compensatory mechanisms which may be attributable to the cerebellum acting as a servo-mechanism for the control of numerous other structures to which it is connected. Yet the underlying pathology may involve diffuse damage to peripheral nerves or posterior funiculi or bilateral lesions affecting the primary sensory neurones in the pathways from nucleus gracilis, nucleus cuneatus, medial lemniscus and thalamus to postcentral gyrus. This leads clinically to defects in joint position sense, involving Golgi tendon receptors, as well as the sensory receptors in muscle, mainly within muscle spindles. This may constitute the basis of the hypothetical Dysequilibrium Syndrome. Some of the proprioceptive fibres from muscle spindles course directly through dorsal grey matter into the ventral grey horn. These different fibres of the two-neurone muscle reflex arc synapsed in the anterior horn cells to constitute the anatomic basis for the muscle stretch (deep tendon) reflexes, classic examples of a local segmental reflex. Whether such abnormalities are solely due to pathological involvement of these pathways or is associated instead with unconscious proprioceptive spino-cerebellar pathways, still remains for objective elucidation. Spino-cerebellar axons end almost exclusively in *the vermis* where they are distributed within two distinct areas: the anterior and posterior target zones. All spinal fibres terminate in mossy fibres in the *granular layer*. A recent clinical expression of pathology therein, with atrophy confined to the vermis (Fig 6) was clearly illustrated on CT scanning in an autosomal recessive form of cerebellar ataxia (Russell and Lingam, 1992).

*Ataxia* in individual limb motions results in irregular misdirected or uncoordinated movements which tends to be aggravated as the target is approached, which it misses "pass-points" or overshoots more or less widely. Such under- or overshooting seen in testing eye-hand coordination, typically reflects *cerebellar* involvement. Adiadokinesia is usually a concurrent manifestation with distortion of normally smooth rhythmic sequence of fingers or hand when carrying out rapid alternating movements. The inability to recognize limb or joint position may be included in the agnosia, with astereognosis more specifically referring to loss of two-point discrimination (with respect to size, shape and texture of an object held in the hand) apart from diminished vibration sense. When due to cerebellar disease, asynergia

is often attended by dysmetria (errors in measuring distance), rebound - marked by failure to inhibit a muscular action, such as when the flexed arm is suddenly released - and sometimes by intention tremor. Hypotonia is typically associated with the asynergia.

Tonic *Cerebellar Ataxia* is the source of *asynergia* - with which hypotonia is typically associated - often attended by dysmetria, and sometimes by *intention tremor, unaffected by visual attention, and characteristically the result of abnormalities of the cerebellar hemispheres..* Nystagmus may co-exist, and/or esotropia. The nystagmus may indeed be the first sign, especially from 3 months onwards, to alert one to suspect oncoming ataxia. This is characterized by marked unsteadiness of head, trunk and limbs, especially in sitting, standing or walking, and is accompanied by dysarthria, or disturbance in articulation, and sometimes by dysphagia, with slowness and difficulty in swallowing.

The flocculo-nodular lobe modulates equilibration and the orientation of head and neck. There are, in fact, important connections between the *flocculo-nodular lobe* and the vestibular nuclei. Lesions thereof produce a characteristic syndrome embodying an inability to stand or even sit without swaying or falling - as extreme expressions of truncal ataxia. This is associated moreover with abnormal head and eye movement including nystagmus. *Anterior lobe* pathology is mainly seen, however, in degenerative disorders of the adult, evoking disturbance in posture, gait and marked truncal hypotonia. Gait ataxia, with unsteady walking and staggering is especially severe, although only mild ataxia of the upper limbs is exhibited in response to testing. *Posterior lobe* function, especially of the large lateral hemispheres, provide a principal servomechanism for coordination of skilled action. Pathology thereof, or rather cerebellar hemisphere disease, leads to limb ataxia ipsilateral to the side of the lesion with irregular movement, loss of muscle coordination (dyssynergia) and loss of ability to measure the range of motion (dysmetonia). Intention tremor is associated, and in general, movements become clumsy and conspicuously uncoordinated.

The cerebellum and its connections comprise the second major control circuit, concerned with the coordination of muscle groups during phasic motor activity, designed to modulate motor activities involved in equilibration, posture, gait and voluntary movements. It especially controls or regulates skilled movement in conjunction with motor regulation by the ganglia motor system. It depends secondarily on cerebellar inputs from proprioceptive, somatic, vestibular, visual and auditory sense organs, whilst cerebellar and striatal outputs interact before reaching the brain stem and motor cortex via relays in ventrolateral or thalamic nuclei.

Complex connections between deep cerebellar neurones via the cerebellar-tectal projection and cells in the region of the superior colliculus (linked to basal ganglia influences via the nigro-tectal pathway) appear to be closely involved. Three fundamental loops have been delineated as the basis of the main cerebellar pathways:

1 *The first via the Dentate Nucleus to the opposite Red Nucleus* and thalamus, thence to the cortex. This loop is completed by axons from the frontal lobe via the internal capsule and cerebral peduncle to the Pontine nuclei which send axons across the midline (via the middle cerebellar peduncle) back into the cerebellum.

2 *Also from Dentate Nucleus to the opposite Red Nucleus* but is completed via the inferior olive which projects back into the inferior cerebellar peduncle. This loop is postulated as coordinating extra-pyramidal with cerebellar functions.

3. This highly specialized *loop connects with ipsilateral Vestibular Nuclei.*

Especially when the vermis is also involved as in the cerebellar hemisphere syndrome, an ataxic dysarthria also results. A random breakdown in articulation is accompanied by irregularities in pitch, loudness and rhythm, and by slowing of speech together with an unusually excessive stress on some syllables or words.

# CONGENITAL HEMIPLEGIA

An unilateral upper motor neurone with corresponding involvement and paresis of the extremities and relative sparing of contralateral limbs, the upper extremities being nearly always affected to a greater extent than lower. Paucity of movement of the often tight-fisted hand may be observed first. But asymmetric responses are especially characteristic, although parents may not appreciate such asymmetry of hand function until 3 to 6 months of age. Perhaps the earliest such manifestation that could be elicited would be an unilateral Moro reflex. Asymmetry of the placing reaction could emerge next... Katona induces unstable movement, akin to a swimming-like motion, as an initial step in his CP diagnostic procedure, when he raises one end of the miniature ramp upon which he places an infant of several weeks of age.

A *difference in reciprocal kicking* may be noted when baby is bathed. *When pulled up to sit* on the traction test, from say 4 months onwards, there is *extension of the hemiplegic leg*. And well before the first birthday or somewhat later, lack of a parachute response on one side only may become a conspicuous sign. This is also clearly demonstrated when rolling him over on a large beach ball which normally elicits a bilateral parachute response. Motor milestones of development, for instance in sitting or crawling, may not be significantly delayed with deferment of the mean age of walking for three or four months.

Signs are not uncommonly preceded by bottom shuffling. An especially sensitive supporting sign in the supine position is a tendency of one lower limb to fall into external rotation at the hip with the foot pointing laterally.

In a recent study of a large cohort of 126 preterm infants by De Vries et al. (1992), five of the six infants who developed hemiplegia showed a delayed NI latency. This delayed latency was defined in both hemispheres in four of them, which is in keeping with the frequent association of upper motor neurone signs on the contralateral side of the body. Indeed, when applying positron emission tomography to infants with hemiplegia following a Grade III haemorrhage, Volpe and colleagues (1982) also found changes of blood flow in the non-affected hemisphere.

Within this category, there is still clinical room for use of the term "plegia" to represent complete paralysis, whilst "paresis" indicates a partial dysfunction. This is especially relevant in describing gradations of hemiparesis, ranging from almost complete lack of function to the mildest degree of functional impairment which is far commoner than is generally recognized.

Immediately after birth and in the neonate, the *tone* of the hemiplegic upper limb is flaccid. Likewise in the acquired form such flaccidity commonly persists for six to eight weeks, when spasticity gradually appears and intensifies. In other words, the hemiplegia is not noted at birth, but after initial hypotonicity and hyporeflexia the deep tendon reflexes become hyperactive, and stretch reflexes become positive on the affected side, and muscle tone increases in the unused arm. The fine movements of the hand are the most affected, especially the pincer grasp of thumb and forefinger extension at the wrist and supination of the forearm. Corresponding changes follow in the leg on the same side, the Babinski remains positive, whilst balance and righting reflexes are asymmetrical. Strabismus and ultimate homonymous hemianopia are also common, affecting between 17 and 27% of congenital hemiplegics. Sparing of the macula has often been demonstrated. This has been ascribed to the vulnerability of the visual pathways to perinatal cerebral oedema. Comparison of posterior cerebral arteries compromises the vascular supply to the occipital lobe. An analogous sequence of change in muscle tone also marks severe diplegia, with initial hypotonia and immobility lasting at least six to eight weeks, the subsequent hypertonicity being often heralded by a phase lasting weeks or months with intermittent momentary increases of tone, this being succeeded by a more continuous hypertonicity, and the assumption on handling, etc., of generalized extensor postures of limbs and trunk. Likewise, before the onset of choreo-athetosis, there is also an initial phase of relative lethargy, immobility and hypotonia, the more severe the underlying damage the greater being the duration of this hypotonic stage.

In the lower extremity of the hemiplegic, dorsiflexion and eversion of the foot are most often impaired. The increased flexor tone is invariably present leading to an hemiparetic posture with flexion at elbow, at wrist, and knees and equinus position of the foot. The deep reflexes are increased along with the positive Babinski. Frequent falls are then typical, and a broad-based gait becomes obvious, sometimes initially obscuring the hemiplegic unilateral limitation of movement. Relative shortening of the affected arm or leg is not usually recognized until 2 or 3 years have lapsed. Indeed congenital hemiplegia is the most likely source of asymmetry of the limbs in a child referred for neurological appraisal.

A mild degree of hemiplegia may thus be overlooked for years. When beginning to walk, the child may first demonstrate a preference for one leg producing an asymmetric gait and loss of associated movements. More careful assessment may have revealed some of the characteristic elements of hemiplegic posture: adduction of the shoulder, slight flexion of the elbow, pronation of the forearm, flexion at wrist and fingers, adduction and slight flexion of the hip and adduction/inversion of the foot.

The affected upper limb remains truly under developed with asymmetry of hands and fingers eventually clearly identifiable. Consequent hand dysfunction may not be appreciated until the second year when hyperextension of wrist and fingers often appears on reaching out for an object. A subtle difference in size of the thumbnails, ordinarily equal until 6 years of age, will eventually expose its larger size on the dominant side, along with cortical sensory loss which is found to be most marked in the hand.

A strong hand preference may provide another early sign, which may be identified by observant parents when the infant reaches out at 5 to 6 months. The asymmetric hand use may first be indicated at 8 or 9 months by difference in finger-grasp, later by difficulty in piling blocks marked by dorsiflexion at the wrist. Poor postural reflexes may also be detectable at 4 months. The postural reflex will highlight failure of the affected arm to extend (or "defend"). The slight aberration of hand movement, of speech and of the relatively unilateral weakness in gait, may be first appreciated subjectively by the child - or by the parents - beyond 5 or 6 years of age.

In the upper limb on the affected side, there is paucity of associated movement with abduction of the arm, flexion at the elbow and pronation of the forearm. Indeed, one of the earliest signs is the increased resistance when passive supinating the forearm on the affected side, recognizing that in normal babies full supination may not occur until 8 months. Characteristically, even before spasticity appears, there is flexion at the wrist with preservation of the primitive grasp reflex and fisting of the hand.

Subsequent gait in the hemiplegic is highly characteristic with a tendency towards an equinus posture of the foot, not uncommonly linked to contractures of the achilles tendon so that the extremity is "functionally longer" on the paretic side. Compensation therefore follows, either by slight flexion of hip and knee on that side, or by circumducting the leg in an arc away from the hip, elevating the pelvic brim whilst dragging the foot slightly, the toes scraping against the floor.

## Associated Movements and Postural Changes

These are frequent accompaniments and indeed constitute an additional handicap. When the normal limb is moved involuntary movements and postural changes follow. Any activity requiring concentration, or running itself, will exaggerate the asymmetric imbalance. The affected side may also participate in "overflow" movement.

In a large proportion of such hemiplegias, the affected limbs may also demonstrate *involuntary movements* especially in the hands. Avoidance responses and athetotic posturing of the hands may then lead to over extension of the fingers and of the wrist when an attempt is made to hold an object. This type of posture recalls that of the parietal lobe syndrome.

# Additional Early Diagnostic Criteria

A major step forward in the understanding of congenital hemiplegia and especially its early diagnosis is represented in the recent meticulous prospective study of five term neonates by the London Hammersmith team led by Lily Dubowitz (1993). Prospective exploration of the evolution of clinical signs in infants with predominantly unilateral brain lesions diagnosed at birth was initiated by cranial ultrasonography and confirmed by neonatal magnetic resonance imaging, followed up serially at 3, 6 and 12 months. Structured neurological examination ensued, exploiting weekly video recordings. In four term infants, *middle cerebral artery infarction* was revealed. One had a basal ganglia lesion. All were hypotonic in the neonatal period, but whilst one had asymmetry of movement, in two asymmetry of tone was not demonstrable for six weeks. Asymmetry of movement eventually emerged in three of the five between 3 and 4 months, with preference for the hand on the side of the lesion by 6 months, becoming more conspicuous by 9 months. Three of the infants first showed fisting and loss of independent finger movement at 9 months. Changes in signal intensity on magnetic resonance imaging were noted in the two infants with middle cerebral artery infarction. In one infant, marked asymmetry of the brain stem was definable at ten weeks, with a milder degree thereof between 5 and 8 months in two others. In the most severe hemiplegic, "marked signs of Wallerian degeneration" were identifiable at 10 weeks. These studies constitute a beautiful illustration of the tremendous potential lying ahead in the understanding of CP and all its entities through the correlation of neuroimaging, neuropathology and precise clinical observation.

# Aetiology

That congenital spastic hemiplegia was predominantly due to cerebral damage at birth was cherished for almost a century since Osler's classical lectures of 1889 largely devoted to hemiplegia. A sequence of comprehensive international surveys from the French series of 185 cases (Goutieres et al., 1972) to that of Hagberg et al in Sweden (1975) and the West German study of Michaelis et al. (1980), switched the perspective towards prenatal influences as decisive or predisposing in about two-thirds of the cases.

In a large series of 1048 low birth-weight survivors, children with and without spastic hemiplegia were identified after 3 years of age. Spastic hemiplegia was found in 16 of 42 subjects of CP and the increased prevalence was related to previous reproductive loss, breech delivery, later birth order, prolonged second stage of delivery, emergency

Caesarean, and low Apgar scores. They concluded that intrapartum events appeared to be closely related to the pathogenesis of hemiplegia in their particular population, although their effects may well have been mediated by postnatal influences.

That CT scanning still occupies an important place in the analysis of underlying cerebral pathology was illustrated by the exploration of 83 subjects of hemiplegic CP (Wiklund, Uvebrandt and Flodmark, 1991). Emphasis was upon *the phase of cerebral maturation* during which the underlying damage had arisen. *Periventricular atrophy* believed to represent periventricular leukomalacia (PVL) was found in 37%. Because of its usual association with hypoxic-ischaemic damage in the immature brain, prenatal timing was presumed. In 17% cerebral malformation could be related to a very early intrauterine lesion. There was therefore strong evidence for a prenatal origin of the hemiplegia in a total of 57%, with a significant proportion due to early congenital malformation. The whole study added support for closely integrating CT analysis of brain morphology with the clinical assessment when evaluating the cerebral basis of partial congenital motor impairment, hemiplegia.

The importance of prenatal vascular factors had already been anticipated however in the 1967 report of Lyon and Robain, with careful correlation of neuropathological and clinical findings, a view confirmed by Goutiere's further studies (1979). Insufficiency of cerebral perfusion, mainly in the third trimester, came more and more to be invoked in the aetiology of hemiplegia. More specific CT scanning supported such vascular patho-physiology: cystic or atrophic changes in the area of the middle cerebral artery (Koch et al., 1980; Kotlarek et al., 1981) or the wedge-shaped cortical lesion of Michaelis et al. (1980) who postulated that newborn with such prenatal lesions were also more likely to suffer perinatal asphyxia in the meticulous study of 226 cases of congenital hemiplegia by Hagberg and Hagberg (1984). Forty-eight percent of their term children with hemiplegia could be envisaged as "prenatally determined... and 27% prenatally predisposed", making up a total of 75% prenatally caused or predisposed. Their conclusions also applied to preterm infants, based upon their deductions that significantly more prenatal risk factors had involved preterm and especially very low birth-weight infants with hemiplegia than had preterm diplegics.

## Acquired Hemiplegia

Spastic hemiplegia believed to be of a vascular or traumatic nature may present at any age although rarely before five to six months. but to accept it as an entity of CP, Kurland (1958) has somewhat academically insisted on the causative insult having arisen between conception and the end of the first month of life, with the hemiparetic motor dysfunction manifest by the age of two years.

Its sudden onset may be heralded by convulsions, in what has been termed "Todd's palsy", or it may emerge abruptly with unilateral paralysis. Trauma, intracranial infection or neoplasm are possible sources other than vascular and anoxic factors which will be discussed subsequently under the subheading of aetiology.

With involvement of the dominant hemisphere, there is also temporary loss of language with some transfer to the undamaged hemisphere. Permanent aphasia is rare.

# "Double" Hemiplegia or
# Parasagittal Cortex Syndrome

Whilst spasticity affecting all four limbs is usually labelled as tetraplegia, interpretation of some particularly severe examples long ago acquired the title of "double hemiplegia". The new data whereby I have linked infarction and/or ischaemia, the parasagittal cortex visualized by MRI has the characteristic clinical pattern of predominantly upper limb spasticity associated with repetitive seizures.

Whilst I believe that "double hemiplegia" represents no more than this special syndrome of tetraplegia, some authorities still retain faith in a double hemiplegia which implies a conjunction of bilateral hemiplegic pathology, presumably a primary conjunction of bilateral upper motor neurone pathology.

Such hypothetical diagnosis, even if it can be more precisely substantiated, is of doubtful practical importance. Substantiation by MRI or contemporary refinements thereof would be more convincing.

It is believed that upper limb involvement is especially severe in cases so diagnosable. The arms then tend to be inwardly rotated and elbows either extended or tightly flexed. Hands are often fisted. Mental handicap is particularly profound in many so-called examples, as well as disabilities that may be associated, such as cortical blindness and epilepsy. Pseudo-bulbar palsy with involvement of speech and of swallowing musculature have also been associated.

# Atypical Hemiplegic and
# Multifunctional Patterns of Hemiplegia

Apart from a disproportionate impairment of speech maturation, associated handicaps may include microcephaly with mental retardation, and even relatively mild ataxia. Signs of mild pyramidal pathology on the apparently normal side may be elicited, so that a presumptive diagnosis of a diffuse or bilateral lesion would be justifiable or even of a double hemiplegia.

Cognitive deficit is already known to be common in less common forms of hemiplegia with the mean IQ being about 20 points lower than the norm. More specific disabilities are also commoner. Of associated ophthal-mological problems, hemianopia may occur in particular.

An increased risk of epilepsy is more firmly associated, apparently related to the severity of the neurological damage, and greater in acquired forms of hemiplegia. The initial seizure may enlarge at any age. In more severe forms focal in onset but with secondary generalisation have on rare occasions benefited by resection of cortex housing eliptogenic focus, or even a hemispherectomy when the foci are multiple.

## Primary Emotional, Behavioural and Psychiatric Associations

Significant emotional and behavioural difficulties characterizing childhood hemiplegia are often overlooked, as is the primary behavioural disturbance associated with CP to which we have previously referred (Chapter 1). Attention has been strongly drawn to this problem, and to commonly underrecognized psychiatric disorder by Goodman (1993) in his extensive study of subjects of hemiplegia between the ages of 6 to 10 years, middle cerebral lesions being a common source. 61% of 149 children manifested problems including inexplicably intense fears, non-compliance temper, aggression, tantrums, and negativism, which substantially interfered with their daily lives. He also emphasized their high incidence of epileptiform reactions, reaching 85% in his series.

## Management

In hemiplegia, the TVR (Tonic Vibration Reflex) is lower in amplitude and more abrupt in onset and cessation, whilst in cerebellar disease it is totally absent. Attempts have been made to exploit such findings in assisting movement patterns through the use of myoelectric potential-activated vibrators.

Petö-inspired management also appears to be particularly effective in restoring function to the affected side and this may be reinforced by application of a Biofeedback approach.

Sporting activities provide both physical and emotional benefits. Skiing is recommended, outrigger ski poles being used to learn. Roller skating also has a contemporary appeal, several hemiplegic children having become expert roller skaters. Swimming is particularly valuable, since buoyancy of the water facilitates the movement of relatively weak musculature.

## Biofeedback Therapy

This is based upon the principle that patients can monitor their own motor performance through selected sensory modalities, auditory or visual. It is conceived that immediate and continuous knowledge of one's own performance may afford instantaneous detection and correction of errors which could serve to reinforce correct adaptation of motor behaviour, and generalize to other functions and life skills without feedback. Thus it has successfully enhanced symmetrical gait in many hemiplegic children (Seeger et al., 1981), apart from improving head and trunk control in other types of CP. EMG biofeedback of selected muscle activity has been explored for muscle re-education in several neurological conditions, and could be usefully applied in selected cases of hemiplegia.

# TREMOR

Rhythmic oscillation of some part of the body is denoted, in particular of the outstretched fingers and hand, or of the neck, mouth and head, or trunk. More conspicuous involvement in this way of the head and neck, a *head-rock*, has also been described as *Spasmus Nutans*, which is made up of a triad of head nodding, and head tilt accompanied by nystagmus, which may be modified by voluntary action, not unusually subduing or eliminating benign essential tremor. This pattern is also a distinctive feature of Pelizeus-Merzbacher disease, when it is accompanied by *pendular* nystagmus as well as clinically manifesting progressive degenerative disorder of the central nervous system, as outlined in a subsequent section on progressive ataxias. Postural tremor rarely, if ever, solely involves the head.

It is rarely consistently present as an isolated phenomenon in either the metabolic or degenerative encephalo-myopathies of childhood, except in their earliest stages. Some month's may elapse before there is spread to other parts of the body, by which time other elements of extra pyramidal or motor ganglia pathology may become manifest.

It may present, however, as a cardinal sign early in Hallevorden-Spatz disease marked by excessive deposition of iron in the central nervous system, or in juvenile Huntington's chorea or juvenile Parkinson's disease. It has also been observed as prominent, but in combination with other salient features, in the genetically-determined Roussy-Levy syndrome or the Charcot-Marie-Tooth form of peroneal muscle atrophy.

In the main, the tremors of childhood take the form of pure action tremors which vary in frequency from five to nine per second and are accentuated during projected movements. It may be attended by classical extrapyramidal or cerebellar signs. However, it is not uncommonly the sole manifestation of a *benign, non-progressive, genetically-determined syndrome,* without any intellectual or other functional deficit of the central or peripheral nervous system. The author has personal experience of seven fathers whose tremor mainly involved fingers, hands, mouth, head, neck from the second or third year of life, who had reared families wherein their disability had been transmitted predominantly but not exclusively to their male progeny. In six of these, there had been unfair initial and insensitive misdiagnosis as learning disability - if not mental retardation - because of their gross inadequacy or distortion of writing. Each had compensated for this in exercising great ingenuity and self-discipline in cultivating skills in fine manipulation culminating in training to become an electrician. In some instances, there had been an initial gradual intensification of the hand tremor, or of that of the mouth, particularly when augmented by intention, during their first two or three years of life.

Those of somewhat more rapid frequency (7 to 9/second), as also expressed as a rhythmic beat in the EMG, may also reflect hyperthyroidism, and rarely of an hypo adrenocorticism, when it may also be accompanied in the child by choreiform movements. It may also be a product of excessive nor-adrenalin secretion, as associated with episodes of undue apprehensiveness in the adrenomedullary neoplasm of phaeochromocytoma.

Apart from genuine fright, fear or anger, particular drugs may be responsible in the adult, such as lithium or the tricyclines. Tremor is also observed in a wide range of degenerative, metabolic or non-metabolic encephalomyopathies, but in no way does it dominate the clinical picture. Thus it may be seen in the hepatic or flapping form (asterixis) more characteristic of liver failure in the adult, and in the hyperammonaemias due to Krebs urea cycle enzyme deficits. Likewise, it may appear in phenylketonuria, Leigh's disease, Nieman-Pick disease, ceroid lipofuscinosis, juvenile Sandhoff's disease with combined deficiency of Hexosaminidase A and B, juvenile Gaucher, in metachromatic or Krabbe's leukodystrophies, or in Hartnup and Refsum's disease. Of the degenerative disorders, tremor becomes a prominent feature in Friedreich's ataxia, Cockayne's dwarf syndrome, neuroaxonal dystrophy, benign familial myoclonus, and ataxia telangiectasia.

Distinctive *intention tremor*, tremor with voluntary activity such as especially typical of lesions in the posterior cerebellar lobe or in cerebellar hemisphere disease. It may, for example, appear in hands and arms during the third year of life in juvenile Sandoff's disease, to slowly spread to trunk and legs. Intention tremor has also been a clinical feature in association with ataxia and myoclonus in biotinase deficiency and linked to hypotonia and general developmental retardation in α-hydroxytrilyric aciduria. In a familial form of "orthochromatic" leukodystrophy with diffuse angiomatosis (van Bogaert, 1970), pronounced tremor was the clinical accompaniment of pyramidal hemiplegia, dysarthria and pseudobulbar symptoms.

# POSSIBLE ACTIVATION OF FUNDAMENTAL CEREBRAL PROTECTIVE MECHANISMS AGAINST NEURONAL DEATH: THE ROLE OF GLUTAMATE RECEPTORS

In this context, it has been possible to demonstrate that the simulation of cerebral palsy entities by neurometabolic and neurodegenerative disorder is not confined to their clinical expressions of disturbed tone, movement and balance. In several disorders, like the *putamen* pathology of glutaryl acyl-CoA dehydrogenase deficiency, we have identified a crucial extension of this simulation even to the pathological bases of these entities. Therefore, it should be of value to apply the same perspectives to both the non-progressive (CP) and progressive clinical disorders on the assumption that there may be pathways of dysfunction, neurometabolic, neuro-traumatic and molecular biological common to them both.

Viewed in this way, the fundamental sequential damage which may or may not finally culminate in neuronal cell death may follow several routes, but all will ultimately converge on a final common pathway. For many, if not all, of these apparently very different conditions it would therefore be relevant to consider here the implications of this exciting new field of molecular biology, especially in relation to the possible role of glutamate receptors in activating fundamental cerebral protective mechanism against neuronal death.

A more fundamental horizon in the limitation of cerebral damage and the prevention of neuronal cell death is opened up by studies in neurotoxicity related to an "excitotonic" hypothesis of neuronal injury apart from its importance in neuronal outgrowth, plasticity and cell to cell interaction. Glutamate and other related excitatory transmitters are envisaged as becoming toxic in their interaction with glutamate receptors thereby releasing a lethal cascade of intracellular events ending in neuronal death. The selective neuronal lesion is more severe in dendrites than in axons, with sparing of glia.

These studies have centred on what could convey neurotoxic properties to an endoglione neurotransmitter, and upon the protective effects of the use of antagonists acting specifically at the level of the glutamate family of neuronal receptors. Three groups of glutamate receptors appear to be involved. Two of them are inotropic receptors affording a binding site and a central intrinsic central ionic channel: one a NMDA (N-methyl-D-Aspartate) receptor subtype, the other a non-NMDA or kainite-quisqualate receptor. The potent protective effects of these antagonists are of considerable potential import. The third class is a metabolic receptor everting its action through second messenger systems by activation of a G-protein.

Basically, a transient over-production of glutamate-receptor synaptic terminals in the immature brain is envisaged as either providing a molecular substrate for increased susceptibility to glutamate receptor agonists, or an heightened synaptic plasticity with consolidation of synaptic connections. Different brain regions and neuronal types show different development profiles of susceptibility to each of the glutamate-receptor agonists. The best glutamate receptor antagonists were first identified as of the NMDA receptor subtype.

The main focus of study has been on the aftermath of fundamental changes in cellular energy metabolism and membrane potential that results from *ischaemic-hypoxic injury*. In the immature brain, such ischaemic-induced injury is expected to be predominantly mediated by NMDA agonists, and in the developed brain a greater degree of injury would be mediated by non-NMDA receptors. Impairment of such basic factors could lead to failure of NA+/K+ATPase and membrane depolarisation, the excitatory process constituting the final common pathway to death of this vital cell.

A similar excitatory process has also been invoked in profound hypoglycaemia, the fundamental neurotoxicity being mediated by NMDA receptors, with aspartate as the endogenous agonist. Only as the membrane is depolarised can the magnesium blockade of the ionic channels be lifted, the receptor being activated, with calcium ions then able to enter the cell. It is the consequent rise in cytosolic calcium which is considered the initiating step in the intracellular events, finally culminating in neuronal death.

The goal of these studies have therefore been focussed on how glutamate receptor blockade can prevent such ischaemia-induced injury. Apart from a potentially powerful influence in profound hypoglycaemia and status epilepticus, a complex interaction between interwoven changes in cerebral energy metabolism, cerebral blood flow, blood-brain barrier function, neuronal depolarisation and glial-neuronal interaction is the product of a secondary outcome of such primary damage. One is left with the hope that a growing understanding of these fundamental intracellular neuronal influences may ultimately be translated into practical clinical guidelines for the early prevention or alleviation of acute and especially ischaemic cerebral damage, such as may be basic to cerebral palsy. In the long term, the preventive implications may be even more relevant to such chronic neurodegenerative disorders asHuntington's chorea and Parkinsonism, not excluding the end result of some inborn metabolic errors.

# THE ROLE OF SUPEROXIDE RADICALS
# EFFECTS OF HYPOXIA AND HYPEROXAEMIA
# EVALUATED IN CULTURED NEURONES

Neuronal cell cultures are valuable tools in the study of mechanisms involved in cell death following hypoxia. It has been learnt from previous studies that neurones and astrocytes reveal differing reactions to hypoxic insult, the neurones proving to be more sensitive than other cell types. Effectively exploiting such techniques has found that amongst the circumstances linking depletion of oxygen supply to brain injury, the accumulation of toxic oxygen-derived free radicals - mainly superoxide radicals - appears to have resulted in membrane peroxidation which has been proposed as an important step in the direction of neuronal cell death.

## References

Allen MC, Capute DJ. (1990) Tone and reflex development before term. Paediatric suppl. 85: 393-399

Anderson U et al. (1989) Reduced glutamate decarboxylase activity in the subthalamic nucleus in patients with tardive dyskinesia (TD). Movement Disorders 4: 37-46

Arens LJ, Peacock WJ, Peter J. (1989) Selective posterior rhizotomy: a long-term follow-up study. Childs Nervous System 5: 148-152

Baird HW, Gordon EC. (1983) Neurological evaluation of infants and children. Spastics International Medical Publication. William Heinemann Medical Books Ltd, London

Byddel GM, Steiner RE. (1982) Nucleate magnetic resonance imaging of the brain. Neuroradiol 23: 231-240

Byers PH, Holbrook K, Marsh GS. (1983) Ehlers Danlos Syndrome. In: Emery AEH, Rimoin DI (Eds) Principles and Practice of Medical Genetics. Churchill Livingstone, Edinburgh. Ch.58.

Crossman AR, Sambrook MA, Jackson A. (1984) Importance of subthalamic nuclear function in movement disorders not restricted to hemiballismus. Brain 107: 579-596

de Long MR, Crutcher MD, Georgopoulos AP. (1985) Primate globus pallidus and subthalamus nucleus: functional organisation. J Neurophysiol 53: 520-543

de Vries LS, Eken P, Pierrat Y, Daniels H, Cassaer P. (1992) Prediction of neurodevelopmental outcome in the preterm infant: short latency somatosensory evoked potentials compared with cranial ultrasound. Arch Dis Child 67: 1177-1181

Dooling EC, Adams RD. (1975) The pathological anatomy of posthemiplegic athetosis. Brain 98: 29-48

Drillien CM. (1972) Abnormal neurological signs in the first year of life in low birth-weight infants: possible prognostic significance. Developmental Med Child Neurol 14: 575

Dubowitz V. (1980) The floppy infant. 2nd Ed. Clinics in Developmental Medicine No. 76. Spastics International Medical Publications. Blackwells, Oxford

Dubowitz LMS, Rutherford MA, Bouza H, Acolet D, Pennock JM, Bydder GM (1993) Early diagnosis of congenital hemiplegia: Prospective study of five full-term neonates. Proceedings 19th Annual Meeting, Br Paediat Neurol Assoc, p 8

Goodman R. (1993) Psychiatric consequences in childhood hemiplegia. Abst Proc British Neurological Association Meeting, Institute of Child Health, London

Goutieres F, Challamel MJ, Aicardi J, Gilly R. (1972) Les hemiplegies congenitales semiologie, etiologie et prognostic. Arch Fran Pediat 29: 839-857

Goutieres F. (1979) Role of circulatory disturbances in the genesis of some prenatal encephalopathies. Proc Europ Fed Child Neurol Soc, 5th Cong. Brussels

Hagberg B, Sanner B, Stern M. (1974) The dysequilibrium syndrome in cerebral palsy. Acta Paediat Scand, suppl. 226

Hagberg B, Hagberg G. (1984) Prenatal and perinatal risk factors in a survey of 681 Swedish cases. In: Stanley F, Alberman E (Eds) The Epidemiology of the Cerebral Palsies. Blackwell, Oxford. p 12.

Hagberg B, Hagberg G, Olow I. (1975) The changing panorama of cerebral palsy in Sweden 1954-1970. Analysis of the general changes. Acta Paediat Scand 64: 187-192

Hagberg B, Hagberg G, Olow I. (1975) The changing panorama of cerebral palsy in Sweden 1954-1970. II. Analysis of the various syndromes. Acta Paediat Scand 64: 193-200

Holmes G. (1917) The symptoms of acute cerebellar lesions due to gunshot injuries. Brain 40: 461-535

Holstege G. (1991) Descending motor pathways and the spinal motor system: limbic and non-limbic components. Progr Brain Res. 87: 307-421

Jüch PJW, Schaufman A, van Willigen JD. (1991) Effect of stimulation of the Locus Coeruleus and other midbrain structures on muscle tone in the rat. 14th Meeting European Neuroscience Association, Cambridge. Europ J Neurosco, Oxford University Press. suppl. 4, p. 303

Koch B, Braillier D, Eng G, Binder H. (1980) Computerized tomography in cerebral palsied children. Dev Med Child Neurol 22: 595-607

Kotlarek F, Rodewig R, Brüll D, Zeumer H. (1981) Computed tomographic findings in congenital hemiparesis in childhood and their relation to etiology and prognosis. Neuropaediat 12: 101-109

Kupferman I. (1979) Modulatory actions of neurotransmitters. Ann Rev Neurol Sci 2: 447-465

Kurland LT. (1958) Descriptive epidemiology of selective neurologic and myopathic disorders. J Chronic Dis 8: 378-418

Lance WJ. (1980) Symposium synopsis. In: RG Feldman, RR Young, WP Koelle (Eds) Spasticity: Disordered Motor Control. Chicago Year Book, pp 485-494

Lange H, Thorner G, Hope A, Schroder G. (1976) Morphometric studies of neuropathological changes in choreatic diseases. J Neurol Sci 28: 410-425

Lyon G, Robain O. (1967) Encephalopathies circulatoires prenatales et paranatales. Acta Neuropathol 9: 79-98

Michaelis R, Rooschutz B, DFopfer R. (1980) Prenatal origin of congenital spastic hemiparesis. Early Human Dev 4: 243-255

Murphy PR, Martin HA. (1993) Fusimotor discharge patterns during rhythmic movements. TINS 7: 273-279

Mycklebust BM, Gottlieb GL, Agarwal BC. (1986) Stretch reflexes of the normal infant. Dev Med Child Neurol 28: 440-449

Osler W. (1889) The Cerebral Palsies of Children. Blakiston, Philadelphia. 13,15,21

Paneth N, Kiely J. (1984) The frequency of cerebral palsy: a review of industrial nationals since 1950. In: Stanley F and Alberman. The Epidemiology of Cerebral Palsy. Clinics in Developmental Medicine No. 87. SIMP with Blackwell Scientific, Philadelphia, Lippincott

Peacock WJ, Arens LJ. (1982) Selective posterior rhizotomy for the relief of spasticity in cerebral palsy. S Afr Mediese Tydskrif Deel 62: 119-124

Peacock WJ, Standt LA. (1991) Selective posterior rhizotomy: Further comments. J Child Neurol 6: 173-174

Russell A, Lingam S. (1992) Hereditary cerebellar ataxia with pathology identifiable in atrophy of the vermis by CT scanning. Unpublished data

Russell A, Perlman M. (1992) Neonatal diagnosis of Riley-Day syndrome. Unpublished communication

Russell A, Shapiro Y. (1994) Fixed "open mouth" syndrome due to prenatal impact upon mandibular growth of congenital myasthenia gravis. Arch Dis Child: in press

Rutherford MA,Pennock JM, Murdoch-Eaton DM, Cowan FM, Dubowitz LM. (1992) Athetoid cerebral palsy with cysts in the putamen after hypoxic-ischaemic encephalopathy. Arch Dis Child 67: 846-858

Saint-Anne Dargassies S. (1977) Neurological Development in the Full-term and Premature Neonate. Excepta Medica, New York

Seeger BR, Caudrey DJ, Scholes JR. (1981) Biofeedback therapy to achieve symmetrical gait in hemiplegic cerebral palsied children. Arch Phys Med Rehabil 62: 364-368

Tirosh E, Jaffe M, Marmur R, Taub Y, Rosenberg Z. (1991) Prognosis of motor development and joint hypermobility. Arch Dis Child 66: 931-933

Tizard JPM. (1949) Osteogenesis presenting with delay in walking. Proc R Soc Med 42: 80

Touwen B. (1976) Neurological development in infancy. Clinics in Developmental Medicine, No. 58. London S.I.M.P. with Heinemann Medical. Philadelphia, Lippincott

Trounce JQ, Fawer CL, Punt J, Dodd KL. (1985) Primary thalamic haemorrhage in the newborn: a new clinical entity. Lancet 1: 190-192

van Bogaert L. (1970) Familial type orthochromatic leukodystrophies. In: PJ Vinken and CW Bruyn (eds) Handbook of Clinical Neurologgy. N. Holland, Amsterdam. Vol. 10, pp 120-128

Volpe JJ, Perlman JM, Hill A, McMenamin J. (1982) Cerebral blood flow velocity in the human newborn: the value of its determination. Pediatrics 70: 147-152

Volpe JJ. (1987) Neurology of the Newborn. Philadelphia, WB Saunders

Walker BA, Beighton PH, Murdoch JL. (1969) The Marfinoid hypermobility syndrome. Ann Intern Med 71: 349-352

Walsh EC. (1992) In: Muscles, Masses and Motion. The Physiology of Normality, Hypotonicity, Spasticity and Rigidity. McKeith Press. p. 113

Westby O, Collinson C, Redgrave D, Dean P. (1991) Deep cerebellar neurons provide tonic excitatory drive for cells in intermediate white layers oif contralateral superior Colliculus. 14th Meeting European Neuroscience Association. Eur J Neurosci, Oxford University Press, suppl. 4, p. 302

Whitlock JA (1990) Neurophysiology of spasticity. In: Glenn MB, Whyte J (Eds) The Practical Management of Spasticity in Children and Adults. Lea and Febiger, Philadelphia

Wiklund LM, Uvebrandt , Flodmark O. (1991) Computerized tomography: 28 preterm infants with hemiplegic CP. Neuropaediat 22: 50-60

Yokochi K, Aiba K, Kodama M, Fujimoto S. (1991) Magnetic resonance imaging in athetotic cerebral palsied children. Acta Paediatr Scand 80: 818-823

# 5

# THE DYSTONIAS

Introduction

What is True Primary Dystonia?

Idiopathic Cervical Dystonia

Dystonia Muscularum Deformans (DMD)

Paroxysmal Dyskinesias with a Dystonic Component

Other Secondary Forms of Dyskinesia associated with Dystonic
Elements

Wilson's Disease
Huntington's Chorea
Hallevorden-Spatz
Manganese Intoxication of Motor Ganglia
MPTP Exposure

## Additional Metabolic Forms of Dystonia Presenting as Progressive Juvenile Dystonia

New Variant of Metachromatic Leukodystrophy underlying 'Idiopathic
Torsion Dystonia'
Inborn Deficiency of Dopamine
Late Infantile or Juvenile Hexosaminadase Deficiency (HexA or alpha-locus
Disorder)
$GM_1$ Gangliosidosis
Juvenile Niemann-Pick Disease
Glutamic Aciduria and Glutaconic Aciduria
Leigh's Disease (Subacute necrotizing encephalopathy)
Fahr's Disease or Familial Strio-cerebellar Calcinosis

## Miscellaneous Diseases Presenting with Dystonia, and only occasionally associated with Choreo-athetosis

Oesophageal Dysmotility in Sandifer's Syndrome
Hereditary Progressive Dystonia
X-linked Dystonia in the Philippines
Dystonia associated with Calcinosis of Basal Ganglia
Familial Striatal Necrosis
Dystonic Seizures
Syndrome of Dystonia, Choreo-athetosis and Pallidal Atrophy
Progressive Syndrome of Dystonia and occasional Choreo-athetosis in
Glutaryl-coenzyme A Dehydrogenase Deficiency
Congenital Cellular Immunological PNP Deficiency

## Possible Therapeutic Approaches

Botulinum toxin
Stereotactic surgical intervention

## Ballismus

## References

# 5

## INTRODUCTION

These represent an important and relatively specific group of movement disorders which are typically progressive, and quite distinct from the classical entities of cerebral palsy which are never progressive. Our clinical need in this context is for a sharper definition of the dystonias as a more or less specific entity of intermittent aberrant muscle tone, movement and posture. Let us first acknowledge that the term "dystonia" has assumed a number of different meanings which have come to be loosely and increasingly applied even in formal neurological and related texts. In the main, it is used as synonymous with involuntary movements characteristically involved in sudden muscular spasms or torsional movements chiefly involving the musculature of neck and trunk as well as proximal muscles of the limbs. In other words, a disorder of movement leading to involuntary twisting distortion and fluctuations of tone, chiefly of proximal parts of the limbs, of oro-facial musculature and to a lesser degree of the trunk. The abnormality of posture may be alternating or fixed whereas the relevant underlying movement disorder is classically intermittent or remittent. Slow spasmodic rotations or torsions, typically producing bizarre postures, are evoked by intention or actively attempted movement whether in the upper limbs on reaching out, in the leg and foot beginning with extension of the big toe, on walking, or in the oro-facial contortions produced on eating or speaking. In essence, the initiated movement precipitates contractions of muscle groups opposing the original movement. Although it usually disappears during sleep, it may persist in response to minor sensory stimuli in severe cases. In early stages, moreover, it is induced by attempted effort, but with subsequent progression torsion spasms or repetitive dystonic movements become spontaneous, intermittent or sustained hypertonus may accompany it, sometimes even developing a rhythmic element.

*Ballismus,* which will be discussed at the end of this chapter, reflects a much coarser large-scale involuntary jerking, flinging or flailing movement of an extremity.

Causation of dystonia may be laid at the door of many different metabolic and non-metabolic factors, although the final common pathway of operation appears to be clearly non-pyramidal and secondarily involves the basal or "motor ganglion", only occasionally confined to other disturbance of movement and tone. In my view, in the light of the impressive accumulation of recent neurobiological data, it is time for a revised conceptualization of all clinical entities defined as movement disorders necessitating a renewed attempt to achieve a comprehensive unified terminology.

To begin with one can accept a definition of movement disorders as that group of neurological dysfunctions in which there is aberrant movement attended either by a paucity of voluntary movement or excess of involuntary movement. Recent neuroanatomical or biological understanding is that underlying their control are the "motor ganglia" components of the basal ganglia which are a coherent set of brain structures, or organization of non-linear neural networks distributed throughout the brain and devoted to processing motor programmes and commands. The main final pathway for the descending information so elaborated in the motor ganglia is the *corticospinal* tract. Additional information is funnelled via the *tectospinal* and *reticulospinal* tracts originating directly in the motor ganglia, pathways mainly devoted to visuomotor integration and gamma motor neural control, and the cerebellum which also acts as a centre for integrating movement commands and the movements themselves.

No implied criticism of pre-existing work is intended. Rather an overdue appeal for clinical clarification which may well have vital preventive and therapeutic implications. The plea should therefore extend first of all to an otherwise lucid and valuable description of the so-called *"transient dystonia of infancy"* (Drillien, 1972; Drillien and Drummond, 1977). This was invoked to account for a transient disturbance in tone patterns or a transient or fluctuating general increase in extensor tone, and corresponding postural aberration, which characterized 35% of

100 infants in their 2-year study who otherwise demonstrated "relative excess of motor delay" and 85% of those displaying behavioural disorder. This fluctuant hypertonic pattern is especially vividly portrayed on vertical suspension with legs adducted, extended and feet in plantar flexion, and with arms either extended, abducted and internally rotated, or flexed across the chest with hands tightly fisted. On lowering to the floor, extension of the toes is followed by a strong extensor thrust as the feet touch the surface. Presumably because of the retained walking reflex, the child begins to walk forward on his toes. Head lag is also initially conspicuous, although in prone the head is held firmly upraised as one would expect with increased extensor tone.

Persistence of several other primitive reflexes may be incriminated, including positive supportive reactions and tonic labyrinthine reactions. But such an involuntary increase in extensor tone, especially of the lower limbs and trunk, is a common enough finding in the early stages of all forms of cerebral palsy. Like the Moro, such hypertonic posturing is precipitated by a loud or sudden noise, an abrupt change of position, or when the head is allowed to fall back in extension. Bearing in mind that this intermittent fluctuation in tone coincides with the period from about 2 to 8 or 9 months when reflexive stepping ceases until supported walking begins, that it marks an irregular low level of the phase of gradual maturation of corticospinal or other related descending tracts reticulo and spinal, or more specifically their maturation of myelogenesis. This maturation involves stages of gradual linkage or intercommunication with the pre-existing spinal locomotor generating unit.

It should already be clear, as well as from subsequent definition, that this is not dystonia but instead reflects an accentuation of extensor tone typically fluctuating in degree and emerging sometime between 2 to 4 months of age to 9 months.

In a proportion of these infants, this clinical pattern may not in fact be transient, and may instead presage the ultimate confirmation of hemiplegia, spastic diplegia, or even of ataxia. Similar features also manifest in one quarter of those infants weighing 1500g or less, but also led on to unequivocal evidence of cerebral palsy in one third of these.

It is also true, however, that although suspicions of CP may entirely resolve in the remainder, there is an aftermath of relatively minor abnormality such as "clumsiness", or facets of learning disability. Indeed, Drillien was prepared to conclude that if abnormal signs still persisted at 9 months, considerable risk of oncoming cerebral palsy could no longer be denied, although he qualifies this by a statement that "in the majority of children manifesting this 'transient syndrome', the abnormal changes of tone will have subsided by 12 to 15 months except in those going on to persistent *hypotonia*, or the rare form of hypotonic cerebral palsy.

Even that outstanding neurosurgeon, Denny-Brown, unwittingly fuelled the semantic confusion that continues to plague the literature on this score. The well-known hemiplegic posture with flexed arm and extended leg was classified by him as "hemiplegic dystonia", whilst the classical flexion posture of Parkinsonism becomes "flexion dystonia". It is surely time to return logically to its original sense as an involuntary non-pyramidal disorder wherein a fluctuant but ultimately persistent hypertonic muscular *torsion* monopolizes the clinical picture. Our quarrel, therefore, is not with Dr. Drillien's highly perceptive neurodevelopmental descriptions, but merely with the category of movement disorder incriminated. It should suffice to simply paraphrase its title to "*a transient fluctuant 'hypertonic syndrome' of infancy*".

# WHAT IS TRUE PRIMARY DYSTONIA?

It is hoped that some repetition and consolidation of the definition can be forgiven. There is an underlying remittent rather than sustained hypertonus, but the specific movement disorder is marked by sudden or slowly developing unwanted involuntary spasmodic muscular contractions. Characteristically, the attempted movement precipitates contraction of muscle groups *opposing* the original movement, and progresses irregularly in a twisting even painful torsion of the muscle groups : whether oro-facial, or of neck, limbs and trunk. These alternating or occasionally parallel contractions of agonist and antagonist muscle groups are typically first evoked by intention: thus an "intention dystonia", with the progressive torsion spreading and becoming more painful. *Any attempt to speak or feed triggers off intense contortions of the oro-facial, masticatory and pharyngeal musculature.*

Not uncommonly the whole pattern is heralded by painful focal hyperextension of the big toes followed by flexion, inversion of the feet, as is also notable as the first anatomical involvement in the dominantly inherited form of dystonia muscularum derformans. Bizarre dystonic postures of the distal extremities may be the outcome. Indeed, the group of *torsion dystonias* have been classified not only in accordance with their age of onset and aetiology, but also particularly because of the affected part or region of the body. For example, either *focal, segmental, multifocal* or *generalized,* with even a distinct group of hemidystonias. Different entities of this as a hemisyndrome have been described, and with underlying unilateral anatomical lesions of motor ganglia components documented by Marsden et al. (1985).

# IDIOPATHIC CERVICAL DYSTONIA

A relatively intense *focal form,* otherwise described as spasmodic torticollis, was studied in a large series of 266 subjects by Jane Chan and colleagues (1991). Trauma often preceded the onset of symptomatology, although an even earlier onset typified those children with a family history of such focal dystonia. Pain was a striking feature in 75%, which may well distinguish this syndrome from all other focal dystonias. Postural hand tremor also coexisted in 23%.

Other focally localized or intensified dystonia includes:
Blepharospasm
Oro-mandibular
Torticollis
Writer's cramp, i.e. action-induced dystonic torsion with contractions of the forearm muscles
Spastic dysphonia:
specifically affecting the vocal cord.

# DYSTONIA MUSCULARUM DEFORMANS (DMD)

This represents the most severe form of dystonia with intense spasms of profound writhing of limbs, neck and trunk with typically grotesque postural distortions of the trunk. Two patterns of inheritance are known. One appears most commonly in autosomal recessive fashion limited to Ashkenazi Jewish families and appearing between 4 and 15 years of age, usually between 8 and 12; the other appearing somewhat later in dominant form in both Jewish and non-Jewish families. Although still predominantly between 9 and 15 years of age, it can make its first appearance in middle adulthood.

Principally, this extreme form of dystonia manifests in late childhood or early adolescence, often initially in one limb, especially in flexion inversion of the foot. It then progresses in a fluctuating or remittent manner to involve the rest of the body in obviously painful torsion spasms which block voluntary movement. At first intermittent, the spasms become more frequent, and finally persist throughout the waking day, ending only in sleep. An hemidystonic pattern may become conspicuous, with the leg extended or flexed at the hip, and the ipsilateral shoulder elevated, or the arm extended and internally rotated.

It is important to be aware of the aggravation of the whole condition by the phenothiazines, particularly chlorpromazine. This has somewhat recklessly been exploited in the detection of heterozygotes (Eldridge, 1970).

Adequate dosage of Diazepam may help to control movement; and anticholinergics, especially Benzhexol, has achieved symptomatic relief when the condition is predominantly unilateral.

# PAROXYSMAL DYSKINESIAS WITH A DYSTONIC COMPONENT

Clinical division of such dyskinesias which may display dystonic posturing, has been suggested within a *kinesigenic* group induced briefly by a sudden movement, or a non-kinesigenic group not so induced.

This form of dyskinesia may follow trauma, including peripheral injuries but especially head injury. *Hypoxia* may be another factor, because of the *especial susceptibility to hypoxia of the globus pallidus*. Drug administration particularly of the phenothiazines or haloperidol have already been mentioned as a source of *tardive dyskinesia*. The neurotransmitters, dopamine, acetylcholine and GABA, and many neuropeptides, are in especially high concentration within the basal ganglia. Drugs that block dopamine receptors, for example antipsychotic agents, are the most prominent offenders responsible for acute dystonic reactions, or tardive dyskinesia with dystonic elements.

Deficiency of glutamate decarboxylase as the precursor of GABA has also been incriminated in primate experiments focusing upon the *head of the caudate nucleus* as the source of this form of paroxysmal dyskinesia.

# OTHER SECONDARY FORMS OF DYSKINESIA ASSOCIATED WITH DYSTONIC ELEMENTS

Particularly when a progressive dystonic state emerges in late childhood or adolescence, or is superimposed upon an apparently established even static CP disorder labelled as chorea or choreo-athetosis fresh diagnostic consideration should be given to a metabolic or hereditary degenerative disease. Specific chemical characteristics of the basal ganglia (Fahn, 1976), and possibly enzymatic and metalloenzymatic needs, render the basal ganglia particularly susceptible to certain metallotoxins, etc. Prominent examples involve the neural or axonal distribution of trace metal deposition.

## Wilson's Disease

This reflects gross *cavitation of lenticular nuclei*, etc. due to excessive deposition of copper. The pigment in the classical Kayser Fleischer ring is a copper salt deposited on the lamina propria of Descemet's membrane. Progressive dystonic postures and torsion spasms, as well as athetosis or choreo-athetosis, may occasionally be major manifestations of Wilson's Disease. But in other cases it is only after protracted general rigidity, that bizarre dyskinesias with dystonic elements and unnatural postures and tonic spasms of limbs are often initiated by a voluntary act. This may extend to the pterygoid muscles when opening of the jaw, or other stereotyped movements may appear. Flagrant dystonic manifestations and choreo-athetosis have been seen early in a few examples, and are distinguished from the diffuse intention myoclonus that may mark the outset.

## Huntington's Chorea

Age of onset in childhood may be between 5 and 12 years, but most cases emerge only in middle adult life. Similar dystonic posturing and torsion spasms may also be rarely exhibited in Huntington's chorea, where the main manifestations are slowness of all movements, maladroitness, and a gait characteristically slow, stiff and short-stepped with the trunk tending to flex. In the form labelled as "pallido-luysian degeneration", large amplitude *ballistic movements* may replace the usual rigidity.

## Hallevorden-Spatz

This autosomal recessive disorder is marked by pigmentary deposits of iron and diffuse axonal swellings (spheroids) in the pallidonigral region. Dystonic postures are superimposed upon rigidity, and choreo-athetotic movements. Each of these ingredients may be the predominant or original sign, the first manifestation developing at any age between 2 and 15 years, whereas the major signs ultimately comprising pyramidal criteria, choreoathetosis, and dementia, make-up a consistent clinico-pathological entity.

Diagnosis during life can only be made tentatively when all major signs, choreo-athetosis, dystonic postures and dementia co-exist.

## Manganese Intoxication of Motor Ganglia

In industrial exposure, manganese intoxication can also produce a characteristic secondary torsion dystonia (Barbeau, 1984).

## MPTP Exposure

Exposure to 1-methyl-4-phenol 1,2,3,6-tetrahydropyridine (MPTP) brings about dystonic manifestations by selectively involving the dopaminergic neurones of the substantia nigra.

# ADDITIONAL METABOLIC FORMS OF DYSTONIA PRESENTING AS PROGRESSIVE JUVENILE DYSTONIA

## New Variant of Metachromatic Leukodystrophy underlying 'Idiopathic Torsion Dystonia'

Initially, transitory episodes of writhing or of *progressive torsional hypertonicity* was dramatically illustrated by the three siblings representing an apparently newly-defined enzymatic or metabolic abnormality underlying so-called *idiopathic* torsion dystonia (Russell and Yatziv, 1985). An 100% deficiency or defect of arylsulfatase A, together with 50% reduction of arylsulfatase of isoenzymes B and C, accounts for failure of breakdown of sulfatides, or sulfate esters of galacto cerebroside, and their aggregation in the Schwann cells of the myelin sheath. This reflects a new variant of metachromatic leukodystrophy confirmed on sural nerve biopsy, but without evidence of intellectual deficit.

Absent ankle reflexes had first drawn my attention to the possibility of a peripheral neuropathy and the significantly slowed motor nerve conduction-velocities on EMG, and a commensurate slowing of conduction velocity in the visually evoked responses, and interference with mid brain evoked potential (Prof. Sohmer), substantiated specific interference with the function of the relevant myelinated axons.

Clinically this was evidenced in the mounting "intention hypertonicity" initially either spontaneous or in response to an intended movement, which parallels and augments the torsion progressively impeding completion of the intended function or postural adjustment. Later this was to emerge spontaneously more and more frequently. This is the clinical hallmark of *dystonia*, characterized by the involuntary and irregularly alternating activation of agonist and antagonist neuromuscular "control", usually by will or intention. Although the prevalence of idiopathic dystonia is unknown, an estimate of 33 per 100,000 population has been suggested in Rochester, Minnesota.

## Inborn Deficiency of Dopamine

An hereditary form of dystonia which is progressive but with clearcut diurnal variations suggestive of a metabolic basis was introduced by Segawa et al. (1976). It is yet another disorder associated with an apparently specific interference with the production of the neurotransmitter *Dopamine* vital to the control of basal ganglia function.

Brain catecholamines stem mainly from Tyrosine through catalysis by tyrosine hydroxylase, the rate limiting step in the synthesis of Dopamine. Interference with this process may derive from defect or deficiency of tyrosine hydroxylase or of decarboxylation of l-dihydroxy phenylalanine (Dopa).

$$Tyrosine \xrightarrow{TH} Dopa \xrightarrow{DC} Dopamine$$

At least in this form, Segawa et al. have shown that the defect can be dramatically circumvented by the administration of this substrate of Dopamine-l-Dopa. So that after *the identification of low dopamine levels in blood (and CSF)*, a therapeutic trial with L-dopa could safely complete the diagnosis.

## Late Infantile or Juvenile Hexosaminadase Deficiency (HexA or alpha-locus disorder)

This may present as progressive dystonia in childhood (Johnson, 1987). Resemblance to dystonia muscularum deformans may be close with respect to the dystonia. But speech is also delayed and elements suggesting dementia together with other atypical features such as hyperreflexia, nystagmus, and low amplitude choreic movements. Hexosaminadase A would be identified as low in serum, leucocytes and cultured skin fibroblasts.

## GM$_1$-Gangliosidosis

Dystonia has also been the presentation in an unusual form of GM$_1$-gangliosidosis.

## Juvenile Niemann-Pick Disease

The presenting features may include dystonia as well as choreo-athetosis.

## Glutamic Aciduria and Glutaconic Aciduria

A prominent feature is dystonia manifesting from early childhood.

## Leigh's Disease (Subacute Necrotizing Encephalopathy)

In 60% of cases the onset is in the first year of life, most often before 3 months, with loss of head control, floppiness, and intermittent abnormalities of respiratory rhythm. Later, difficulties in walking, *ataxia*, dysarthria and nuclear or supranuclear oculomotor paralysis become manifest. It is upon this complex pattern, together with axial hypotonia and bilateral pyramidal involvement, that dystonic or tonic torsion spasms become prominent. Serum and urinary lactate levels are elevated.

## Fahr's Disease or Familial Strio-Cerebellar Calcinosis

Isolated perivascular strio-cerebellar calcification has been described by Fahr in association with a slowly progressive familial leuco-encephalopathy including mental retardation. This involvement in the main of lenticular and dentate nuclei has been associated with a diversity of type and timing of movement disorder including choreo-athetosis, ataxia and dystonia.

The movement patterns have typically been mixed so that intermittent dystonic postures may be superimposed upon a more constant choreo-athetosis. The disorder has therefore been outlined under the heading of Progressive Entities of Choreo-athetosis.

# MISCELLANEOUS DISEASES PRESENTING WITH DYSTONIA, AND ONLY OCCASIONALLY ASSOCIATED WITH CHOREO-ATHETOSIS

Twenty-five other diseases in which dystonia is prominent have been defined by Fahn and Eldridge (1976), whilst Hagberg and colleagues (1979) have reviewed a further series of neuro-metabolic disorders producing dystonia. Some especially interesting examples are listed below:

## Oesophageal Dysmotility in Sandifer's Syndrome

The associated "silent" gastro-oesophageal reflux has been linked with dystonic posturing. In this instance, intermittently simulating a dystonic entity. Even gross posturing of this kind has been totally overcome by effective anti-reflux surgery (Puntis et al., 1989).

## Hereditary Progressive Dystonia

Hereditary Progressive Dystonia with diurnal fluctuations has been reported by both Schenke and Krushke (1975) and Segawa et al. (1976).

# X-linked Dystonia in the Philippines

X-linked dystonia in the Philippine Islands was introduced by Lee et al. (1976).

# Dystonia Associated with Calcinosis of Basal Ganglia

Dystonia, one form thereof associated with calcification of the basal ganglia reported by Caraceni et al. (1974).

# Familial Striatal Necrosis (Hawke and Donohue, 1950)

This progressive disorder was first described in five children of two families and was first manifest between 2 and 6 years of age. The disturbance of gait was first conspicuous mainly ascribed to spasticity or rigidity of the limbs upon which athetotic and dystonic movements were superimposed. Dysarthria and dysphagia also became manifest. Pyramidal signs were detected in several. It is important to note that autopsy exposed necrotic lesions strictly confined to the striatum, i.e. caudate nucleus and putamen. Evidence of necrosis has been claimed by Bargeton-Frakas et al. (1964) as being recognizable in CAT scans taken in Leigh's disease.

# Dystonic Seizures

A description introduced by Hishikawa et al (1973), These seizures are induced by movement.

# Syndrome of Dystonia, Choreo-athetosis, and Pallidal Atrophy

Onset is between 5 and 15 years of a disorder characterized by *torsion spasms*, associated with *athetosis* and occasional choreic movements. Starting on one side of the body, it later becomes generalized. An important aetiological aspect, is that pathology is restricted to *atrophy of the globus pallidus* (Jellinger, 1968).

# Progressive Syndrome of Dystonia and Occasional Choreo-athetosis in Glutaryl-coenzyme A Dehydrogenase Deficiency

Two of the 11 examples more recently studied by Hoffman et al. (1991) specifically exhibited dystonic movement. Even these were associated with athetosis although to a lesser degree than in seven others. The condition has consequently been outlined more fully under Progressive Choreo-athetoid Disorders. In particular, the *excessive glutaric acid levels* in urine, plasma and cerebral spinal fluid are equally diagnostic. Likewise, a therapeutic trial of a low-protein diet, complemented with a low lysine and tryptophan formula, followed by a combination of riboflavin and lioresall (a parachlorphenyl analogue of GABA) should be worthwhile (Brandt et al., 1979).

## Congenital Cellular Immunological PNP Deficiency

At least one genetically-determined example of *spastic tetraplegia manifesting episodic dystonic spasms* conspicuously linked to *pain* in both hands and feet, was associated with a proven specific immunological defect due to PNP *(pyruvate nucleoside phosphorylase) deficiency* (Stoop et al., 1977). Specific biochemical parameters were an *abnormally low plasma uric acid*, and excessive urinary excretion of purine nucleosides.

# POSSIBLE THERAPEUTIC APPROACHES

*Benzodiazepines* especially *Diazepam*, may afford some symptomatic relief in adequate dosage (1-5 mg). Rapid dystonic movements may particularly respond to *Clonazepam*. Likewise, *anticholinergics* blocking muscarine receptors may be helpful (Rosenbloom, 1981). They are still in the process of being tested in various forms of dystonia. Benzhexol (Artane) is the agent most commonly exploited, starting with 2 mg increasing to 8.0 mg or more, although a higher dosage level, up to 30 mg daily, is considered to be necessary to be truly effective in significant dystonia.

*Anticonvulsants*, including combinations with neuroleptics, are of particular value in the *kinesigenic* type of paroxysmal choreo-athetotic dyskinesia which may show dystonic posturing. *Baclofen* (or Lioresal) has been effective in some patients, and is believed to act by virtue of interference with release of glutamate from corticostriatal (and other) fibres, which may be responsible for neuronal degeneration in susceptible individuals carrying the HD gene or by counteracting the effect of glutamate at glutamate receptors.

## Botulinum Toxin

For the focal dystonias listed, investigations continue to evaluate the role of local intramuscular and subcutaneous injections of Clostridium Botulinum type A toxin, especially in blepharospasm. It produces muscle "paralysis" by blocking the release of acetylcholine from motor neurones. It is already being used to treat strabismus and essential blepharospasm. It has also been exploited to treat torticollis and facial spasm. Larger doses (up to 40 ng) are prescribed for larger muscles rather than the 3 ng used in ophthalmology.

## Stereotactic Surgical Intervention

In selected cases of progressive neurological dysfunction in DMD, stereotactic neurosurgery, producing specific lesions in the ventrolateral nuclei of the thalamus (cryothalamotomy), has achieved the most effective results. Another novel future approach may be in the surgical *transplantation* of tissue into the brain, such as has been utilized in Parkinson's disease to replace the missing neurotransmitter, dopamine. Implants of embryonic nigral tissue to subprimates have, for example succeeded in reversing some features of nigral degeneration.

# BALLISMUS

I have added this outline of ballismus, and its implications, because of its probable relevance to children with paroxysmal movement disorder superimposed upon choreo-athetosis for whom the issue of possibly associated dystonia has been raised. This more exaggerated movement expression may also be confused with dystonia but more typically comprises very large scale choreic movement. These large amplitude excursions effect violent tossing or flailing movements. Like dystonia, however, it begins suddenly in proximal muscle groups, spreading thence to involve the whole limb or a major part of it. There is conspicuous irregularity in both location, and lack of any rhythmicity. The upper limbs may be thrown violently upwards, and indeed all movements may be so unexpectedly violent as to be self-injurious. It most often manifests as a hemi-syndrome, *hemiballismus*, such as seems to be characteristic of basal ganglia involvement and appears to be due to a lesion in the *contralateral subthalamic nucleus,* and possibly of its dopaminergic projections. A basis of multiple small infarctions (lacunes) in the contralateral striatum has also been suggested. Precipitation of this form of dyskinesia by the recent ingestion of a drug, such as phenothiazine or haloperidol, has to be taken into consideration.

Ballismus has also appeared intermittently in association with choreo-athetosis in primary degeneration of the Corpus Luysi (Melamud and Demmy, 1960). Another family with hereditary ballismus attributed to this neuropathology was long ago reported by Rakonitz (1933).

## References

Barbeau A. (1984) Manganese and extrapyramidal disorders. Neurotoxicol 5: 13-36

Bargeton-Frakas E et al. (1964) Encephalopathie infantile familose avec necrose bilaterale et symetrique des corps stries. J Neurol Sci 1: 429-445

Brandt NJ et al. (1979) Treatment of glutaryl CoA dehydrogenase deficiency (glutaric aciduria): experience with diet of riboflavin and GABA analogue. J Pediat 94: 669-673

Caraceni T, Broggi G, Avanzini G. (1974) Familial idiopathic basal ganglia calcification exhibiting features of DMD. Neurology 12: 357-359

Chan J et al. (1991) Idiopathic cervical dystonia. Movement Disorders 6: 119-126

Denny-Brown DE. (1949) Interpretation of the electromyogram. Arch Neurol Psychiat 61: 99-128

Drillien CM. (1972) Abnormal neurological signs in the first year of life in low birth-weight infants: possible prognostic significance. Dev Med Child Neurol 14: 575

Drillien CM, Drummond MB. (1977) Neurodevelopmental Problems in Early Childhood. Blackwell Scientific Publications Oxford. pp 243-245

Eldridge R. (1970) The torsion dystonias. Literature review and genetic and clinical studies. Neurology (Minneapolis) 20: 1-78

Fahn S. (1976) Biochemistry of the basal ganglia. Adv Neurol 14: 59-85

Fahn S, Eldridge R. (1976) Definition of dystonia and classification of the dystonic state. Adv Neurol 14: 1-5

Hagberg B, Kyllerman M, Steen G. (1979) Dyskinesia and dystonia in neurometabolic disorders. Neuropädiat 10: 305-320

Hawke WA, Donohue WK. (1950) Bilateral symmetrical nerosis of corpora striata: report of fatal case and reference to a possible syndrome of corpora striata. J Nerv Ment Dis 113: 20-39

Hishikawa Y, Furuya E et al. (1973) Dystonic seizures induced by movement. Arch Psychiat Nervenka 217: 113-138

Hoffman GF, Trefz FK, Barth PG et al. (1991) Glutaryl coenzyme A dehydrogenase deficiency: a distinct encephalopathy. Pediatrics 88: 1194-1203

Jellinger K. (1968) Progressive pallidumatrophy. J Neurol Sci 6: 19

Johnson WG. (1987) Neurological disorders with hexosaminidase deficiency. In: Paediatrics Update. Ed AJ Moss. Elsevier, New York, Amsterdam pp. 91-103

Lee LV et al. (1976) Torsion dystonia in Panay. Adv Neurol 14: 137-150

Marsden CD, Obeso JA, Zarranz JJ, Lang AE. (1985) The anatomic basis of symptomatic hemidystonia. Brain 108: 463-483

Melamud N, Demmy N. (1960) Degenerative disorder of the subthalamic nodes. J Neuropathol Exp Neurol 19: 96

Puntis JWL, Smith HL, Buick RG, Booth IW. (1989) Effects of dystonic movements on oesophageal peristalsis in Sandifer syndrome. Arch Dis Child 64: 1311-1313

Rakonitz E. (1933) Die Eigenerkrankung des Corpus Leysi. Z Neurol Psychiat 144: 255

Rosenbloom L. (1981) Chronic central nervous system disease in childhood. In: Recent Advances in Pediatrics. D Hall (Ed). Churchill Livingstone, Edinburgh, London and New York. pp 213-230

Russell A, Yatziv S. (1985) A metabolic basis of idiopathic torsion dystonia: a new variant of metachromatic leukodystrophy. World Pediat Child Care 1: 25-29

Schenke E, Kruschke U. (1975) Familial progressive dystonia with diurnal fluctuation. Klin Wochenske 53: 779-780

Segawa A, Hosaka A, Miyagawa F. (1976) Hereditary progressive dystonia with marked diurnal fluctuation. Adv Neurol 14: 215-233

Stoop JW et al. (1977) Purine nucleoside phosphorylase deficiency associated with selective cellular immunodeficiency. New Engl J Med 296: 651-655

# 6

# THE REVOLUTIONARY ROLE OF ADVANCES IN NON-INVASIVE NEURO-IMAGING PATHO-PHYSIOLOGY

The Potential of Neuro-imaging

Serial Computed Tomography Scanning (CT)

Positron Emission Tomography (PET)

Single Photon Emission Computerised Tomography (SPECT)

$T_C$-99 in HM-PAO SPECT in Identifying Hypoperfusion as Basis for Cerebral Dysfunction

LFDG-PET Images Correlated with MRI in the Study of Cerebral Glucose Metabolism

Application of Magnetic Resonance Imaging (MRI) to the study of Cerebral Patho-Physiology and Blood Flow

Magnetic Resonance Spectroscopy (MRS)

Encephalo Scintigraphy

Somatosensory Potentials

Other Electrophysiological ("Multi-Modality Evoked Potentials) Assessments

Conclusions

References

# 6

# THE POTENTIAL OF NEURO-IMAGING

To recapitulate, several major causes of cerebral mortality have been related to the timing of gestation, and the patho-physiological situation which may then encompass the *pre-term* infant before or during birth as distinct from the perinatal or postnatal circumstances which may focus their impact upon the full term infant. Periventricular or intraventricular haemorrhage can be visualized as the first impact leading to intracerebral involvement in the preterm infant, although in either primary or secondary association with hypoxic-ischaemic-encephalopathy whether in the preterm or in the asphyxiated term infant.

An urgent broadening and intensification of in-depth patho-physiological research is mandatory in the analysis of these and related underlying phenomena and factors of cerebral blood flow, of cerebral perfusion or of focal haemorrhage and infarction are crucial on the one hand, and the myelinoclastic and other destructive and metabolic sequelae of hypoxic-ischaemic and other encephalo-pathic damage on the other hand.

*The new generations of neuro-imaging* are already showing an unprecedented and almost revolutionary acceleration of applications to these problems. Major advances in our understanding of cerebral palsy have already resulted, especially in the clinico-pathological diagnostic clarification of different entities. These first products we shall try to sum up in Chapter 7, but the technological evolution from CT or ultrasonography (US), to magnetic resonance imaging (MRI), magnetic resonance spectroscopy (MRS), and thence to positron emission tomography (PET) and single photon emission computed tomography (SPECT), will be touched on below.

Basically, both MRI and MRS exploit the magnetic properties of the nucleus of biological chemicals such as $^1$H, $^{18}$C, $^{19}$F, $^{23}$Na and $^{31}$P. Exposed to a strong magnetic field, these nuclei resonate with a specific oscillating magnetic field in the radio frequency range of several megahertz. At such resonant frequency, such low energy radio waves are repeatedly absorbed ("Excitation") and then emitted after a time characterizing each tissue ("Relaxation"). Unusual safety levels without known biological hazards are attributable to NMR signals beyond a million-million times less energetic than x-rays or gamma rays.

The remarkable and exquisite images of MRI depends upon the distribution of the body's most abundant nucleus: the hydrogen nucleus or proton. Both tissue water and fat share a relatively high proton concentration of 20 to 50 moles/kg. but each tissue comprises an unique concentration of protons and widely differing relaxation times. The net magnetic signal in a tissue slice is displayed sometime after proton excitation.

As a basis for spectroscopy, these fat and water protons are abundant but easily distinguishable by different $T_1$ and $T_2$ relaxation times. Large tissue voxels are chosen to achieve enough signal chemical information in the form of a chemical spectrum. An image is evolved of the general region of interest, the tissue region being selected (so-called Depth-resolved spectroscopy).

The image reconstruction stemming from all these techniques are all based upon the same mathematical principle that the data garnered in a plane from, through or on a subject from multiple perspectives around the subject allow reconstruction of a slice of the data in a plane through the subject embodying these signals.

More precise commentary upon each technique and its applications will now follow, to be subsequently elaborated in Chapter 7.

# SERIAL COMPUTED TOMOGRAPHY SCANNING (CT)

As already noted, the high incidence of periventricular and intraventricular haemorrhage (PVH-IVH) has reached 35-45% in the preterm (Tarby and Volpe, 1982). *Using real-time ultrasonography, a* study of 460 infants with birth-weight below 2000 gms (McMenemin et al., 1984) exposed an incidence of 39% of PVH-IVH. Likewise, in the skilled hands of Tarby and Volpe, this high incidence had already been recorded (1982) as reaching 35-45% in the preterm.

A British physicist, Dr G N Hounsfield was awarded the Nobel Prize for evolving this technique as the greatest technical advance in neurological diagnosis in the 60 years since the contrast procedures of air-encephalography and angiography had been introduced. A narrow beam of radiation is emitted by the x-ray tube as it passes in a series of scanning movements through an arc of 360° around the child's head. Its

sensitivity to small variations in x-ray absorption co-efficients between intracranial content allows visualization of the cortex, white matter, internal capsule and corpus callosum as well as ventricles and subarachnoid spaces.

Its accuracy has been enhanced by using an intravenous contrast medium which sharpens the contrast between tissue densities. High grade scanners can now also construct sections of coronal, sagittal or oblique planes from axial planes which clarify details in the region of the pulmonary and even internal auditory meatus.

Further analysis of the predictive role of serial ultrasonography for CP in infants at birth-weight below 1200 g was undertaken in 116 infants by the team of Bozynski and colleagues (1988). Serial real time sonography was performed on days one, five and 21, then monthly until term-corrected age. 48 infants revealed intraventricular haemorrhage with three showing periventricular leukomalacia. When re-examined at 12-18 months corrected age, 12 had CP whilst 38 were classified as "suspect".

A clear association was established between risk groups based on sonography at term and the ultimate failure of the cranial CT scanning to become normal by term-corrected age was highly predictive of CP. Apart from that the duration of mechanical ventilation was considered the best index of suspect neuromotor status.

Serial ultrasonography was also effectively applied in the study of 232 neonates of <32 weeks gestational age by Sinha et al. (1990). Ultrasound brain scans carried out shortly after birth, daily for the first week and twice weekly thereafter, exposed the periventricular echogenicities progressing to periventricular leukomalacia. A technical mechanical sector scanner with a 7.5 MHz probe was used. Periventricular echogenicities were even revealed within 2 hours of birth in nine babies and 30 other babies subsequently developed similar lesions.

In 192 infants who had required mechanical ventilation, serial sonographic abnormalities also proved highly predictive of CP, independent of $PCO_2$ measurements. A significant relationship was established (Graziani et al., 1992) between vaginal bleeding during the third trimester, low Apgar scores and maximally low $PCO_2$ values during the first three days of life, and

large periventricular cysts (in 41 cases) and 43 examples of CP. The severity of intracranial haemorrhage in the mechanically ventilated was significantly associated with gestational age and maximally low $PCO_2$ and pH, but not with Apgar scores and maximally low $PO_2$.

$PCO_2$ values of less than 17 mmHg during those first three days were associated with an increased risk of moderate to severe PV echodensity, large PV cysts, and Grade II-IV intracranial haemorrhage.

Those with intracerebral involvement predominantly ischaemic and leading to cystic periventricular leukomalacia have produced the vast majority of all the neurologically impaired infants with PVH-IVH. The two possible pathogenic mechanisms we should therefore address in seeking to prevent or limit such intracerebral pathology comprise either a localized extension of blood from germinal matrix or lateral ventricle into previously normal white matter, or secondly, intracerebral penetration by haemorrhage or infarction as no more than one facet of a larger primary lesion. The basic nature of the parenchymatous involvement was studied by Volpe (1989). Diffuse cerebral changes confirmed by CT scanning are common and may obscure some critical elemental damage. Infarction, for instance, may well precede the subependymal bleed, let alone its extension intracerebrally. Techniques based upon the newer imaging methods, *magnetic resonance imaging* (MRI) and positron emission tomography (PET) have been applied to the measurement of regional cerebral blood flow, cerebral perfusion, and possibly related patterns of auto-regulation in term infants with hypoxic-ischaemic encephalopathy, and to the definition of the associated brain damage.

# POSITRON EMISSION TOMOGRAPHY (PET)

This technique applies the principle of CT imaging to kinetic tracers of short-lived positron emitting radionucleotides that are incorporated into basic physiological processes. These nucleotides are at the lower end of the periodic table with short half-lives which are cyclotron or accelerator generated. Because PET demanded proximity to a cyclotron to prepare short-life isotopes, and moreover entailed the use of radiation, it remained largely a research tool. Recently, it involved the intravenous injection of a positron-emitting isotope - usually 15O-labelled water. The interaction to produce two gamma rays is detected externally by a circular array around the head. A measure can thereby be achieved of regional cerebral blood flow largely proportional to the rate of cerebral metabolism. The images it produces furnish the most dramatic illustration of neonatal regional cerebral perfusion. In the process, it has exposed, *widespread cerebral ischaemia in babies preceding or in parallel with small periventricular haemorrhage,* emphasizing that such haemorrhages first revealed on ultrasonography reflect a much more widespread disturbance of cerebral blood flow.

Promise lies ahead for extension of the use of PET even for the assessment of functional capacity in areas of speech, hearing and vision, although it is mainly dependent upon the concentration of active blood flow in cortical areas controlling these functions. It may become possible to diagnostically interpret variations in such localization and intensity during the active operation of functional tests. When the cortex is exposed at operation, for instance, in recent surgical intervention for intractable epilepsy, consequent changes in colour of corresponding cortical surfaces could even be visualized during tongue movement or in the naming of objects.

Ethical issues of risk to the infant firstly in the course of transportation and secondly from radiation exposure, remain to be justified on the individual merits of each case. Nevertheless, the brilliant images already provided by this method (Volpe et al., 1983) have been of dramatic practical import in the exposure of a pattern of neonatal regional cerebral perfusion. At the same time an even more important finding has been the revelation thereby of widespread and simultaneous cerebral ischaemia even though the associated periventricular bleeds have been relatively small. And this basis may well have even greater relevance to the aetiology of cerebral palsy. Continuous recording of the neonatal cerebral circulation has become a justifiable goal in particular circumstances. The reconstructed PET images can give information about regional blood flow, oxygen extraction or utilization by glucose uptake.

Positron emission tomography has been applied with the PET VI tomograph. The cranial ultrasound scan in a typical case confirms bilateral subependymal haemorrhage and IVH, much more marked on the left, with haemorrhagic intracerebral involvement on the left confined to frontal white matter: (a) *on the side opposite to the intraparenchymatous lesion*, the highest blood flows were laterally in the region of adjacent fronto-temporal cortex (Sylvian), and in some slices within basal ganglia zones; (b) *in the midline*, highest blood flows are in adjacent right and left medial frontal and occipital cortex and with particular significance; (c) marked decreases in regional blood flow in the hemisphere containing intraparenchymal blood. In keeping with this finding, a blood clot in the left frontal white matter has been continuous with extensive non-haemorrhagic softening of the posterior fronto-parietal and occipital white matter.

According to the topography of the abnormality of cerebral blood flow shown by PET, the lesion involves periventricular white matter especially vulnerable to ischaemic damage in the preterm. The topography is also compatible with ischaemia in the distribution of the *middle cerebral artery*. But the timing or precise causation of the ischaemia remains to be established. Using PET an impressive degree of ischaemia was demonstrable posterior to the haemorrhagic lesion. The sick preterm is in any case especially susceptible to ischaemic cerebral damage which may often be *secondary to systemic*

*hypotension* because of the pressure-passive cerebral circulation. The secondary effects of blood in lateral ventricle, cerebral parenchyma or subarachnoid space are also to be considered. Furthermore, the cerebral blood flow is just as high in the basal ganglia as in the cerebral cortex. Likewise, additive roles in impairing cerebral perfusion must be weighed in relation to postnatal hypoxaemia, acidaemia, hypercarbia or brain oedema. Further in-depth measurement through PET adaptations, of *regional cerebral blood flow, blood volume* and *oxygen consumption and metabolism* via *infra-red spectroscopy*, would be of especial help in clarifying some of the fundamental issues involved, including the possibility, even *probability, of failure of auto-regulation*. Current observations, therefore, support the concept that the haemorrhagic intracerebral involvement in severe PVH-IVH is the secondary component of a larger primary ischaemic phenomenon with underlying failure of cerebral perfusion, and possibly associated disruption of *cerebro-vascular* and *cerebro-metabolic factors* interrelated with an hypothetical physiological mechanism of auto-regulation.

To comprehend the relevance to related problems of cerebral ischaemia and haemorrhagic fluctuations in cerebral perfusion, studies have been focussed upon how they may derive from underlying disturbance in the hypothetical physiological balance of auto-regulation in preterm or term neonate. Whether such a phenomenon could be dependent upon myogenic factors controlling arterial diameters, or upon regulation by the autonomous nervous system, invites fuller study. The mechanism may cease to function under the influence of hypoxia. It has been suggested that in the very sick preterm, that auto-regulation has failed and been replaced by a precarious pressure-passive situation. The correlationship between intracranial pressure (ICP), mean arterial pressure (MAP), cerebral blood flow (CBF) and cerebro-vascular resistance (CVR), has been represented simply in the following equation:

$$CBF = \frac{MAP - ICP}{CVR}$$

The technique is also promising for metabolic studies using oxygen-15 or deoxyglucose labelled with fluorine-18. Fluorodioxyglucose (FDG) has been frequently used to study cerebral glucose metabolism in diverse disorders particularly when associated with seizures, or in the dementias. Rubidium - behaving metabolically like potassium - is generator produced proving to be superior to thallium in the crucial differentiation of ischaemic (still with tissue viability) from infarcted muscle.

# SINGLE PHOTON-EMISSION COMPUTERISED TOMOGRAPHY (SPECT)

In this technique which is becoming increasingly available, gamma-emitting radio labelled compounds are injected into the circulation. Usually these are small lipophilic molecules remaining in place long enough to be monitored by a computer-controlled rotating gamma camera. Both SPECT and PET utilize thallium activated sodium iodide crystal detectors which emit a flash of light when struck by a photon.

SPECT provides a measure of regional blood flow largely proportional to the rate of local metabolism. Somatosensory potentials are recordable after electrical stimulation of a nerve such as the median nerve and can be recorded from the skin surface over the spinal cord or contralateral cerebral cortex. It may be abnormal in multiple scleroma and also in degenerative conditions such as Friedreich's ataxia.

A stationary SPECT system employs stationary detector rings. Its principal application has been in the brain where fast imaging times have permitted studies of cerebral blood flow with Xenon 133. Its use of tagged receptors such as HMPAC and iodoamphetamine have already been applied in studies of epilepsy, schizophrenia, Alzheimer's disease and Huntington's chorea.

Rotating SPECT systems, have exploited 1-131 iodoamphetamine and $T_c$-99 in HMPAO as below in so-called receptor studies of brain functions. These have already been applied in the diagnosis of stroke, Alzheimer's disease, schizophrenia and migraine, or for the localization of epileptic foci. Its images have also proved useful in monoclonal antibody studies applied to the characterization and localization of cerebral or bony metastases.

# T$_C$-99 IN HM-PAO SPECT IN IDENTIFYING HYPOPERFUSION AS BASIS FOR CEREBRAL DYSFUNCTION

The role of hypoperfusion in relation not only to the severity of motor problems in CP but also bearing upon the associated disabilities upon which the child's ultimate outlook may so much depend, was explored in 13 children with CP (13 months to 12 years of age) by Denays et al. in 1990. This constituted an initial exploitation of the technique of single photon emission computed tomography (SPECT) with techyelin-99m hexamethyl propylene amine oxime (HM-PAO). In all the hemiplegic children, hypoperfusion was demonstrated in the hemisphere contralateral to the motor deficit. Where the di- or tetraplegia was moderate, there was bilateral hypoperfusion in the superior motor cortex. In those with severe or tetraplegia, the reduced perfusion involved inferior motor prefrontal and parietal cortices.

# LFDG-PET IMAGES CORRELATED WITH MRI IN THE STUDY OF CEREBRAL GLUCOSE METABOLISM

PET linked to the use of FDG(2-deoxy-2(18F) fluoro-D-glucose) (Kerrigan, Chugani and Phelps, 1991) has opened up an important avenue of study of intrinsic cerebral glucose metabolism. This has first been focussed on four different entities of cerebral palsy. FDG-PET images were correlated with MR imaging or computed tomography. The distribution of metabolic impairment often extended beyond the area of anatomic involvement. In spastic diplegia, PET revealed focal areas of cortical hypometabolism and in the absence of apparent structural change. In the choreoathetoid, marked hypometabolism was confined to the thalamus and lenticular nuclei, but the pattern of cortical metabolism was relatively normal. The infantile hemiplegic showed symmetrical cerebellar glucose metabolism with absence of crossed cerebellar hypometabolism (diasolusis) contrary to its persistence in adult patients with acquired cerebral lesion. Swift metabolic recovery in the infant, possibly attributable to developmental plasticity, is offered in explanation. Whether the degree of cortical sparing on the one hand, and of a potential learning disability be predicted in this way remains to be explored.

*Transcephalic impedance measurement* of the impedance pulse and cardiac synchronous pulsations from the heads of newborn babies related to changes in cerebral blood volume, have also been researched for this purpose by and Costeloe and Rolfe (1989). Its use, initially pioneered in the USSR to detect either hydrocephalus secondary to shunt obstruction or large IVH, or changes related to birth asphyxia, has been largely superseded by ultrasound and other imaging techniques.

Significant variability in the height of the pulsatile impedance signal may even attend increasing acidosis (Weindling et al., 1986). *Recent improvements in pulsed Doppler technology* have facilitated further evaluation of such impedance measurements.

A kindred technique, the use of (1231)iodoamphetamine (IMP) or (99mTc)hexamethyl propylene amine oxyme (HM-PAO) being linked to brain single photon emission computed tomography (SPECT) was also tested in a neonatal study by Denays et al in 1989. In the first place, some subcortical periventricular and Sylvian lesions and all the parasagittal lesions were visualized in SPECT studies but had not been identifiable in ultrasound scans. Moreover, in the presence of subependymal and/or intraventricular haemorrhage, only SPECT could localize parenchymal abnormality. It was claimed by Denays and his colleagues that its potential clinical value was substantiated insofar as it facilitated the neurodevelopmental outcome being closely related to the site, the extent and the number of cerebral lesions. Long term clinical follow-up is nevertheless inescapable to more precisely define which SPECT abnormality leads to which neurological deficit.

# APPLICATION OF MAGNETIC RESONANCE IMAGING (MRI) TO THE STUDY OF CEREBRAL PATHO-PHYSIOLOGY AND BLOOD FLOW

The proton can extract energy from this applied magnetic field. On removal of this applied field, its magnetic effect fades although persisting long enough for measurement and the amount of energy removed from the field is a measure of the number of nuclei present. The rate at which the nuclei lose their energy provides data on their environment. Nuclei with cold numbers of protons or neutrons act as magnets under the influence of a strong magnetic field - of radiowave emission - they align themselves with the field. When a second weaker field - alternating at high frequency - is applied, the nuclei resonate.

Focus in MRI is based upon the detection of signals from water protons. The magnetic axis of the protons is perturbed by a radio signal at a specific frequency. When the protons relax back into alignment with the strong magnetic field, the tiny radio signal is then emitted being recorded in two planes: in line with the magnet T19 or at right angles T2.

The technical nature of this signal, its repetition time (tR) and time from pulse to echo (tE), are adjusted to achieve maximal definition of the tissue contrast in the reconstructed image.

A most obvious advantage over the CT scan in this context is the better differentiation between grey and white matter. Mainly this is because grey matter contains more hydrogen in the form of water than white matter and the hydrogen atoms are less bound in fat and large molecules. In other words, MRI exploits the magnetic properties of the hydrogen proton widely diffused throughout the body, with each hydrogen nucleus behaving as a small magnet. This has been adapted as the basis of *images of the spatial distribution of these signals*, in the process giving excellent anatomical detail.

One sharp illustration of the superiority of MRI over normal cerebral computed tomography is identifying and localising the white matter lesions in the watershed zones of arterial territories in cerebral palsy as was shown in the convincing study of van Bogaert et al. in 1991. In two subjects with spastic diplegia in whom CT scans had been negative, MRI clearly exposed bilateral lesions either in the subcortical regions or in the occipital periventricular regions. Likewise, unilateral pathology in the periventricular region was revealed in the child with congenital hemiplegia. MRI is now more and more contributing to the more precise diagnosis and even timing of the nature and extent of hypoxic/ischaemic damage, and indeed of any disordered embryogenesis, even including arteriovenous malformations (Kendall and Demaerel, 1992). How effectively its serial use, supported sometimes by MR spectroscopy, can help in the prediction of neurodevelopmental outcome has already been suggested by the serial MRI follow-up from birth by the Hammersmith team (Dubowitz LMS et al., 1992) of their seven examples of congenital hemiplegia. It is now recognized as the most sensitive modality for monitoring progress. Intra-uterine infection can also be best depicted by MRI, although CT may be more effective in showing any associated calcification. Technical refinements in MRI studies of diffusion and flow imaging, etc. will no doubt help to increase our understanding of cerebral perfusion and its autoregulation in the human foetus, and the potential for effective intervention to prevent lesions leading to CP.

A valuable retrospective analysis of the effective contribution of MRI in this field was also pursued by Truwit et al. (1992) on 42 patients. In 11 preterm, MRI demonstrated the periventricular white matter damage characterising hypoxic-ischaemic damage (82%). Of the 29 born at term, they defined three pathological patterns:

1. Gyral anomalies, polymicrogyria in particular believed to consistently reflect mid-second trimester injury.

2. Isolated PV:, reflecting late, second or early third trimester damage.

3. Watershed cortical or deep grey nuclear damage characterising late third trimester, perinatal or postnatal injury.

Of especial import is their conclusion that in 16 (55%) of 29 full-term subjects, the MR findings were implicit of intra-uterine brain damage. Developmental anomalies emerged in over half of these, nearly twice the rate recorded in prior studies solely using computerised tomography.

209

A development in the application of magnetic resonance imaging to fundamental neuroscience has been the location of increased nerve cell activity in living brain. It now provides a method of *functional brain mapping* through visualization of activated regions. Termed "*BOLD*", or *Blood Oxygen Level Dependent* Imaging, it can detect increases in blood flow to active areas of the brain by measuring changes in the amount of oxygen bound to haemoglobin. Increased flow is identified in searching for pockets of high oxygen blood.

# MAGNETIC RESONANCE SPECTROSCOPY (MRS)

*MR Spectroscopy* adds the detection of signals from a range of metabolites, permitting the non-invasive cerebral study of energy status, neuronal loss or damage, and of phosphate movement, and a widening span of abnormal biochemical changes basic to metabolic disorder.

In application to the study of cerebral blood flow, it is firstly essential to differentiate between stationary and moving nuclei. Measurement of *blood velocity* has followed and therefrom the computation to blood flow estimation. Exploiting so revolutionary a technique in this field, it has been possible to determine velocity within the internal jugular vein (Singer and Crooks, 1983). Once velocity is thereby measurable, the computation of blood flow should be feasible, although not yet achieved in the newborn. A fascinating development of this technique which has already come to have relevance in cerebral palsy research, is this remarkable adaptation in conjunction with spectroscopy. The way will progressively be opened for *non-invasive biochemical and metabolic investigation within the immature brain*. Blood gas and pH changes which influence fluctuations in CBF, can already be assayed. The principal factors are therefore related to such vital practical indices as the partial pressure of $CO_2$ ($PaCO_2$) and of oxygen ($PaO_2$). When $PaCO_2$ rises, for example, there is vasodilatation of cerebral vessels and a fall in CBF. Conversely, vasoconstriction and a rise in CBF accompanies a falling $PaCO_2$.

# ENCEPHALO SCINTIGRAPHY

Methods of circulatory radio-encephalography and encephalo scintigraphy were applied in a study of 103 children with CP in order to identify changes in cerebral blood flow (Akopian, Pshel'la and Khobba, 1988). Basing their intervention on the predominant disorder in the cerebral blood flow in the microcirculatory arterial and venous systems, they even claimed to have been able to use vasoactive drugs to achieve haemodynamic correction.

# SOMATOSENSORY POTENTIALS

These are measurable after electrical stimulation of a nerve such as the median nerve, and are recordable from the skin surface over the spinal cord or contralateral cerebral cortex. It may be abnormal in multiple sclerosis but also in degenerative conditions such as Friedreich's ataxia.

# OTHER ELECTROPHYSIOLOGICAL ("MULTI-MODALITY EVOKED POTENTIALS) ASSESSMENTS

In eight children with severe athetoid CP (ACP) the correlationships were studied between specific clinical features in CP, and a broad range of electrophysiological assessments as well as all-night polygraphic data. These included:

(a) Short latency somatosensory evoked potentials (SSEPs)
(b) Auditory brainstem responses (ABRs)
(c) Electrically elicited blink reflexes (BRs)
(d) All night polysomnographic examination (PSG).

A significant illustration of their use was in post-icteric ACP following severe neonatal hyperbilirubinaemia. The absence of ABR was documented. In most, there were also gaze abnormalities and a significant reduction in rapid eye movements during REM sleep as observed on PSG. In two cases, prolongation of the interpeak latency, N13-N20, of SSEP existed concurrently with disturbed later components of BR. In most, furthermore, impairment was observed of phasic submental muscle contractions during sleep.

These multimodality evoked potentials together with PSG, proved to be useful in assessing brain stem dysfunction in ACP. It has also been suggested as of possible help in elucidating the pathogenesis of episodic sudden death in CP.

# CONCLUSIONS

The above techniques can thus provide information as to cerebral blood pressure and volume as well as average flow. Intracranial pressure monitoring on a continuous basis is now practicable using a non-invasive sensor. When linked to arterial pressure it can complete a comprehensive pattern of the variables related to the basic issue of cerebral perfusion. Spectral analysis of Doppler ultrasound signals has made feasible the measure of blood velocity in single vessels.

As already mentioned, electric impedance techniques supported by the newer techniques of positron emission tomography and MRI can permit continuous monitoring of parameters expressing cerebral blood flow, volume and cerebrovascular resistance.

But as yet, there is no ideal technique for the full study of cerebral perfusion. Nevertheless, valuable insight can be derived from the available methods outlined. They can offer data on pressure, volume and flow, etc. The continuous measure of intracranial pressure with a non-invasive sensor applied to the anterior fontanelle still hinges upon the simple equation linking this with the arterial pressure cited earlier:

$$CBF = \frac{MAP - ICP}{CVP}$$

It can help to provide basic values relevant to cerebral perfusion. Of tracer methods for estimation of CBF, only that using Xenon 133 is now of relevance, and can solely provide data on intermittent average flow estimates. The measure of regional cerebral blood flow by Xenon-133 inhalation and single photon emission computed tomography was applied by Tandorf and Vorstrup in 1989 to ascertain the relationship between hypoxic-ischaemic encephalopathy and CP. The mean cerebral blood flow value in 20 CP patients aged 6-19 years was $67\pm11$ (ISD) ml/100 g/min, identical to that in nine normal children. Nonetheless, in 16 of these children there

were focal hypoperfused areas in the tonograph flow map. In the seven preterm infants, these were mainly in posterior watershed areas (often solely in one hemisphere). In the 13 term infants, both the asymmetrical and symmetrical hypoperfused areas were in the anterior as well as posterior watershed areas. Some children had larger low flow areas in frontal and fronto-parietal lobes. But sadly enough, poor concordance between the location of low flow areas and the clinical findings was the interpretation of these workers.

*Jugular venous occlusion plethysonography*, which can add additional variables on concurrent changes in CBF is only advisable in healthy full-term babies. But spectral analysis of Doppler signals can still be very helpful in the measure of blood velocity in single vessels, and in the further derivation of estimates of volumetric flow which also dictates simultaneous ultrasonography. Although this does not allow for continuous long-term monitoring, *electrical impedance techniques comes to the rescue* with the practical possibility of thereby providing indices of CBF, cerebral blood volume and cerebro-vascular resistance (CVR). And as already outlined, information provided by PET and MRI methods can helpfully reinforce a clinical portrait of cerebral perfusion, an understanding of which should lead to feasible methods of preventing the patho-physiology thereof and concurrently the prevention or arrest of the patho-physiology of cerebral ischaemia-hypoxia with or without focal GLH/IVH.

# References

Akopian AV, Pshel'la V, Khobba VD. (1988) Characteristics of cerebral blood flow in children with cerebral palsy during the dynamics of treatment. Zh Nevropatol psikhiat 88: 50-53

Bozynski ME et al. (1988) Cranial ultrasonography and the prediction of cerebral palsy in infants weighing less than or equal to 1200 gms at birth. Dev Med Child Neurol 30: 542-548

Costeloe K, Rolfe P. (1989) Techniques for studying cerebral perfusion in the newborn. In: Perinatal Brain Lesions. Eds. KE Pape and JS Wiggleworth. Blackwell Scientific Publications, Oxford, London.

Denays R et al. (1989) Brain single photon emission computed tomography in neonates. J Nuclear Med 30: 1337-1341

Denays R et al. (1990) Cerebral palsy: initial experiences with Tc-99m HMPAO SPECT of the brain. Radiology 175: 111-116

Dubowitz LMS, Rutherford MA, Bouza H, Acolet D, Pennock JM, Bydder GM (1992) Early diagnosis of congenital hemiplegia: Prospective study of five full-term neonates. Proceedings 19th Annual Meeting, British Paediatric Neurology Association, Institute of Child Health. p.8

Kendall BE, Demaerel P. (1992) Imaging of pediatric and congenital brain disease. Curr-Opin-Radiol 4: 28-37

Kerrigan JF, Chugani HT, Phelps ME. (1991) Regional cerebral glucose metabolism in clinical subtypes of cerebral palsy. Pediat Neurol 7: 415-425

McMenemin JB, Shackleford GD, Volpe JJ. (1984) Outcome of neonatal intraventricular haemorrhage with periventricular echodensities. Ann Neurol 15: 285

Singer SR, Crooks LE. (1983) Nuclear magnetic resonance blood-flow measurements in the human brain. Science 221: 654-656

Tarby TJ, Volpe GD. (1982) Intraventricular haemorrhage in the premature infant. Pediat Clin N Am 29: 1077

Truwit CL, Barkovich AJ, Koch TK, Ferriero DM. (1992) Cerebral palsy: MR findings in 40 patients. Am J Neuroradiol 13: 67-78

van Bogaert P, Baleriaux D, Christophe C, Szliwowski HB. (1991) MRI of patients with cerebral palsy and normal CT scan. Paed Neurol 7: 426-428

Volpe JJ. (1989) Positron emission tomography in the study of regional blood flow in the premature infant with major intraventricular hemorrhage and in the term newborn with asphyxia. In: P Evrard, A Minkowki (Eds) Developmental Neurobiology, vol 12, pp 225-238. New York, Vevey/Raven Press Ltd.

Volpe JJ, Herscovitch P, Perlman JM, Raichle MF. (1983) Positron emission tomography in the newborn: extensive impairment of regional cerebral blood flow with IVH and haemorrhagic intracerebral involvement. Pediatrics 72: 589-601

Weindling AM, Rolfe P, Tarassenko L, Costeloe K. (1986) Cerebral haemodynamics in the human newborn studied by the elctrical impedance method - clinical considerations. In: Neonatal Physiological Measurements. Ed. Rolfe P. Butterworths 137-144

# 7

# UPDATE ON NEURO-IMAGING AND THE LOCALIZATION OF A SPECTRUM OF NEUROPATHOLOGY UNDERLYING THE DIFFERENT ENTITIES OF CEREBRAL PALSY

## The Continuing Importance of Ultrasonography in both Diagnosis and Prognosis

Intraparenchymatous Areas of Increased Echogenicity and Venous Infarction
Doppler Ultrasonography and Hypoxic-Ischaemic Encephalopathy (HIE)

## MRI in the Localization of Underlying Neuropathology

MRI Emphasis upon Prenatal Origin of CP in Term Infants
MRI Visualization of Periventricular Leukomalacia by US and MRI
MRI Spectrum of Neuropathology Differentiated According to Preterm and Term Birth
Focal Parenchymatous Haemorrhages
MRI Exposure of Parasagittal Cortical and Subcortical Involvement

## Neuro-imaging Findings Especially MRI Underlying Spasticity or Hypertonic Cerebral Palsy

Contrasting Preterm versus Term Hypertonic CP Sources
Continuous "Hyperintensity Areas": MRI
Contribution of Computed Tomography

## Spastic Diplegia with Defects of Visual Perception

Associated Disturbances in MRI Localization of Neuropathogenesis

## Cerebro-cortical Dysgenesis and MRI Identification

Agenesis or Partial Agenesis of the Corpus Callosum
Neuroectodermal Defects
*Neuroectodermal Dysplasia*
*Neuroectodermal Proliferation and Migrational Disturbances*
Localization of Cerebral Dysfunction or Aberrant Cerebral Metabolism by use of PET or its SPECT Modification

## Choreo-Athetosis

MRI Localization of Basal Ganglia Pathology
*The Globo-Luysian Group and the Thalamo-Putaminal Group*
*Fahr's Syndrome*
*Basal Ganglia Haemorrhage*

## Cerebellar and Related Pathology Underlying Ataxic Syndromes: MRI Localizations

## Focal Epileptogenic Areas: MRI in their Identification

## Ultrasound Foetometry or Foetal Sonography

Prenatal Destructive Brain Lesions and Foetal Serial Abdominal Sonography

## Spastic Hemiplegia

MRI findings Underlying its Identification and Possible Pathogenesis

## References

# 7

# THE CONTINUING IMPORTANCE OF ULTRASONOGRAPHY IN BOTH DIAGNOSIS AND PROGNOSIS

An excellent analysis of the contemporary use of ultrasonography was recently provided by Anthony and Levene (1993). They still consider real-time ultrasonography as the imaging modality of choice in the neonatal unit. In their own studies, this has applied to the differentiation of intraventricular haemorrhage (IVH) from periventricular lesions, haemorrhage and leukomalacia. Certainly it has also proved helpful in distinguishing between IVH, 95% of which occurs within 120 hours of birth, and the intraparenchymatous areas of increased echogenicity which may emerge either immediately adjacent to the lateral ventricle or clearly separate from it.

## Intraparenchymatous Areas of Increased Echogenicity and Venous Infarction

Such lesions are now being increasingly identified as due to *venous infarction*, and attributed to impeded venous return from the area of parenchyma affected by listension of the ipsilateral ventricle by IVH. These lesions are often unilateral, breaking down later to form a communicating porencephalic cyst, which in turn is often associated with a *contralateral motor deficit* but good cognitive outcome.

A second form of such parenchymatous echogenicity is triangular with its apex only 3 mm from the superolateral limit of the ipsilateral lateral ventricle. Ascribed to ischaemic damage, these areas degenerate into discrete echo-free cavities representing cystic periventricular leukomalacia. The cysts eventually resorb and ultimately end in *cerebral atrophy*.

What is known as a prolonged "flare" is an echogenic area persisting for more than two weeks. Cerebral palsy (CP) is the result in 8-17% of this phenomenon, although it is conceivable that such a finding might be correlatable with a less severe form of motor impairment than CP. *When a structural defect or deficiency* is under suspicion, however, especially in areas less accessible to ultrasound such as cortex or posterior fossa, Anthony and Levene recommend that the ultrasound image be supported by a CT scan. Disorders of diverticulation such as *holoprosencephaly*, septo-optic dysplasia disturbances of migration and sulcation, and both lissencephaly and schizencephaly may come within this category, although MRI may nonetheless be more helpful in their diagnosis.

## Doppler Ultrasonography and
## Hypoxic-Ischaemic Encephalopathy (HIE)

The term abbreviated as HIE has advisedly been repeatedly used in out text as almost synonymous with "asphyxia". Doppler ultrasound, and its extension to interpret the Doppler signal from the circle of Willis have been recently shown to provide valuable information on this patho-physiological basis underlying the genesis of CP (Anderson and Mawk, 1988). Hopefully, this can yet prove to be sufficient to permit valid prognostic prediction. One hopes that it may at least come to be adequately helpful in serially evaluating the progression of ventricular dilatation and/or hydrocephalus. Likewise, the influences of shunting or other therapeutic interventions during and after ventilation.

The areas of brain concerned are thus clearly visualized by ultrasound and the scanning readily achieved from the cotside. On the other hand, whilst MRI can afford better resolution, its relative inaccessibility is a major disadvantage. The value of ultrasonographic imaging, therefore, has been adequately vindicated over the past decade for the sick infant being ventilated, etc. and in most neonatal units not only for diagnostic purposes but also as prognostic parameters of neurological outcome.

# MRI IN THE LOCALIZATION OF
# UNDERLYING NEUROPATHOLOGY

Confirmation of the localization of underlying cerebral pathology is proceeding stepwise in relation to the different entities of cerebral palsy. There has been a sequence of refinement of neuro-imaging technique from ultrasonography (US) to computed tomography (CT) and then magnetic resonance imaging (MRI) and positron emission tomography (PET). Other growing developments of SPECT have been touched upon in Chapter 6. This updating, correlated with autopsy findings, will mainly highlight the spectrum of neuropathology in CP so far identified, especially through the application of MRI.

The neuropathological categories making up the relatively specific entities of CP can be interpreted as follows:

Selective neuronal necrosis

Local and multifocal ischaemic brain necrosis

Periventricular leukomalacia

Parasagittal cerebral injury

Status marmoratus of basal ganglia and thalamus

Although such pathological states frequently overlap, the nature of the noxious factor - whether haemorrhagic or hypoxic-ischaemic - the gestational age of the foetus

218

or neonate and the correlated clinical manifestation, will tend to highlight the dominance of one.

In the meticulous *MRI study of Truwit et al.* (1992) focussed upon 40 CP patients of ages from 1 month, the outcome was subdivided according to gestational age. The findings of the seven born prematurely revealed periventricular white matter damage, apparently reflecting hypoxic-ischaemic damage in 82%. Of 29 born at term however, three major patterns were separable:

1. *Gyral anomalies*, mainly suggesting poly microgyria - and compatible with *mid-second trimester* damage.
2. *"Isolated"* periventricular leukomalacia - believed to reflect *late second or early third trimester injury*.
3. Watershed *cortical or deep grey nuclear damage* compatible with *late third trimester* perinatal or postnatal damage.

## MRI Emphasis upon Prenatal Origin of CP in Term Infants

The important overall conclusion is that *CP in term* infants was often the outcome of *prenatal factors*. Thus in 16 or 55% of the 29 CP patients born *at term the findings were interpreted as reflecting intrauterine brain damage, in over half of which MRI exposed developmental anomalies, i.e. nearly twice the rate of prior studies employing CT scanning.*

*The features most likely to predict ultimate cerebral palsy* have been furthermore listed as follows:

1. Cavities within the occipital zone.
2. Involvement of multiple regions of the brain.
3. Lesions larger than 1 cm in diameter.
4. Cavities clearly associated with *subcortical* leukomalacia.

Extensive or severe cystic leukomalacia with cysts well displayed at the *periventricular* margins and in *subcortical* regions, has been particularly documented as the product of hyperbilirubinaemia in preterm infants (Ikonen et al., 1992). Its significant role in CP, especially in the preterm infant, was also highlighted in a retrospective analysis of CT scans in 76 infants with cerebral palsy (Schouman-Claeys et al., 1989). It appeared in 45% of their preterm series, or 88% of the total series. The lesions proved to be *mainly posterior*, generally bilateral and symmetrical. The contours of the lateral ventricles were affected, becoming straight and angular, also associated with ventriculomegaly in 85%. In about 6%, localized juxta ventricular hypodensities could be identified.

The significance of *transient periventricular densities* was analysed in a study of the evolution of such findings by the London Hammersmith team of de Vries, Regev, Pennock, Wigglesworth and Dubowitz (1988). The neurodevelop-mental outcome in 53 of the infants showing such PV ultrasound densities was compared with 92 of 107 infants whose ultrasound scans were normal. *Four of the 53 infants* with transient periventricular densities developed spastic diplegia in comparison with 8 of the

92 children with normal ultrasound scans. On the other hand, *24 of these child subjects developed so-called transient "dystonia"*, a term which I have nonetheless questioned in Chapter 5, whereas this apparent disorder of tone appeared in only 8 of the 92 children with normal ultrasound. Persistence of the densities (for more than 10 days) and their presence in the trigone, were particularly related to subsequent problems. Autopsy findings substantiated the previous impression that these echodensities represented *the milder end of the spectrum* of periventricular leukomalacia (PVL) which has increasingly become a truly *predictive index of cerebral palsy in the preterm*. Diminution of PV white matter is invariable as a possible reflection of an underlying mainly *myeloclastic* disorder. It is consistently indicative of leukomalacia, firstly because of its peri-trigonal localization of white matter damage and its accompaniment by prolongation of $T_2$ relaxation.

# MRI Visualization of Periventricular Leukomalacia by US and MRI

Its ultimate outcome was initially followed by ultrasonography, as illustrated in the analysis by Shortland et al. (1988) of 46 cases. In the process he presented four common areas of periventricular distribution. PVH was specifically studied on $T_2$-weighted MRI in 21 infants of less than 12 months of age by Konishi and colleagues (1990). In four, round foci of PVH surrounded the frontal and occipital horns of the lateral ventricle. It is important to realise that 14 infants showing continuous PVH had developed spastic diplegia or tetraplegia, and that its extent appeared to reflect the severity of the brain damage.

Of 399 preterm infants of gestation less than 35 weeks studied more recently by Kadoi in 1992, MRI identified lesions indicative of periventricular leukomalacia in all 28 preterm infants who presented with spastic diplegia.

In the first place, PV high intensity areas were definable on $T_2$-weighted images.

There was decreased volume of PV white matter, associated with irregularity of the ventricular wall, and apparently related dilatation of the lateral ventricle. The functional significance of the *thinning of the posterior body of the corpus callosum* often associated remains unclear.

The histopathology of underlying PVL was initially classified into four ultrasonographic stages by Lily Dubowitz and co-workers in 1985:

1. Initial echogenicity consistent with haemorrhage.
   The direct evidence of haemorrhage on MRI may persist for up to 2 months because of imaging of blood breakdown products.
2. Normalization.
3. Development of cysts.
4. Resolution of cysts with development of periventricular atrophy and ventricular enlargement.

In other sites or forms of white matter disease, such as Alexanders, pathology may be identifiable by MRI solely in the frontal lobes. Another form of periventricular white matter damage reproduced in later childhood may be the result of intrathecal methotrexate use in leukaemia.

# MRI Spectrum of Neuropathology Differentiated According to Preterm and Term Birth

The precision of neuropathological identification achieved by high resolution MRI is illustrated in the recent identification thereby (Truwit et al., 1992) of cerebral abnormality in 93% of their 40 child subjects of cerebral palsy. Their findings were related to CP subjects of preterm or term birth.

## 1. In the Preterm

A diminution of periventricular white matter was invariable in the preterm, and was consistently indicative of leukomalacia in respect of the *peri-trigonal localization of white matter damage* and/or its accompaniment by prolongation of $T_2$ relaxation. *The focus of pathology* therefore appears to be *myelinoclastic*.

The relatively *small brain stems* in three examples were also identifiable. Volpe's interpretation (1992) was that this reflected *selective necrotic changes* affecting the neurones of *inferior olivary nuclei and ventral pons* wherein the principal neuronal injury in the preterm is believed to occur.

## 2. In Term Infants

These were clearly distinctive insofar as there was developmental evidence of *disrupted neuronal migration* in *31%* of their 29 term infants. Consequent focal disturbances of the cortex, including an "abnormally thick" cerebral mantle, ends either as *polymicrogyria*, which could be postulated to originate at approximately the fifth month of gestation, or as *pachygyria* expected to originate in the fourth month. Moreover, a larger proportion, 59%, comprised an apparently heterogeneous aggregation of abnormalities. Diminution of cerebral myelin was prominent. Likewise, cortical thinning or atrophy, and/or infarction and/or hydrancephaly and/or multicystic encephalomalacia. The separate group of lesions of the basal ganglia and thalamus was also distinctive. The resulting abnormal signal intensities in basal ganglia and thalamus (in 6 cases in Truwit's series), and discrete *cystic formation in the putamen* in at least two, separated a special group correlatable with choreo-athetosis.

The timing of the PVL and its basic ischaemic origin, could be gauged to occur either in the third trimester or in the perinatal period. Approximately 50% of the examples with myelin diminution did not show evidence of underlying PVL. In only eight were there long $T_2$ signals and in only nine was the diminution of myelin *peritrigonal*. An hypothetical developmental disturbance of neurones with secondary anomalous maturation to explain the 19 term infants exhibiting diminution of myelin could be dated between the latter months of pregnancy to some stage of the first year of life (Fig 15). A *secondary* disturbance in myelin deposition because of impaired axonal formation was suggested, the latter possibly related either to the migrational defect, or to an intrinsic derangement of neuronal outgrowth, or to a prior neuronal injury with later stunting of axonal development.

## Focal Parenchymatous Haemorrhages

In general, the ability of MRI to measure the extent of these and the above lesions in both term and preterm infants has proved to be superior to both CT and US. Localization of these focal lesions - as identified by MRI - has been primarily parieto occipital, as a vascular border zone area and a common location histopathologically for focal ischaemic lesions. Serpiginous lesions at the junction between cortex and subcortical white matter (Fig 8) were especially significant in four of the cases of Keeney et al. (1991). This area is also a delicate vascular border zone incorporating acute bending of meningeal arteries.

## MRI Exposure of Parasagittal Cortical and Subcortical Involvement

The selective vulnerability of cerebral areas such as the parasagittal cortex was first identified on CT. It has since been sometimes acknowledged as the cardinal ischaemic lesion of the *term infant*. Further support for this recognition has stemmed from PET in the straying cerebral blood flow. This was highlighted by Volpe and co-workers (1983) in its application to 17 "asphyxiable" term infants during the acute phase of illness. This again emphasized the relative decrease in cerebral blood flow to parasagittal regions. Indeed their values were at 25 to 50% lower than those for the Sylvian cortex.

Their conclusions are important, that the topography of the PET abnormality in cerebrovascular watershed regions - considered to reflect tissue injury - indicate basically ischaemic injury. The characteristic arterial border and end-zones in the cortical and subcortical parasagittal areas - *mainly in the posterior cerebrum* - appear to be the site of the basic patho-physiology. Such zones are particularly vulnerable to falls in cerebral blood flow especially likely in the newborn with secondary *systemic hypotension*, associated with impairment of vascular autoregulation during and after perinatal asphyxia. Neonatal seizures were exhibited by 11 of these infants during the first postnatal day, and spastic tetraparesis was the outcome. It has been presumed furthermore that the parasagittal distribution of damage explains the clinical pattern of motor defect, *proximal limb weakness* characterizing 13, and the *upper limbs being affected more than the lower*, as characterizes severe tetraplegia of a type sometimes labelled as "double hemiplegia". Repetitive seizures are also a characteristic sequel. Brain lactate levels rise after the insult, although this may be preceded by the onset of epileptiform reactions and secondary cytotoxic oedema. These phenomena have been confirmed in experimental reproductions of this lesion in foetal sheep (Tan, 1992).

When the correlationship with radio-nuclide brain scanning was evaluated, a striking pattern of increased tissue uptake of the radionuclide was measured in the parasagittal regions bilaterally, and posteriorly more than anteriorly.

More recently (Keeney et al., 1991), MRI has proved superior in localization of this distribution of injury than radionuclide scanning in prospective observation upon ischaemic lesions affecting 100 high risk neonates. A close correlation with disturbance of cerebral blood flow was also clear. At autopsy in one such infant softening was apparent bilaterally in the parasagittal parietal cortex. This involvement extended into periventricular white matter whilst neuronal sections exposed regions of softening in the *parasagittal cerebral cortex* and *subcortical white matter*, especially posteriorly. Occasional cortical neurones showed eosinophilic cytoplasm and/or pyknotic nuclei. Similar cellular changes may be found in the caudate nucleus as well as in the ventral pons, and the Purkinje cells of the cerebellum.

That parasagittal cerebral ischaemia is a frequent pathological consequence of perinatal hypoxic-ischaemic brain damage

was also supported by findings in *technetium-enhanced brain scanning* and *by PET*, but an example of parasagittal infarction has already been documented by Pasternak in 1987. His serial CT scans showed that the *major structural injury was a symmetrical wedge-shaped haemorrhagic infarct* in the border zones between the distribution of the anterior and middle cerebral arteries. This type of lesion is similar to that documented in experimental animal studies including foetal primates. The major impact of extracortical injury was on basal ganglia and cerebellar areas that may also be within arterial border zones likely to be vulnerable to ischaemic injury.

Parasagittal as well as Sylvian and peri-ventricular lesions, hitherto not diagnosable by ultrasound scans, are particularly well visualized in SPECT studies (Denays et al., 1989). And in neonates with subependymal and/or intraventricular haemorrhage, the existence of parenchymal injury was only identified by SPECT. It has thus been clearly shown that [123I] IMP or [99mTc]HM-PAO Brain SPECT has potential clinical value since the neurodevelopmental outcome is related to the site, the extent and the number of cerebral lesions.

Consequent upon hypoxic-ischaemic insult in the preterm infant, MRI also frequently reveals *hippocampal damage*. Indeed, cerebral cortical neurones, especially those of the CA1 region of the hippocampus (Sommer's sector) are especially vulnerable to necrotic sequelae. In the preterm, the subiculum of the hippocampus is thus the principal site of neuronal injury, along with the inferior olivary nuclei and the ventral pons. Apart from that involvement, predominant damage in the preterm encroaches upon periventricular white matter to produce leukomalacia.

As also outlined in Chapter 4, its pathophysiology in the term infant is related mainly to the distribution of excitatory synapses mediated by the excitotoxic amino acid, glutamate. It is postulated that hypoxic-ischaemic damage leads to both increased release from nerve endings and decreased uptake by presynaptic neurones and by astrocytes. Hence the toxic accumulation of extracellular glutamate. So that current studies confirming implication of glutamate receptor blockers, calcium channel blockers or free radical scavengers may in due course prove to be of major therapeutic or even preventative benefit.

In the context of a metabolic end-point, and the localization under discussion, *regional circulatory factors* may also play a contributory pathogenic role. After all, cortical neuronal injury tends to be more intense in arterial border zones, in those in the depths of sulci and in the parasagittal region of the cortex. The motor outcome is typically a spastic tetraparesis.

Involvement of the caudate nucleus, putamen, globus pallidus and thalamus leading to status marmoralus and choreoathetosis is apparently related to both transient maturational dependent density of glutamate receptors and the vulnerability of neurones undergoing differentiation in the perinatal period.

A clinical syndrome identified with neonatal parasagittal ischaemia especially includes characteristic hip-shoulder weakness, but also incorporates profound cognitive impairment and microcephaly. The predominance of the parasagittal injury in CT scanning certainly confirms the selective vulnerability of this region.

# NEURO-IMAGING FINDINGS ESPECIALLY MRI UNDERLYING SPASTICITY OR HYPERTONIC CEREBRAL PALSY

MRI has rapidly usurped US and CT scanning in the identification of US and CT-undetectable white matter lesions mainly involved in producing spastic diplegia or tetraplegia whether in periventricular zones or in the vulnerable watershed zones of arterial territories below the cortex, such as in parasagittal regions. Its reliability has extended to congenital anomalies, enhancing the recognition of such lesions, and their prevalence, as well as contributing strikingly to our understanding of the role of neuronal migrational and other patho-embryology such as holoprosencephaly in the prenatal genesis of CP. Even in the often comparable cerebral changes associated with neurometabolic disorders simulating different entities of cerebral palsy, MRI has also proved to be the most sensitive modality to date for monitoring such progressive and metabolic changes.

The cardinal findings have been illustrated in a number of retrospective and prospective studies completed during the past three to four years. The principal damage identified in an MRI analysis of 34 children with spastic diplegia between 2 and 10 years of age by Yakochi et al. (1991) included *dilatation of the trigone, atrophy of the peri-trigonal white matter* and prominent deep cortical sulci. In addition, *periventricular high-intensity areas* in the white matter adjacent to the trigones and bodies of the lateral ventricules were frequently seen. The suggested interpretation is that they are sequelae to periventricular leukomalacia, and that only the extent and degree of residual white matter correlates with the severity of disability.

In 1990, Feldman, Scher and Kemp et al. in an MRI investigation of 15 children of 8 months or older, had already shown the *increased white matter signals* on $T_2$-weighted images, but attention was also drawn to *ventricular enlargement* adjacent to the regions of abnormal white matter in 12 children with hypertonic cerebral palsy. Three of these also manifested significant sensory impairment. In addition to the structural abnormalities, maturational defects, especially *delayed myelination*, were also identifiable, or a combination of both, from the age of 8 months in all nine infants in whom Byrne et al. (1990) found subsequent

development of CP. Eight months indeed appeared to be the earliest age at which MRI findings correlate well with a later adverse neurological outcome. Other MRI studies reported in 1990 confirmed similar findings.

The MRI investigation (Koeda et al., 1990) applied to 18 children with *spastic diplegia* was aimed at clarifying differences in lesions between preterm and term infants with spastic diplegia, 11 preterm and 7 term. *The preterm infants* all showed similar abnormalities in the PV white matter representing high intensity in $T_2$-weighted imaging. The lesions appeared to represent PVL and pathological *dysmyelination*. The extent and degree thereof correlated well clinically with spastic diplegia. In the seven term infants, PVL was clarified in one, whereas brain anomalies were exposed in two, eg *schizencephaly* in one and *coprocephaly* in the other.

It has been suggested that spastic diplegia of the preterm is not only a clinical but also a pathological entity. A study of 21 infants less than 12 months of age were shown to have PV hyperintensity (PVH) on $T_2$-weighted MRI. Ten had suffered neonatal asphyxia, six intracranial haemorrhage, two meningitis and three apnoea. PVL was classified according to extent. In four there were round foci of Picot surrounding frontal and occipital horns of the left ventricle, in 17 continuous PVH and in 14 others spastic diplegia or tetraplegia.

## Contrasting Preterm versus Term Hypertonic CP Sources

That MRI can also serve to differentiate the cerebral pathological entities underlying cerebral palsy of preterm origin from that of term or of perinatal source in either was also well illustrated by its application (Koeda et al., 1990) to 18 victims of spastic diplegic CP, 11 of preterm and 7 term birth. In all the preterm, it exposed similar abnormality of the periventricular white matter (represented by high intensity in $T_2$-weighted imaging, and low intensity in $T_1$

imaging). These lesions were interpreted pathologically as PVL and "dysmyelination".

On the other hand, the *spastic diplegics of term birth* showed diverse lesions including one with PVL, and two with brain anomalies (schizencephaly and corpo-cephaly). The significant conclusion was that the preterm birth is both a clinical and pathological entity.

## Continuous "Hyperintensity Areas": MRI

The significance of hyperintensity areas of periventricular distribution (on $T_2$-weighted MRI) (PVH) was specifically studied in 21 infants less than 12 months of age (Konishi et al., 1990). Ten of these infants had suffered neonatal asphyxia, intracranial haemorrhage in six, and three apnoea. In four of these, round foci of PVH

surrounded the frontal and occipital horns of the lateral ventricles. It is of importance that 14 infants showing continuous PVH had developed spastic diplegia or tetraplegia, and that the extent of PVH appears to reflect the severity of neonatal brain damage.

## Contribution of Computed Tomography

In a retrospective analysis of CT scans in 76 children with CP but without any severe intellectual handicap, CT abnormalities were exposed in 63%, and in the preterm the proportion rose as high as 88%. This highlights the ominous role of PVL in CP since it appeared in 45% of this series of preterm.

The lesions are *mainly posterior*, and generally *bilateral and symmetrical*, affecting contours of lateral ventricles which become straight and angular whilst being associated

with ventriculomegaly in 85%. In a few cases (6%) there were localized juxta-ventricular hypodensities. Cognitive and intellectual sequelae were more severe in those whose CT examination was abnormal. They were also more pronounced when the longitudinal fissure of the cerebrum is enlarged.

The ultimate sequelae in other large series of periventricular leukomalacia were also significant. In the MRI analysis of 30 infants suspected of having suffered perinatal asphyxia by Steinlin et al. (1991), *severe cortical necrosis* was diagnosed in 11 children on the basis of $T_2$ hyperintensity areas in white matter with blurred limits to the cortex in the early MRI exposure. Of these eleven, eight were to manifest *severe* CP and three of moderate degree.

In another series of 95 full-term and preterm infants undergoing MRI monitoring by Cioni et al. (1992) until at least 12 months of corrected age, 32 demonstrated severe neurological outcomes, mainly of cerebral palsy sometimes associated with mental retardation and/or cerebral disorder of visual perception. *At 12 months of age*, the principal categories of abnormal images were within the white matter and area of cortical atrophy, including cystic lesions, ventriculomegaly with irregular outlines, high intensity areas in the long tracts, and evidence of delayed myelination.

# SPASTIC DIPLEGIA WITH DEFECTS OF VISUAL PERCEPTION

## Associated Disturbances in MRI Localization of Neuropathogenesis

In conditions producing spastic diplegia or tetraplegia, *the optic radiation* will be vulnerable as it passes through the posterior limb of the internal capsule. The upper fibres run directly through the subcortical white matter of the occipital lobe to the *upper lip of the calcarine sulcus* on its medial aspect. The cortical areas lying above and below the calcarine sulcus comprise the *visual cortex*.

In the series of 12 such children in whom visual disturbance was associated with spastic diplegia (Koeda et al., 1990), *the underlying lesions were identified by MRI in ten*. In these, the pathology was localized to periventricular white matter which extends to the semiovale centre as well as to the subcortical white matter of parietal and occipital lobes.

Anatomically, these lesions corresponded to the *superior longitudinal bundle* and the vertical occipital bundle, comprising vertical neuronal columns, the functional correlates of which are best demonstrated in the visual cortex. The mechanism underlying the disturbance of visual perception is therefore suggested as a "disconnection" or interruption by one of the pathogenic lesions hitherto described at some stage of these higher visual pathways.

# CEREBRO-CORTICAL DYSGENESIS AND
# MRI IDENTIFICATION

Dorsal induction marks the third or fourth weeks of gestation, the neural plate folding to produce the neural tube. Failure to close at the cephalad end may lead to anencephaly or encephalocele, whilst failure to close caudally results in myelomeningocele.

The mesencephalon then divides to face the telencephalon, with failure at this stage resulting in prosencephaly. The germinal matrix generates the neurones which migrate to form the cortex. Interruption of such migration or failure to form such normal cortical layers brings about heterotopia. The gross anatomical malformations are readily demonstrable by MRI, including holoprosencephaly, Dandy-Walker syndrome and other conditions.

## Agenesis or Partial Agenesis of the Corpus Callosum

May also represent a complete or partial agenesis of the cingulate gyrus and of the septum pellucidum - development of which depends or follows evolution of the corpus callosum. Another striking anatomical association is the presence of a longitudinal bundle embodying nerve fibres unable to cross to the opposite hemisphere via the corpus callosum which has failed to appear.

Two principal versions of their clinical manifestation may obtain. Firstly, in that described by Erdlinger and colleagues in 1972. Seizures and mild to moderate mental retardation are associated. The second version encompasses many morphological anomalies of the cerebrum comparable to the neuroectodermal defects of proliferation and migration to be next outlined. These mainly include disorders of cellular proliferation and migration leading to micropolygyrus, heterotopias of grey matter and other migrational disorders which may arise in one instance as a result of materno-foetal infection such as with cytomegalovirus. An X-linked disorder of this kind linked to severe intellectual retardation and seizures was documented by Menkes, Phillipart and Clark (1964).

In addition, each of several chromosomal anomalies may be an important source. Curiously enough this includes the three trisomy syndromes of 4p, 8 and 13. There is scientific interest in that even an inborn metabolic error may be associated either as source or sequel of agenesis of both corpus callosum and cingulate gyrus. Lactic acidaemia may be one such, and another is a valine metabolic defect due to deficiency of 3-hydroxy isobutyryl CoA diacyclase. Accumulation of methacrylyl CoA is one outcome.

Both the partial and complete forms may be identified by either CT scanning, or more comprehensively by MRI.

228

# Neuroectodermal Defects

## Neuroectodermal Dysplasias

This group of neuroectodermal or neurocutaneous syndromes are characterized by specific changes in both skin and nervous system which both derive from ectoderm, including Neurofibromatosis, Tuberous sclerosis and Sturge-Weber disease. They are all clearly definable by MRI.

## Neuroectodermal Proliferation and Migrational Disturbances

These must in general originate during the peak period for neuroepithelial proliferation and migration in the human cerebral cortex. Primarily these defects lead to abnormalities in the form and architecture of the cerebral hemisphere. These anomalies range from failure of gyral formation (lissencephaly) through formation of abnormally large gyri (pachygyria) to numerous abnormally small gyri (polymicrogyria). These gyral anomalies are compatible in timing with mid-second trimester damage.

MRI has also served to dramatically reveal major migrational defects as the outcome of specific prenatal infections. Two groups of such cases deserve special attention. Firstly the 1991 report by the Japanese team of Sugita et al. of two child victims of the prenatal rubella syndrome and of an impressive series of six with cytomegalovirus. Cranial MRI with $T_2$-weighted spin-echo and inversion recovery sequences was able to clearly identify parenchymal lesions and much more effectively than CT in the following patterns:

1. Migrational defects leading to oligo-pachygyria in two cases.
2. Periventricular hyperintensity in four cases.
3. *Subcortical* hyperintensity in five.
4. Delayed myelination in four.
5. Cerebellar hypoplasia in two.

Moreover, a clear correlation was demonstrated between the degrees of disability and MRI abnormality. The MRI elucidation of major migrational defects was even more convincingly demonstrated by Hayward et al. in 1991 in five examples of congenital cytomegalovirus encephalopathy. The defects were consistent anatomically with the spectrum of lissencephaly-pachygyria, hitherto occasionally ascribed to chromosomal abnormality or unknown early prenatal insults. The neuroradiological delineation was of "broad flat gyri, shallow sulci, and incomplete opercularisation". The associated white matter and myelin pathology were exposed in the white matter hypodensity of CT scans or increased signal intensity on long-TR MRI scans, along with the apparently related ventriculomegaly and periventricular calcifications. MRI thus achieves superior definition of the nature and extent of gyral and white matter abnormalities resulting from the effects of severe cytomegalovirus infection upon neuronal growth, maturation and development. These two major reports in one year of a considerable series of migrational cortical dysgenesis as the basis for severe spastic tetraplegia certainly suggests that this underlying pathogenesis may be much commoner than hitherto suspected.

## Localization of Cerebral Dysfunction or
## Aberrant Cerebral Metabolism
## by use of PET or its SPECT Modification

Apart from morphological changes, specific functional defects, including those of perfusion and autoregulation may be identifiable and measurable by new technical methods, especially of PET and the related valuable research tool: c = 99m HMPAO SPECT. Thus in a study of 13 children with CP (Denays et al., 1990) it has been possible to demonstrate *localized cerebral hypoperfusion*, remarkably relatable in localization to the underlying dysfunction. *In all children with hemiplegia*, for example,

SPECT revealed *hypoperfusion* in the hemisphere contralateral to the motor deficit. In mild diplegia, the SPECT findings were negative, whereas in patients with moderate di- or tetraplegia, there was bilateral hypoperfusion in the superior motor cortex. This correlationship with clinical severity is an especially challenging result, with reduction of perfusion extending to the superior and inferior motor cortex as well as the prefrontal and parietal cortices in patients with severe di- or tetraplegia.

# CHOREO-ATHETOSIS

## MRI Localization of Basal Ganglia Pathology

The major constituents of athetosis have been described in Chapter  . In the main they constitute a variety of involuntary movements leading to impairment of postural stability and to oral motor dysfunction.

Of underlying cerebral pathology, CT served to reveal no more than non-specific abnormalities such as *ventricular dilatation* and *cortical atrophy*. Lesions specifically concentrated within basal ganglia or thalamus, and typically ascribed to acute ischaemic or hypoxic processes, have recently been clearly demarcated through MRI.

A recent study of 22 athetoid children between the ages of 2 and 12 years by Yokochi et al. (1991), using a slice thickness of 7 mm, illustrates the more precise localization of cerebral damage in athetotic CP to the basal ganglia and thalamus which MRI has made possible. In six of these, symmetrical high intensity areas involved both the *putamen and thalamus*. In five these areas were confined to the thalamus and *the putamen* was solely affected in one, mainly in its dorsal parts. In another six, the symmetrical high intensity areas were periventricular, mainly peritrigone and in the dorsal part of the body of the lateral ventricles.

More specifically in 10 of 11 children in whom *thalamic* pathology was identified, it was mainly in the lateral and middle parts thought to represent the *ventro-lateral nucleus*. They were also able to recognize *status marmoratus*, the excessive but abnormal myelination in the basal ganglia and/or thalamus hitherto usually attributed to perinatal hypoxic-ischaemic damage. Other lesions in the globus pallidum were reported as "status demyelination" showing *reduced densities of myelinated fibres* in damaged gliotic structures thought to reflect bilirubin encephalopathy. Where the lesions had been limited to cerebral white matter in this series, a mild motor developmental defect was the only outcome. The postulated causative factors strongly lent towards perinatal asphyxia, 16 cases being so identified, with attribution to perinatal jaundice in two.

A recent clarification of status marmoratus was achieved on high-field MRI by Menkes and Curran (1993). It is worth pointing out that prior CT scanning had failed to show more than non-specific abnormality such as ventricular dilatation and focal cortical damage. In the analysis of severe athetoid CP by Hayashi et al. in 1991, they divided them neuropathologically into two groups on the basis of neuro-image findings, especially of MRI. Their study included ten patients described as having suffered perinatal asphyxia on the basis of abnormal blood pH, Apgar scores and neonatal period. Subsequent development of severe choreiform movements, or a mixed picture of choreo-athetosis and dystonia, and in four of them a seizure disorder, were related to characteristic focal high signal on

$J_2$-weighted images in the *posterior putamen* and *antero-lateral thalamus*. Borderline mental retardation marked two of them, profound retardation only in one. Menkes also suggested that the scan may appear normal despite the cerebral palsied child's mild to moderate extrapyramidal movements. This may not hold true when progressive refinement of neuro-imaging techniques can eventually ensure the even more precise delineation of pathology in the basal ganglia.

An even more discrete localization of cerebral pathology was achieved in the nineties by the Hammersmith team of Rutherford, Dubowitz et al. especially as recorded in 1992, in three children in whom the athetoid element was already manifest during the first year of life. Symmetrical bilateral cystic lesions were confined to the posterior putamen in all three following upon haemorrhage into the basal ganglia associated with what was presumed to be hypoxic-ischaemic encephalopathy.

### The Globo-Luysian Group and the Thalamo-Putaminal group

The major sites in the first group were in the globus pallidus and subthalamic nucleus, whereas in the second group they were in both thalamus and putamen although with more widespread and often fibrillary gliosis extending into the central grey matter of the midbrain. The subthalamic nuclei were described as predominantly devastated. Severe perinatal jaundice and neonatal asphyxia had been the principal causative factors. Clinically, in the first group, rigid spasticity had been demonstrable in parallel with fluctuating athetosis, whereas in the thalamo-putaminal group, variations in hypertonicity accompanied a milder degree of athetosis.

## Fahr's syndrome

A rare condition associated with idiopathic cerebral symmetrical calcification, has also been subjected to a more recent analysis through CT scanning, even though the intracranial calcification on radiography has long been well known.

Its clinical manifestation may be of an extrapyramidal disorder which is characterized by an encephalopathy associated with cerebral calcifications, particularly prominent in the basal ganglia. Its deposits mark the *caudate*, and *putamen*, as well as the dentate nuclei, similar to those in hypoparathyroidism, the internal capsule being relatively spared. Now known as *Fahr's syndrome*, it has hitherto been described as *familial strio-cerebellar calcinosis*.

Clinical manifestations are in keeping with slowly progressive basal gangliar involvement, ranging from simple generalized rigidity to athetosis. Dystonic manifestations and cerebellar ataxia have also been reported. Occasionally it presents from infancy whether or not associated with mental retardation. Familial occurrence has been frequent. A similar localization and calcification occurs in mitochondrial encephalomyopathy, as well as in disorders involving calcium metabolism such as hypoparathyroidism or pseudohypopara-thyroidism.

A substantial personal series of 14 examples was presented by Billard et al.

(1989). They proposed a four group classification:

1. An autosomal recessive inheritance is claimed with dwarfism, retinal degeneration and optic atrophy as the principal features. An unknown underlying process embodies symmetrical patchy demyelination, associated or followed by the calcification. Some cases have an early onset and rapid evolution.
2. *An isolated congenital encephalopathy* which has produced a *cerebral palsy syndrome* not hitherto reported. A causative basis of sporadic non-progressive anoxo-ischaemia or viral prenatal disease has been suggested.
3. Encephalopathy has been associated, microcephaly and persistent cerebro-spinal fluid lymphocytes.
4. This time, the inheritance of the disorder with basal ganglia calcification appears to be autosomal dominant.

A striking illustration of a similar basal ganglia involvement simulating athetotic cerebral palsy has been identified in a progressive metabolic disorder associated with athetosis. This has been found in glutaryl acyl CoA dehydrogenase deficiency. Cystic degeneration within the striatum was visualized through MRI.

## Basal Ganglia Haemorrhage

The prospective MRI study of 100 high risk neonates by Keeney, Adcock and McArdle (1991) included five term infants with bilateral haemorrhagic lesions of the basal ganglia. *Punctate hyperintensity* on $T_1$-weighted images and hypointensity on $T_2$-weighted images were reported, all nuclei of the basal ganglia being involved especially caudate and putamen. The thalamus was only occasionally involved in three of the five, and one infant also demonstrated lesions of the PV white matter.

Follow-up imaging in four of the five revealed "residual calcification in one, cysts in two and resolution of the lesions in one. Athetotic CP was the expected neuro-

developmental outcome. Apart from PVL in 12 of Keeney et al's study (1991), other pathogenic lesions associated with hypoxic-ischaemic encephalopathy and detectable by MRI included multicystic encephalomalacia (in five), and focal parenchymal haemorrhage (in 15 infants) but not associated with intraventricular haemorrhage.

# CEREBELLAR AND RELATED PATHOLOGY UNDERLYING ATAXIC SYNDROMES: MRI LOCALIZATIONS

The term Ataxic CP has been applied to a wide range of very different conditions manifesting first with hypotonia, and the ataxia emerging after either 18 months or so or after several years. The recent application of MRI to five non-progressive ataxic subjects by Immamura and his colleagues (1992) has thrown an interesting light on cerebro-cerebellar pathology underlying these differences.

The typical clinical course in each began with hypotonia, usually identified from 4 to 7 months of age. Floppiness and hypotonia was clearly in evidence from 7 months of age in the first child, a girl of 3 years, with ataxia and some hypertonicity in the legs being first observed beyond 18 months of age. *Generalized atrophy of the cerebellum*, especially in the anterior-superior, was identified on MRI. Slight *atrophy of the pons* was also associated.

In the second child, a girl of 8, first manifesting ataxia at 17 months of age,

there was a similar MRI finding of cerebellar atrophy also of the anterior-superior part. The third child, a boy of 10, had been hypotonic from early infancy, but ataxia only manifested from 4 years of age. Here again dwarfism and bilateral cataracts coexisted in a case proving to be an example of Marinesco-Sjogren syndrome. Again linked to that of the pons, a generalized spino-ponto-cerebellar atrophy was identifiable. This finding was replicated in the fourth child, whose initial hypotonia had been unmistakable from 4 months. The fifth child, whose head-nodding and bilateral nystagmus were also first observed at 4 months, was lacking in speech development, but did not show ataxia until 8 years of age. MRI revealed *agenesis of the anterior medullary velum* and *cranium bifidum*.

In the MRI of two ataxic children assessed in 1993 by Russell and Lingam at the London Hornsey Centre for Cerebral Palsied Children there was an important isolated finding of what was defined as *"atrophy"* rather than agenesis or hypoplasia of the vermis, the synaptic terminus of the spino-cerebellar tract. It remains for us to clarify the precise nature of such defects.

Ataxic cerebral palsy associated with mental retardation, microcephaly and deafness was the sequel in nine children from 2 months to 8 years (Boesch et al., 1989) who had suffered congenital cytomegalovirus infections. These were comparable to the five examples reported more recently by Hayward et al. (1992) whose cases manifested spastic tetraplegia and underlying lissencephaly.

In contrast, in the cases of Boesch et al. (1989) oligopachygyria was the developmental lesion identified, together with other principal features exposed on MRI as follows:

Dilated lateral ventricles, and subarachnoid space

Delayed/pathological myelination

Paraventricular cysts (the cysts were adjacent to the occipital horns of the lateral ventricles, separated therefrom solely by a thin membrane)

Intracranial calcification was also identified on MRI, although CT scanning is more effective in revealing such calcifications.

# FOCAL EPILEPTOGENIC AREAS: MRI IN THEIR IDENTIFICATION

Localized developmental gyral anomalies detected by MRI were studied by Guerrini et al. (1992) in ten patients (mean age: 15 years 6 months). Two groups of such major malformation were identified:

1. Seven with unilateral "macrogyric" insulo-opercular changes. One died early in life, revealing exclusive microgyria, six had mental retardation and epilepsy with focal neurological signs.
2. Three with abnormal gyri, bulging grey matter and ventricular deformity. Focal cortical dysplasia was associated with intractable complex partial seizures underlying focal EEG anomalies closely correlated with a well-defined eliptogenic zone that was identifiable by MRI.

CT brain scans were used by Wiklund et al. (1991) in a population-based study of 83 children born at term, classified to reflect the phase of cerebral maturation during which the underlying pathology originated. The most common finding proved to be *periventricular atrophy* (regarded as representing PVL) in 37%. Cerebral maldevelopment due to a very early intrauterine lesion was exposed in 17%, and cortical/subcortical lesions in 16%. In other words, the CT findings indicated *a prenatal origin in 57%*. Imaging portrayal of brain morphology provided by CT brain scanning also therefore emerges as an important adjunct to clinical assessment.

# ULTRASOUND FOETOMETRY OR
# FOETAL SONOGRAPHY

Recognition of an underweight foetus by ultrasound foetometry (Hohenhauer, 1980) was one facet of its potential use.    Hohler (1985) provides an excellent analysis of its application in the diagnosis and monitoring of intra-uterine growth retardation.

## Prenatal Destructive Brain Lesions and
## Foetal Serial Abdominal Sonography

*Foetal brain injury*, although strongly suspected, may be asymptomatic or exhibit few clinical signs during the neonatal period.  On the other hand, in the study of Soher et al. (1991) six neonates were presented in whom radiological and neurophysiological studies indicated *the foetal onset* of destructive brain lesions, CP being subsequently documented in all six. In two, the maternal histories were apparently significant of either placental bleeding or toxaemia during the second or third trimester.  In both, *serial abdominal sonography* clearly documented foetal porencephaly which had presumably resulted from intraventricular haemorrhage. There were no neurological or other abnormal signs at birth.  However, four subsequently showed isolated seizures at 8-30 hours of life.  CT within the initial 30 hours confirmed the cerebral pathology. Initial documentation of cerebral lesions by foetal sonography, or CT scanning during the initial 30 hours, timed the lesions to the antepartum period.    Neurological examination and neuro-imaging in the immediate newborn period is recommended for neonates believed to have such cerebral lesions based upon maternal sonography or even upon the evidence of isolated seizures.

There could be a helpful role for such serial maternal foetal sonography where there is evidence of chronic foetal distress and a foetal heart rate pattern suggesting the genesis of cerebral palsy.

In the analysis of suspected perinatal antecedents in 75 infants with cerebral palsy by Shields and Schifrin (1988), CP arose in association with acute intrapartum asphyxia in 8% and traumatic delivery in 11%.  On the other hand, there was evidence of *chronic foetal distress in 35%*.  This was mainly defined on the basis of *an unique pattern of foetal heart rate* which consisted of a normal baseline rate but persistently absent variability and mild variable deceleration with overshoot.  This pattern was often found in association with postmaturity and intrauterine growth retardation (a situation comparable to that which was found in the    intrauterine growth deficiency of Russell).

A prenatal cine-scanning of the foetal movement pattern may one day come to establish whether and in what way some early manifestations of cerebral palsy arise. Hypertonicity could be expressed by conspicuous restraint of limb movement

235

whilst abnormal floppiness could also be linked to severe limitation of foetal movement and the earliest reflection of underlying hypotonia. Likewise, intermittent tremor of hand and arm when apparently reaching out may be the very first recognizable indication of early atactic involvement.

# SPASTIC HEMIPLEGIA

## MRI Findings underlying its Identification and Possible Pathogenesis

CT findings sufficed to clarify evidence of unilateral cortical or subcortical cerebral maldevelopment in 18% of the 28 preterm infants with hemiplegic CP who underwent CT analysis by the Wiklund, Uvebrandt and Flodmark team in 1991. When the findings were classified in accordance with a system devised to reflect the phase of brain maturation during which the pathogenesis of hemiplegia is likely to have arisen, periventricular leukomalacia was diagnosed in 50%, being labelled as PV atrophy, although considered to represent PVL, in 37%.

Other studies, detailed in Chapter 6, highlighted the possibly associated pathogenic mechanism in terms of unilateral cerebro-cortical *hypoperfusion,* demonstrable through a specific positron emission tomographic extension of the SPECT technique.

## References

Anderson JC, Mawk JR. (1988) Intrauterine arterial duplex Doppler wave form analysis in infants. Childs Nerv Syst 4: 144-148

Anthony MY, Levene MI. (1993) Neonatal cranial ultrasound. In: Recent Advances in Paediatrics. Churchill Linvingstone, Edinburgh, London 6: 85-102

Billard C et al. (1989) Encephalopathy with calcification of the basal ganglia in children: A reappraisal of Fahr's syndrome with respect to 14 new cases. Neuropediatr 20: 2-9

Boesch C et al. (1989) Magnetic resonance imaging of brain in congenital cytomegalovirus encephalopathy. Pediatr Radiol 19: 91-93

Byrne P, Welch R, Johnson MA, Darrah J, Piper M. (1990) Serial magnetic resonance imaging in neonatal hypoxic-ischaemic encephalopathy. J Pediat 117: 694-700

Cioni L et al. (1992) Neuroimaging and functional outcome of PVL. Behav Brain Res 49: 7-19

Denays R et al. (1989) Brain single photon emission computed tomography in neonates. J Nuclear Med 30: 1337-1341

Denays R et al. (1990) Cerebral palsy: initial experiences with Tc-99m HMPAO SPECT of the brain. Radiology 175: 111-116 de Vries LS, Regev R, Pennock JM, Wigglesworth JS, Dubowitz LM. (1988) Ultrasound evolution and later outcome of infants with periventricular densities. Early Hum Dev 16: 225-233

Dubowitz LMS, Bydder GM, Muskin J. (1985) Developmental sequence of periventricular leukomalacia correlation of ultrasound, clinical and nuclear magnetic resonance function. Arch Dis Child 60: 349-355

Erdlinger G et al. (1972) Agenesis of the corpus callosum: a behavioural investigation. Brain 95: 327

Feldman HM, Scher MS, Kemp SS. (1990) Pediat Neurol 6: 276-302

Guerrini R et al. (1992) Epilepsy and focal gyral anomalies detected by MRI: electroclinico-morphological correlations. Dev Med Child Neurol 34: 706-718

Hayashi M, Satoh J, Saramoto K, Morimatsu Y. (1991) Clinical and neuropathological findings in severe athetoid cerebral palsy: a comparative study of globo-Luysian and thalamo-putaminal groups. Brain Dev 13: 47-51

Hohenhauer L. (1980) Intrauterine Wachstumskuroen fur den deutchen Sprachraum. Z. Geburtsh Perinotol 184: 167

Hohler CW. (1985) Ultrasound diagnosis of intrauterine growth retardation. In: RC Sanders, AE James Jr. (Eds) Principles and Practice of Ultrasonography in Obstetrics and Gynecology. Appleton-Century-Crofts, Norwalk, connecticut. p 157

Ikonen RS, Janas MO, Koivikko MJ, Laippala P, Kuusinen EJ. (1992) Hyperbilirubinaemia, hypocarbia and periventricular leukomalacia leukamenia in preterm infants: relationship to cerebral palsy. Acta Paediat 81: 802-807

Immamura S et al. (1992) Ataxic cerebral palsy and brain imaging. No-To-Hattatsu 24: 441-448

Keeney SE, Adcock EW, McArdle CB. (1991) Prospective observations of 100 high risk neonates by high field (1,5 Tesia) magnetic resonance imaging of the central nervous system. I. Lesions associated with hypoxic-ischaemic encephalopathy. Pediatrics 87: 431-438

Koeda T et al. (1990) Spastic diplegia: comparative study. Preterm vs. term infants. Neuroradiol 32: 187-190

Koeda T et al. (1990) Disturbances of visual perception and the lesions in spastic diplegia. No-To-Shinkel 42: 759-763

Konishi Y, Kuriyama M, Hayakaior K et al. (1990) Periventricular hyperintensity detected by magnetic resonance imaging in infancy. Pediat Neurol 6: 229-232

Menkes JH, Curran J. (1993) Clinical and magnetic resonance imaging in children with extrpyramidal cerebral palsy. Proc 19th Meeting British Neurology Association, Institute of Child Health, London

Menkes JH, Phillipart M, Clark D. (1964) Hereditary partial agenesis of the corpus callosum. Arch Neurol 11: 198

Pasternak JF. (1987) Parasagittal infarction in neonatal asphyxia. Ann Neurol 21: 202-203

Russell A, Lingam S. (1992) Hereditary cerebellar ataxia with pathology identifiable in atrophy of the vermis by CT scanning. Unpublished data

Rutherford MA, Pennock JM, Murdoch-Eaton DM, Cowan FM, Dubowitz LM. (1992) Athetoid cerebral palsy with cysts in the putamen after hypoxic-ischaemic encephalopathy. Arch Dis Child 67: 846-858

Schouman-Claeys L, Picard A, Lalande G, Kalifa G, Lacert P, Brentanos E, Frija G. (1989) Contribution of computed tomography in aetiology and prognosis of cerebral palsy. Br J Radiol 62: 248-252

Cerebral Palsy Entities

Shields JR, Schifrin BS. (1988) Perinatal antecedents of cerebral palsy. Obstet Gynecol 71: 899-905

Shortland D, Levene MI, Trouncer J, Ng Y, Graham M. (1988) The evolution and outcome of cavitating periventricular leukomalacia in infancy: a study of 46 cases. J Perinatal Med 16: 241-246

Steinlin M et al. (1991) MRI following severe perinatal asphyxia. Pediat Neurol 7:

Tan WKM. (1992) Suppression of post-ischaemic epileptiform activity. Ann Neurol 37: 672-682

Truwit CL, Barkovich AJ, Koch TK, Ferriero DM. (1992) Cerebral palsy: MR findings in 40 patients. Am J Neuroradiol 13: 67-78

Volpe JJ. (1992) Brain injury in the premature infant - current concepts of pathogenesis and prevention. Biol Neonate 62: 231-242

Volpe JJ, Herscovitch P, Perlman JM, Raichle MF. (1983) Positron emission tomography in the newborn: extensive impairment of regional cerebral blood flow with IVH and haemorrhagic intracerebral involvement. Pediatrics 72: 589-601

Wiklund LM, Uvebrandt F, Flodmark O. (1991) Computerized tomography: 28 preterm infants with hemiplegic CP. Neuropaediat 22: 50-60

Yokochi K, Aiba K, Kodama M, Fujimoto S. (1991) Magnetic resonance imaging in athetotic cerebral palsied children. Acta Paediat Scand 80: 818-823

# SECTION II:

## NEUROPATHOPHYSIOLOGY

SECTION II

# 8

# DYNAMIC IMPLICATIONS OF NEUROPATHIC EVIDENCE, AND POSSIBLE PREVENTIVE IMPLICATIONS

Implications of Neuropathic Evidence

Periventricular/Intraventricular Haemorrhage

Subependymal/Germinal Matrix Haemorrhage

Primary Thalamic Haemorrhage

Intracerebral Haemorrhagic Involvement

Role of Cerebral Blood Flow

**Cerebral Blood Flow Velocity and the Doppler Technique**

Continuous Wave Doppler Ultrasound

**Haemodynamic Factors and Anoxic Damage**

**Preventive Applications**

**References**

# 8

# IMPLICATIONS OF
# NEUROPATHIC EVIDENCE

*Pre*natal or *peri*natal anoxia or ischaemia are prominent aetiological factors of cerebral damage. But haemorrhagic lesions of differing location and severity, germinal cell layer, peri and intraventricular, can also be crucially pathogenic, whether in association or not with the hypoxic-ischaemic factors. Metabolic abnormality in the neonate including *hypoglycaemia* may also play a part, as well as disorders of cerebral perfusion resulting from cerebral oedema and fluctuations in the way of hypotension or hypertension, possibly linked to failed auto-regulation of blood flow. These may or may not be superimposed upon cerebral dysgenesis such as stem from disorders of gyration, including polymicrogyria, or the sequelae of developmental or leukomalacic sequelae, such as *porencephaly*. These patho-physiological phenomena may participate directly and indirectly by induction of such ependymal matrix haemorrhage, and/or infarction in the area of the caudate nucleus or putamen, apart from other destructive hypoxic-ischaemic periventricular consequences such as leukomalacia.

In studies of the pathogenic role of periventricular haemorrhage and related bleeds, therefore, the variety of lesions represents a spectrum ranging from a small germinal layer haemorrhage (GLH) (Fig 7), through periventricular (PVH) and intraventricular haemorrhage (IVH) to varying degrees of parenchymal involvement such as may ultimately underlie different clinico- pathological entities of cerebral palsy. Indeed, most follow-up studies have indicated that such poor neuropathic outcome has been mainly associated with parenchymal lesions, conjoined with white matter damage linked to periventricular leukomalacia which is likely to constitute the major pathogenic factor.

Venous drainage of developing white matter is mainly via the thalamo-striate venous system, and this involves the subependymal matrix adjacent to the highly vascularized caudate nucleus. By the time the foetus attains potential viability towards the end of the second trimester, there is already a well-developed vascular bed supplying central parts of the cerebrum such as the thalamus and caudate nucleus.

Critical bleeds may occur in these areas, especially involving the striatum and subthalamic nuclei which are fundamentally involved in the future control of posture and movement, and likely to be the source of choreo-athetoid forms of cerebral palsy. Damage to intervening corticospinal pathways are more likely to be expressed in the spastic diplegias. The changing structure and functional anatomy of such cerebral components, and their associated vascular systems, will thus be reflected in a variable yet constant pattern of vulnerability to adverse influences including anoxic-ischaemic, interwoven with the direct and destructive effects of haemorrhage.

In practical terms, therefore, the site and extension of the initial bleed should remain a focus of primary prevention, particularly in the perspective of the probably associated hypoxic-ischaemic factors. In other words, the ultimate aim of prevention is how to prevent or minimise the initial bleed and limit its extension. Studies into its origin, both experimental and human, has led to the relevant matrix bed of capillaries and fine vascular spaces (Fig 7). And the strategy of prevention or limitation of that primary bleed is likely to focus on one or more vulnerable sites, and upon

haemodynamic changes that may well be operative. A delicate depression or *loss of autoregulation* of blood flow attributable to initial hypoperfusion related in turn to asphyxial hypotension, has been postulated. Restoration of normal blood pressure, or even transient hypertension after that initial local hypotension, may be the source of crucial impact upon capillary and fine vascular fragility or of some other mechanism. As already emphasized, the potential role of the choroid plexus as full-term approaches, and its vulnerability to such haemodynamic stresses should also be an especially worthy target of in-depth study.

# PERIVENTRICULAR/INTRAVENTRICULAR HAEMORRHAGE

These appear predominantly in premature infants, its incidence in infants less than 1500g being 40%. In 80% of these cases, the haemorrhage originating in the germinal matrix and periventricular zone extends into the intraventricular system. And in 15-25% of those infants, there is an associated cerebral or intraparenchymatous haemorrhage which strongly influences the prognosis. When co-existing with a severe (Grade III) haemorrhage, the expected mortality is 57% - more than half - with morbidity for major motor dysfunction or CP in the survivors reaching 87%.

The outcome depends upon either or both the severity of the haemorrhage and any association with an intra-parenchymatous bleed. The recent study by

Lin, Goh, Brown and Steers (1993) attempting to evaluate the topographical neurological distribution, patterns of abnormal tone and related functional neuromotor impairment in 33 children with previous grade 3 or 4 IPVH of mean gestational age 30.9 weeks (range 25-40 weeks) and mean birth-weight 1743 g (range 866-3600g), is more specific about the outcome. The neurological examination was at 4.7 years and neurological signs were equally distributed between the grade 3 and 4 IVH groups in 23 out of the 33 cases. The largest single distribution was in the form of hemiparesis in eight of the 23 children, in which tone was assessed as normal in seven, followed jointly by spastic diplegia and triplegia in six cases each, and tetraplegia in three cases. Grade 4 IVH, however, tended to produce asymmetrical syndromes: hemiparesis in seven out of eight cases and triplegia in five out of six.

## SUBEPENDYMAL/GERMINAL MATRIX HAEMORRHAGE

Unilateral or bilateral, this is the basic and commonest form of pre- and perinatal cerebral haemorrhage, again mainly in the preterm, especially in the region of the head of the caudate nucleus or with caudothalamic localization. At times, small haemorrhages, of less than 5 mm diameter, can be visualized in the preterm brain which are *difficult to distinguish from the normally echogenic choroid plexus*. Haemorrhage in this section may extend medially if not anteriorly or supero-laterally into the ventricle. Occasionally, however, it may extend inferiorly into the thalamus. *Subependymal cystic areas* often replace the original haemorrhage, and these could simply represent liquefaction of the haemorrhage, if not related to eventual periventricular leukomalacia.

A less common entity in the preterm is haemorrhage directly *into the choroid plexus*. This would be suspect should the choroid plexus be larger and more irregular than

## Germinal Matrix Haemorrhage and Hypoxia/Ischaemia

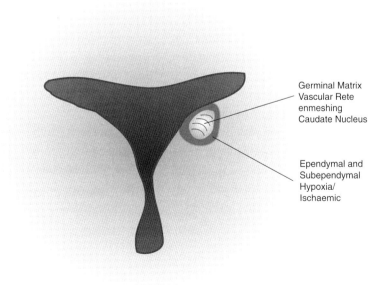

Germinal Matrix Vascular Rete enmeshing Caudate Nucleus

Ependymal and Subependymal Hypoxia/ Ischaemic

anticipated in the absence of a subependymal haemorrhage. There is a gradual reduction in size of the germinal matrix, so that when close to term, or beyond 32 weeks when the matrix is no longer in evidence, choroid plexus bleeding becomes the most common site (Fig 3). Even in the preterm, haemorrhage into the choroid plexus is believed to be the source in 25% of those with IVH (Hambleton and Wigglesworth, 1976). The site of origin of this haemorrhage is related to the gestational age. Before 28 weeks the germinal layer matrix overlies the body of the caudate nucleus, and the haemorrhage often involves this site. But between 28 and 32 weeks, the commonest focus of haemorrhage is within the matrix where it overlies the head of the caudate nucleus at the level of the foramen of Monro (Fig 7). Current evidence indicates that the haemorrhage originates in endothelial-lined vessels which after 28 weeks resemble mature capillaries, making up the vascular bed of the matrix. A more precise localization of the haemorrhage to its capillary-venule junctions has been suggested. A constant sequel is infarction with disorganization of the gelatinous matrix and destruction of adjacent cellular elements. Whether the infarction has an ischaemic or venous source, or is secondary to the haemorrhage rather than primary is not resolved.

The concept of subependymal haemorrhage as an initial bleed extending towards periventricular and intraventricular sites, therefore, has important preventive implications. Especially important would be the prevention of such periventricular haemorrhage, and of the periventricular leukomalacia consequent upon it, if not of the preceding or underlying ischaemic-hypoxic situation.

# PRIMARY THALAMIC HAEMORRHAGE

This specific clinical syndrome is associated with an unilateral thalamic haemorrhage (Fig 8). Although generally benign, it may penetrate into the lateral ventricle. It usually presents in the second week of life in a previously well infant who then has an acute onset of seizures and eye signs deviating towards the side of the lesion. The haemorrhagic localization can be clearly seen by ultrasound. Abnormal neurological signs may prevail for some time, but it is reassuring to learn that the majority have a good neurological outcome even by 18 months.

This lesion can be clearly distinguished from the lesion of *bright bilateral thalami* seen in asphyxiated infants who present at birth with a grave prognosis for neurological outcome.

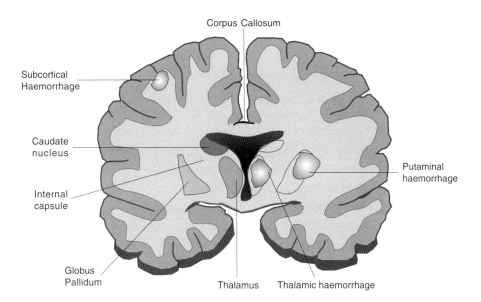

## Thalamic, Putaminal and Subcortical Haemorrhages

Corpus Callosum

Subcortical Haemorrhage

Caudate nucleus

Internal capsule

Globus Pallidum

Putaminal haemorrhage

Thalamus    Thalamic haemorrhage

# INTRACEREBRAL HAEMORRHAGIC INVOLVEMENT

Usually unilateral, and located dorsal and lateral to the lateral ventricle, this is one consequence in 15-20% of the more severe instances of IVH (Guzzetta et al., 1986).

The sequence of events leading to serious parenchymal haemorrhagic involvement is clearly, therefore, of primary preventative import. Bleeding penetrates from the germinal matrix, or from the ventricular cavity into the periventricular white matter to produce venous haemorrhagic infarction. Unilateral intraparenchymal *echodensities* on cranial ultrasound can illustrate this, as well as the acute distention of blood of the lateral ventricle. This may obstruct venous outflow to contribute to the acute venous infarction. Periventricular leukomalacia is also inevitably associated. It may follow obstruction to branches of the thalamo-striate veins by an initial subependymal bleed followed by secondary venous infarction. Another hypothesis supports a somewhat different sequence, that the dangerous parenchymal spread is secondary to a subependymal bleed into an area of PV leukomalacia already consequent upon ischaemia or other factors already frequently established in utero. The spread itself may also conceivably represent an extending process of venous infarction that may arise either secondarily to intraventricular haemorrhage, or primarily following ischaemic or subsequent bleeding into the damaged area, as well as into the adjacent ventricular system.

*Haemodynamic researches* have recently been focussed on an exploration of this sequence of events leading to a primary bleed within the capillary vascular bed, or a subependymal haemorrhage from one or more vulnerable sites, or to the critical lesion of periventricular leukomalacia per se. And its localization and that of the subependymal matrix particularly encroaches upon the region of the head of the caudate nucleus, and to a lesser extent upon the thalamus and its subthalamic nuclei. If the critical damage is within the confines of periventricular leukomalacia, it may emerge either before or after subependymal or germinal layer bleeding. A pathological extension of the leukomalacia would then be through its cystic changes, even to the extent of porencephalic dimensions which may not appear for one or two months. Within the basal ganglia themselves, spongiform changes may become grossly prominent. In the now rare circumstances of a kernicteric basis, there is also underlying degeneration within the basal ganglia associated with bilirubin impregnation of neurones in a pattern appropriate to the form of cerebral palsy characterizing this syndrome, leading to a triad of mental defect, deafness and athetosis.

# ROLE OF CEREBRAL BLOOD FLOW

Partly on the basis of experimental studies it is believed that abnormalities in cerebral blood flow could produce this sequence of cerebral damage. Germinal matrix haemorrhage in the beagle puppy can follow systemic hypertension with and without initial hypotension. The consequent increase of cerebral blood flow is secondary to raised perfusion pressures, or cerebral hyperfusion in the sick "asphyxiated" preterm infant where the cerebral circulation is apparently pressure-passive. Infarction which is probably primary to the periventricular leukomalacia is envisaged as a consequence of cerebral ischaemia secondary to systemic hypotension. But tissue ischaemia may also be secondary to raised venous pressure, itself subsequently producing infarction.

# CEREBRAL BLOOD FLOW VELOCITY
# AND THE DOPPLER TECHNIQUE

The velocity of blood flow in the anterior central artery, but not tissue perfusion, is measurable by the Doppler technique applied via the anterior fontanelle.

Two types of Doppler systems have been applied to study of the cerebral circulation: Continuous wave and Range-gated Doppler Ultrasound (Altman and Volpe, 1987).

## Continuous Wave Doppler Ultrasound

A bidirectional pencil-shaped probe is applied over the anterior fontanelle and oriented towards the pericallosal or terminal branch of the anterior cerebral artery. Arterial pulsations of advancing flow are detected by simultaneous aural (with an audio headset) and visual recording.

The pulse range-gate Doppler technique is able to selectively detect blood flow in a specific area. Exploiting this technique, the velocity can be measured from a small area within a vessel at a selected depth. Incorporating this instrument into a conventional ultrasound imaging instrument, and the specific vessel or for example arteries at the circle of Willis can

then be directly visualized through refinement of the linked ultrasonography, it will at last become practicable to measure the total volume of blood flow rather than solely its velocity.

The ultrasound beam virtually "looks down the barrel" of the vessel. Quantitation has used the pulsatility index (PI) to allow meaningful comparison of serial estimates of blood flow velocity. Serial measurements of PI may also reflect fluctuations in cerebral perfusion as well as cerebrovascular resistance. Cerebral blood flow as measured by positron emission tomography proved to be related to cerebral blood flow velocity (with a correlation coefficient of Q7).

# HAEMODYNAMIC FACTORS AND
# ANOXIC DAMAGE

The "global" variety of anoxic damage involves all structures of the cerebrum, although in respect of this factor, as distinct from haemorrhagic events, the basal ganglia and the cerebellum are usually spared. In neuro-imaging the affected areas are of low density equivalent to or lower than that of

normal white matter. These can be diagnosed with ease. As early as twenty-six weeks, infants die or survive with severe brain damage which may be expressed as severe generalized atrophy or a generalized cystic encephalomalacia. Such changes are typically complete by two to four weeks. If hydrocephalus should supervene because of haemorrhage or other reason, the damaged brain offers little resistance to the increased pressure, rapidly leading to gross ventricular dilatation. Diffuse cystic changes can be seen to be associated on CT.

Haemodynamic changes near the time of birth which are especially relevant appear to include hypotension swiftly followed by a local hypertensive impact. One hypothesis is that episodes of hypotension impair cerebral perfusion and oxygenation at the boundary zone between the medullary artery branches entering the white matter from the cortex and the thalamostriate artery branches supplying the ependyma, and the immediate periventricular white matter. This phenomenon has been supported by evidence presented by Sinha and colleagues (1985) of a significant association between clinical conditions causing hypotension and the development of PVL. So that *maintenance of an adequate or stable blood pressure* becomes a vital consideration in the prevention of the sequence of bleeding which can end in parenchymatous damage. That is, apart from cortical foci, which may sometimes lead to multiple areas of cortical scarring as well as *PV leukomalacia underlying ultimately severe cerebral palsy.* Intraventricular haemorrhage most often appears to reflect an extension of an initial subependymal haemorrhage. The significance of patho-physiology of movement and postural function stemming from damage to caudate, putamen, subthalamic and other related basal ganglia components (globus pallidus and substantia nigra), becomes a crucial area of study through the prenatal stage onto perinatal events.

# PREVENTIVE APPLICATIONS

An important facet with strong preventive implications, would be the possibility of *identifying the infant at extreme risk* for IVH, for instance with fluctuating blood pressure and cerebral blood flow velocity prior to the occurrence of the haemorrhage. Could the impending cerebral damage be averted by appropriate intervention? Fluctuating blood flow velocity and systemic blood pressure influences may have marked underlying changes in cerebral perfusion pressure and perhaps to blood flow.

Such change of perfusion and low flow, could give rise to tissue ischaemia and infarction, haemorrhage ensuing subsequently during hyperperfusion and raised blood pressure. In an impressive study of 50 ventilated preterm infants of less than 1500g, at especially high risk for IVH such as those suffering from the respiratory distress syndromes, Max Perlman and his colleagues (1983) showed a specifically aberrant pattern of cerebral blood flow velocity in 23, fluctuating systolic and diastolic pressures being identified as a valid predictor, at 12-24 hours of life, of subsequent IVH. Concomitant serial measure of arterial blood pressure exhibited fluctuations identical to those in the cerebral circulation. Twenty-one of the total of 23 cases subsequently developed IVH, whereas it emerged in only 7 of the 27 infants demonstrating a stable pattern. Pathogenesis of the fluctuant pattern appears to derive from changes in intrathoracic pressure associated with events such as attempts to breathe out of synchrony with the ventilator.

Logical application of these dramatic results led the Perlman team to attempt to prevent IVH by endeavouring to eliminate such fluctuations in cerebral blood flow velocity by the abolition of distressing respiratory effort via paralysis with *pancuronium*. None of the paralysed group developed severe IVH, although 5 of the 14 did produce a lesser degree of IVH. *IVH overtook all ten of the non-paralysed group.*

Other cerebro protective mechanisms to control the associated or primary hypoxic-ischaemic damage demand urgent exploration. Testing in the experimental animal has included the scavenging manipulation of free radicals just referred to, blockade of excitatory neurotransmitters, immunomodulation and the effects of hypothermia. *Near infrared spectroscopy (NIRS)* may provide the effectively direct measure required to monitor cerebral oxygenation and foetal haemodynamics during labour. The practical possibilities of being able to more precisely delineate the indications for a broadening of the preventive or therapeutic role and timing of *maternal hyperoxygenation* in this context, to which we have already referred in relation to *intra-uterine growth retardation* (Chapter 1), also remains to be addressed.

## References

Altman DS, Volpe JJ. (1987) Cerebral blood flow in the newborn infant: Measurement and role in the pathogenesis of PV and IV haemorrhage. Adv Pediat 34: 111-138

Guzzetta FF, Shackelford GD, Volpe S, Perlman JM, Volpe JJ. (1986) Periventricular intraparenchymal echodensities in the premature newborn. Critical determinant of neurologic outcome. Pediatrics 78: 995-1006

Hambleton G, Wigglesworth JS. (1976) Origin of intraventricular haemorrhage in the preterm infant. Arch Dis Child 5: 651-659

Perlman JM, McMenamin JB, Volpe JJ. (1983) Fluctuating cerebral blood flow velocity in the respiratory disress syndrome. Relation to the development of IVH. New Engl J Med 309: 204-209

Sinha SK, Davies JM, Sims DG, Chiswick ML. (1985) Relation between periventricular haemorrhage and ischaemic brain lesions diagnosed by ultrasound in very premature. Lancet 2: 1154-1156

# 9

# SIGNIFICANCE OF CEREBRAL VENTRICULAR DILATATION, IN RELATION TO PERIVENTRICULAR HAEMORRHAGE AND NEUROPATHIC OUTCOME

Implications of Cerebral Ventricular Dilatation

Prenatal Hydrocephalus

Colpocephaly

References

# IMPLICATIONS OF CEREBRAL
# VENTRICULAR DILATATION

In earlier clinico-pathological analyses related to the opportunities provided by ultrasound techniques (Palmer et al., 1982), neuropathogenic emphasis was placed upon ventricular dilatation mainly as consequent upon germinal layer and intraventricular haemorrhages (IVH) (Palmer et al., 1982). These have been estimated to occur in about half of very low birth-weight and pre-term infants (Papile et al., 1978; Thorburn et al., 1981). Of the 39 preterm infants studied by Palmer and her colleagues, 11 revealed ventricular dilatation as well as IVH. In five, the preceding haemorrhage had been moderate or Grade II, whilst the prior IV haemorrhage had been large or Grade III in five. Ultrasound scanning had enabled not only the early diagnostic identification of such haemorrhage, but also the serial monitoring of its evolution and resolution, as well as of the changes in ventricular size to which these workers had been alerted (Palmer et al., 1982). On the basis of ultrasound measurements at the level of the body of the lateral ventricle, ventricular dilatation was considered to have been defined if the ventricular index (distance between lateral ventricle and falx on an axial scan through the temporo-parietal region) increased from normal values to above the 97th centile for gestational age (Levene and Starte, 1981), or if the distance from roof to floor of the lateral ventricle (Levene, 1981) exceeded 6mm.

Of importance also were the pre- and perinatal complications that appeared to especially mark the subjects of ventricular dilatation. In all infants showing evidence of both intraventricular haemorrhage and ventricular dilatation, this had been preceded by the especial stresses of the respiratory distress syndrome, recurrent apnoea, proved sepsis, or necrotizing enterocolitis (Palmer et al., 1982) although one of these had preceded IVH alone in over half, and in one third of the controls. Each such clinical situation provides opportunities for primary preventive approaches towards most of the peri-natal group of causes of cerebral palsy.

*Hypertonia* was considered a significant sequel in the series of Palmer et al. (1982), recorded in their tabulation in 2 of 12 examples solely of IVH, and in 3 of 9 examples with ventricular dilatation in association with IVH. Of the survivors in this group, neurological abnormality was definable in 8 of 14 examined at one year. Five showed mild hypertonia. Of especial significance in the light of my emphasis upon understanding the basis of associated disabilities in different clinico-pathological entities of cerebral palsy, is their record of suspected *hearing* or *visual impairment in 4 of 12 instances solely of IVH*, and in as much as *4 examples out of 9 when linked to ventricular dilatation*. Hypotonia was instead confirmed on neurodevelopmental examination at 12 months of age in 2 of 14 cases showing solely IVH, and in 2 of 10 examples also with ventricular dilatation. The especially significant aspect was that 10 victims of large IVH and dilatation of ventricles revealed major neuropathic handicap, including profound sensori-neural deafness and visual impairment. In one infant in whom cerebral atrophy had been exposed alongside ventricular dilatation, overt evidence of spastic tetraplegia had preceded death at four months. *Hemiparesis emerged in at least half of the infants showing significant ventricular dilatation.* Indeed, the conclusion of Palmer and colleagues (1982) was that in those infants who developed either transient or persistent ventricular dilatation after IVH, a high incidence of serious neurological abnormality, even reaching 60%, is to be expected. They believed this to be irrespective of the size of the preceding intraventricular haemorrhage. This contrasts with the study of the Thorburn team (1981) which supported the view that the size of the initial haemorrhage was the principal determinant of neuropathic outcome. Although at least three reports (Robinson and Desai, 1981; Ment et al., 1982; Fitzhardinge et al., 1982) have failed to substantiate this, several other studies have supported an adverse relationship between the severity of periventricular haemorrhage and ultimate neurodevelopmental consequences. Fifty-six infants of the extreme preterm series of Catto-Smith et al. (1985) were examined at the corrected age of 2 years by multidisciplinary testing including cerebral ultrasonography and the Bayley indices of mental and psychomotor development. Periventricular haemorrhages were identified in 61% (34), germinal bleeds in 12 (22%), intraventricular haemorrhage in 18 (32%), extending intracerebrally in 4. Six or 19% of the 31 survivors manifested cerebral palsy, 4 with tetraplegia, and a mental developmental index below 50 in

three of these. Only one survivor with no periventricular haemorrhage suffered a major disability compared with 11 (55%) of survivors with PVH. The incidence of major disability amongst those with lesser or no haemorrhage (3 of 19 or 16%) was lower than those with more severe haemorrhage, 9 of 12 or 75% (p <0.02, Fisher's exact test).

In a study of 154 consecutive survivors of birth-weight 500-1500 g (Kitchen et al., 1990), of 39 in whom serial cranial ultrasonography had detected abnormality, CP was confirmed in only 7 (17.9%). These included, however, ventricular dilatation with or without cerebrovascular haemorrhage. They claimed furthermore that this degree of ventricular involvement had the highest positive predictive value (40%). An Australian analysis (Tudehope et al., 1989) of 153 very low birth-weight babies with CP, with 146 survivors being assessed at 2 years, the prevalence of ventricular dilatation was 19.9% (4.1% necessitating a ventriculo-peritoneal shunt).

The possible bases for the weighting of the neuropathic outcome by the ventricular dilatation per se was also touched upon by Thorburn et al. (1981). They suggested that it may reflect a more generalized cerebral abnormality by virtue of compression of the cerebral mantle with consequent reduction in the cell population, akin to an hydrocephalic element of which there is only very occasional evidence. A particularly strong predictive correlationship between ventriculomegaly and CP was drawn by Feldman, Scher and Kemp (1990). In an MRI series of 15 children (8 months and older) in whom increased white matter signal on $T_2$-weighted images with ventricular enlargement adjacent to those regions of abnormal white matter, 12 manifested CP with significant sensory impairment in five.

Noting, however, that the ventricular dilatation can be a transient phenomenon, it has been questioned whether, or to what degree, it has any primary pathogenic role. Is it rather a secondary reflection of anoxic/ischaemic white-matter disintegration, with or without associated severe intraventricular or periventricular haemorrhage? Its tendency to persist after PVL supports the latter hypothesis. So does the added definition of cerebral abnormality underlying CP achieved by Schouman-Claeys et al. (1989) in a retrospective analysis of CT scans in a series of 76 children with CP without any associated severe intellectual handicap. In highlighting the pathogenic role played by periventricular leukomalacia in CP, the CT scanning revealed that the abnormalities, generally bilateral, symmetrical and posterior, were concentrated upon the contours of the lateral ventricles which become straight and angular, and were accompanied by ventriculomegaly in as many as 85% of these children. On the other hand, it has already been emphasized that unilaterality of the ventricular dilatation has been exposed on ultrasonography of hemiplegic CP, whilst it was possible to demonstrate crossed cerebellar diaschisis in five of 25 hemiplegic children studied by a SPECT technique using N-isopropyl-p-1-123-iodoamphetamine (Hamano et al., 1991). Unilateral lesions in the periventricular region were also shown on MRI to be the underlying basis of congenital hemiplegia by van Bogaert et al. (1991).

# PRENATAL HYDROCEPHALUS

The ultrasound identification of prenatal hydrocephalus through measure of the biparietal diameter estimated by repeated ultrasonic examination, is usually belated, and at a mean fetal age of 30.5 weeks or more. The integrated growth curve of pre- and postnatal cranial growth modified by Evrard (1984) could be usefully exploited in such studies, and indeed in any phase of the natural history of prenatal brain disorders.

Plotting the progression of lateral ventricular dilatation has long provided an important clinical use for real-time neonatal cranial ultrasound. Levene (1981) has related ventricular dimensions to the range of normal values for a given gestational age through measurements in the coronal plane at the level of the foramina of Monro. Holt (1989) has refined these dimensions by expressing ventricular size vs bi-parietal diameter as a ratio: that for mild dilatation to severe ranging from <0.4 to >0.6 respectively. Cohen, Haller and Pollark (1990) have attempted to reinforce this process by pursuing the evolution of fenestrations in the septum pellucidum through serial scanning in infants with post-haemorrhagic hydrocephalus. Such early scanning, from 4 days to 23 weeks after first recognizing the hydrocephalus, would not only clearly differentiate such an acquired threat from congenital absence of the septum but could accelerate the opportunity for prophylactic and therapeutic intervention.

Not only could critical nerve tracts on a periventricular course be subjected to growing pressure effects exerted by distending lateral ventricular walls, but vascular distortions within and adjacent to them could contribute to disturbances of flow and supply towards important visual and auditory pathways so often gravely involved in cerebral palsy.

Dislocation of the choroid plexus in the lateral ventricles, or evolution of the ratio between the lateral ventricular diameter and thickness of the cerebral mantle, may also permit earlier diagnosis of prenatal primary hydrocephalus. Albeit rare, it may derive from areas of cerebral spinal fluid resorption, apart from subnormal permeability of subarachnoid spaces, or failed opening of the foramina of Magendie and Luschka.

# COLPOCEPHALY

In neuro-imaging it must be recalled that an abnormal ventricular configuration with unduly large occipital horns of the lateral ventricles may be due to colpocephaly (Bodensteiner and Gay, 1990). This is ascribed to persistence of the foetal configuration of the lateral ventricles. This in turn is associated with multiple aspects of disturbed or arrested development of the brain, including in particular a diminution of thickness of white matter in the posterior portion of the centrum semiovale.

## References

Bodensteiner T, Gay CT. (1990) Colpocephaly: Pitfalls in the diagnosis of a pathological entity. J Child Neurol 5: 166-168

Catto-Smith AG, Yu VYH, Bajuk B, Orgill AA, Astbury J. (1985) Effect of neonatal periventricular haemorrhage on neuro-developmental outcome. Arch Dis Child 60: 8-11

Cohen HL, Haller JO, Pollark A. (1990) Ultrasound of the septum pellucidum. Recognition of evolving fenestrations in the hydrocephalic infant. J Ultrasound Med 9: 377-383

Feldman HM, Scher MS, Kemp SS. (1990) Pediat Neurol 6: 276-302

Fitzhardinge PM, Flodmark O, Fitz CR, Ashby S. (1982) The prognostic value of computed tomography of the brain in asphyxiated premature infants. J Pediat 100: 476-481

Hamano S, Nara T, Nizaki H, Fukushima K, Imai M, Kumagai K, Maekawa K. (1991) Crossed cerebellar diaschisis demonstrable by SPECT in hemiplegic children. No To Hattatsu 23: 58-64

S23-S31

Kitchen WH et al. (1990) 5-year outcome of infants of birth-weight 500-1500gms; relationship with neonatal ultrasound. Am J Perinatol 7: 60-65

Levene MI (1981) Measurement of the growth of the lateral ventricles in preterm infants with real-time ultrasound. Arch Dis Child 56: 900-904

Levene MI, Starte DR. (1981) A longitudinal study of post-haemorrhagic ventricular dilatation in the newborn. Arch Dis Child 56: 905-910

Ment LR et al. (1982) Neonates of <1250 grams birth weight: prospective neurodevelopmental evaluation during the first year post-term. Pediatrics 70: 392-396

Palmer P, Dubowitz LMS, Levene MI, Dubowitz V. (1982) Developmental and neurological progress of preterm infants with intraventricular haemorrhage and ventricular dilatation. Arch Dis Child 57: 748-753

Papile LA, Burstein J, Burstein R, Koffler H. (1978) Incidence and evolution of subependymal and intraventricular haemorrhage: a study in infants with birthweights <1500 gms. J Pediat 92: 529-534

Robinson RO, Desai NA. (1981) Factors influencing mortality and morbidity after clinically apparent IVH. Arch Dis Child 56: 478-480

Schouman-Claeys L, Picard A, Lalande G, Kalifa G, Lacert P, Brentanos E, Frija G. (1989) Contribution of computed tomography in aetiology and prognosis of cerebral palsy. Br J Radiol 62: 248-252

Thorburn RJ et al. (1981) Prediction of death and major handicap in very preterm infants by brain ultrasound. Lancet 1: 1119-1121

Tudehope DI et al. (1989) Neonatal cranial ultrasonography as prediction of 2-year outcome of very low birthweight infants. Aust Paediat J 25: 66-71

van Bogaert P, Baleriaux D, Christophe C, Szliwowski HB. (1991) MRI of patients with cerebral palsy and normal CT scan. Paed Neurol 7: 426-428

# 10

# THE ELEMENT OF ISCHAEMIC/ANOXIC DAMAGE

The Element of Ischaemic/Anoxic Damage

Associated Hypocapnia and Hypotensive Factors in Relation to Severe
    PV and IV Haemorrhage

Degrees or Phases of Cerebral Anoxia

Anoxic/Ischaemic Encephalopathy

The Underlying Neuronal Changes

Pathogenesis of these Forms of Selective Neuronal Necrosis

Subcortical Leukomalacia in Association with Localized or Generalized
    Cerebral Atrophy

**Hypoxanthine Secretion in Hypoxic-Ischaemic-Induced Periventricular Leukomalacia (PVL)**

**Concurrent Factors in Cerebral Energy Metabolism**

**Possible Implications for Therapeutic Intervention**

**References**

# 10

# THE ELEMENT OF
# ISCHAEMIC/ANOXIC DAMAGE

Evidence grows that prenatal or perinatal anoxia may be a primary if not the predominant aetiological factor in cerebral palsy. Because of differences in vascular anatomy with gestational maturity of the brain, the site of predominant hypoxic-ischaemic injury is likely to vary with gestational ages. The associated major factor, however, may nevertheless be haemorrhage: germinal layer (GLH), periventricular (PVH) and/or intra-ventricular (IVH). These especially characterize the *preterm* baby, although PVH does occur in the *term* infant. PV leukomalacia, as an interwoven sequel of these two major aetiological factors - one possibly *predisposing* to the other - has to be seriously considered in the pathogenesis of CP.

Foetal hypoxia and hypercapnia leads to prolonged partial asphyxia with brain damage resulting from an arterial oxygen reduced by 90% for more than 25 minutes (Myers et al., 1969). Cerebral oedema in the parasagittal strip of the cerebral hemispheres is part of this pattern, extending from the paracentral region posteriorly into the parietal lobe. Islets of ischaemia and necrosis in the oedematous areas will leave behind focal cortical damage. When asphyxia is prolonged, the generalization of the oedema brings about increasing intracranial pressure, flattening of gyria, and falling cerebral perfusion.

During hypoxia, usage of glucose ketone bodies is limited so that energy is supplied through anaerobic glycolysis leading to lactic acidaemia. Consequent acidosis may accentuate brain injury by impairing vascular autoregulation inhibiting glycolysis and further direct brain injury with ischaemia superimposed on hypoxia. The process is augmented by heightening brain acidosis, by increasing lactate and carbon dioxide, leading to further impairment of cerebral blood flow.

The localization and consequently the type of permanent residual damage of hypoxic-ischaemic encephalopathy may differ in the preterm and term. In the preterm, damage is thus mainly located in the germinal matrix in the periventricular region with sparing of the cortical mantle. Residual peripheral damage in the cerebral cortex and underlying white matter is, however, the major focus of damage in the full term infant. But in trying to comprehend the underlying patho-physiology in order to evolve a more rational approach to the management of the hypoxia and ischaemia occurring together if the intrauterine phase or in the perinatal asphyxia of the full-term neonate, the relative contributions of hypoxia, ischaemia and cerebral oedema require exhaustive evaluation.

Fitzhardinge et al. (1982) were unable to correlate "low density" in the imaging of the premature brain with subsequent abnormal development at 18 months of age. Even from 32 to 36 weeks there are still difficulties (Fitz, 1989). In the diagnosis of anoxia by this technique, atrophic or encephalomalacic changes occur quite rapidly being complete or at least severe in 2 to 4 weeks. The central less affected tissues retain relatively normal density, whereas in *global oedema* the remainder of the brain can approach the density of CSF. If hydrocephalus should supervene because of haemorrhage or other reason, it is believed that the damaged brain offers little resistance to the increased pressure, so that there is rapid ventricular expansion. Diffuse cystic changes such as emerge within the PV leukomalacia are easily visualized on CT.

Intra-cerebral calcifications may also be visible on follow-up by CT scanning of anoxic damage, although they appear to be more consistently demonstrable after "primary" haemorrhagic lesions. The phenomenon of *reactive hypervascularity* has also been observed after severe anoxia, as reflected by increased density of the central grey matter.

# ASSOCIATED HYPOCAPNIA AND HYPOTENSIVE FACTORS IN RELATION TO SEVERE PV AND IV HAEMORRHAGE

But despite enhanced survival of premature infants, reports nevertheless appeared in 1989 by both Hagberg and colleagues and Riikonen et al. of cerebral palsy affecting increasing numbers of these survivors.

Periventricular leukomalacia proves to be the most important neuropathic lesion associated with their spastic diplegic manifestation. I have indicated the possibility that bleeding stemming from the highly vascular matrix enmeshing the caudate nucleus or striatum could initiate the periventricular infarction or allied damage leading to the leukomalacia. On the other hand, this central bilateral lesion in white matter arises at a point furthest from the arterial blood supply, supportive of anoxia/ischaemia as the primary aetiological factor rather than one predisposing to or associated with haemorrhagic lesions. Although it is likely that hypotension is an important causative factor (Trounce et al., 1988), the leukomalacia itself is not consistently associated with hypotension. That *hypoxanthine*, which was shown by Sangstad (1988) to be a valid plasma marker of cellular hypoxia, fails to rise in jugular or sagittal sinus blood during hypocapnia, supports the deduction that it alone cannot bring about cerebral ischaemia. Nevertheless, it is postulated that *when hypocapnia*, which has been related to a cerebral vasoconstrictive response, *is superimposed upon hypotension*, cerebral blood flow velocity would be reduced sufficiently to heighten the risk of cerebral ischaemia.

A recent therapeutic advance has introduced a new and possibly preventable aetiological factor in terms of peri- and intraventricular haemorrhage. Two large multicentre trials (European Collaborative Study, 1988; Horbar et al., 1990) have exposed a significantly increased risk of severe periventricular and intraventricular haemorrhage associated with the intratracheal administration of the surfactant Curosurf (porcine-form) in infants suffering the respiratory distress syndrome. In the Collaborative European Study, an unexpectedly high incidence of severe intraventricular haemorrhage (26%) was recorded in spite of significant reduction in mortality and bronchopulmonary dysplasia. Associated factors of hypotension (Miall-Allen et al., 1987) and fluctuations in cerebral blood flow velocity (Perlman et al., 1983), each appear to play a part.

To help obviate the summation of such factors, a slower continuous infusion of the surfactant without physical disturbance of the infant has been suggested alongside the use of an endotracheal connection with a side-arm for the infusion, etc.

# DEGREES OR PHASES OF CEREBRAL ANOXIA

These have been descriptively divided into three:

1. The most severe or "global" form is diagnosable as early as 36 weeks of gestation, wherein the density of affected areas is equivalent to, or lower than that of normal white matter. All structures of the cerebrum are involved, sparing the basal ganglia, thalamus and cerebellum.

   Cisterns and subarachnoid spaces are more compressed than in the normal neonate. Where the damage is less pronounced, "strands" of gyral grey matter suggest sulcal haemorrhage. Recovery cannot be expected when the underlying severity of brain damage is visualized as marked generalized atrophy, or a generalized cystic encephalo-malacia.

2. A second or less severe form: This is visualized as an increased prominence of white matter showing extensions into grey matter, and to the cortical surface in some areas.

   Indeed, such extensions through the cortex suggests anoxic damage in a 36 week infant. Central structures and cerebellum are spared. This is comparable to the normal appearance at a lower gestational age.

   Follow-up CNS examination will be abnormal in most, and major neurologic defects are to be expected in survivors.

3. A third gradation of anoxic damage, primarily involving the *central basal ganglia* and thalami, is uncommon. These structures normally stand out as denser than the adjacent white matter even in the premature, whereas a lowered density is easily overlooked.

These structures appear to be often damaged in older children as a result of metabolic abnormality such as hypoglycaemia or carbon monoxide poisoning.

Hypoglycaemia per se appears to play a more frequent and more fundamental cerebral role in the newborn who has faced anoxic insult. The associated primary or secondary atrophy was unexpectedly diffuse in two examples studied by Hirabayashi et al. (1980). The outcome is usually equal to that of *focal central infarction*, if not of a generalization of significant atrophy. No long-term follow-up of infants with CT evidence of mild or equivocal anoxic injury has been reported to date.

Nor has unilateral damage of this hypoxic character been as yet demonstrated by either ultrasound or CT. Although O'Brien et al. (1979) using radionucleotides without ultrasound or CT correlation in a group of 85 full-term asphyxiated infants was able to identify *unilateral middle cerebral artery abnormality* in 6 of 56 atypical or abnormal scans. This pattern showed a *higher correlation with clinical abnormality* than any other, making up 17% of abnormal children on follow-up. *Even though focal infarcts* are more commonly associated with, or ascribed to, birth trauma, they probably occur in utero, the ultrasonography usually showing increased echogenicity with or without haemorrhage, which should be identifiable on CT. The *middle cerebral artery* is usually involved. A *delayed onset of haemorrhage* may arise in such infarcts. Such bleeding is typically within the gyri, and is most likely the product of initial *petechial bleeds into necrotic tissue*.

# ANOXIC/ISCHAEMIC ENCEPHALOPATHY

This may be suffered by infants of any gestational age with a wide variety of pathological pattern, and differing clinical presentation. Periventricular leukomalacia may be regarded as one form. Differing patterns of damage may be characterized by a common pathogenesis of *selective neuronal necrosis*. *Infarction* may underlie this, and there may be herniation of the uncus or cerebellum through the tentorium. The cortical ribbon often shows pallor, although the centrum semi ovale and thalamus are intensely congested. *Foci of congestion* are also often visible in midbrain and medulla. *Old* lesions may be characterized by *foci of calcification*, abnormal *pallor*, and a *firm consistency* suggesting advanced myelination. They may also be evidenced by a range of gross morphological alterations, including Ulegyria, status marmoratus or cystic encephalomalacia. Some degree of *ventricular dilatation*, likewise frequently indicative of *loss of cerebral tissue*, is also associated.

Isolated ventricular dilatation was also exposed as underlying CP in two children in further MRI exploration.

Further MRI exploration of the cerebral effects of hypoxic-ischaemic encephalopathy in 15 term infants was reported by Byrne et al. (1990). This was carried out serially during the neonatal period and at 4 and 8 months of age, and then compared with their neurodevelopmental outcome at 18 months of age. Cerebral palsy was the result in nine, with abnormality of tone and delayed motor milestones suggestive of CP in two. The principal abnormal feature in all nine who developed CP, however, was delayed myelination, or structural abnormalities, or a combination of the two. These were likewise detected at the age of 8 months in all nine. An important conclusion was that the earliest time at which MRI findings correlate with later neurological outcome *appears to be 8 months.*

Ultrasonography was also used to define the evolution of transient periventricular densities in 59 infants (de Vries, Regev, Pennock and Wigglesworth, 1988). Spastic diplegia ensued in four of them, after developing what was called transient dystonia, whereas only 8 of the 92 children with normal ultrasound scans produced this finding. Persistence of the densities for more than ten days, and the presence of such densities in the trigone were of more serious prognostic import.

Of the patterns of *selective neuronal necrosis, several* have been defined:

(i) A *descending* pattern: this classical pattern involves *cortex, white* matter and *thalamus.* Underlying brain swelling may also bring about secondary infarction.

(ii) An *ascending* pattern: involving neurones of spinal cord, brain stem, midbrain and thalamus which may spare the cortex. This *"lesion"* is seen after *acute forms* of total anoxia, or *anoxic/ischaemic stress* such as that due to *compression of a collapsed umbilical cord* or neonatal cardiac arrest.

(iii) *Pontosubicular* pattern: damage is to the subiculum of the hippocampus, and especially in deep areas of grey matter eg. *thalamus.* In white matter, this resembles PV leukomalacia.

# THE UNDERLYING NEURONAL CHANGES

Early: Pyknosis of nuclei with shrinkage of cytoplasm associated with oedema.

Old: Loss of neurones following prolonged asphyxia during birth in term infants, likely to be associated with swelling of an oedematous brain in infants dying within a few days.

# PATHOGENESIS OF THESE FORMS OF
# SELECTIVE NEURONAL NECROSIS

Primary processes leading to the basic anoxic/ischaemic brain damage are (1) hypoxia or anoxia, or (2) failure of the cerebral circulation. The mode and sequence of their development appear to influence the associated or consequent pattern of *selective neuronal necrosis*. This is illustrated in the prolonged hypoxia of birth asphyxia, when a sequence of anaerobic glycolysis and lactic acidosis leads to breach of the blood-brain barrier, failed cerebral perfusion and ultimate neuronal necrosis. The pattern of such failure of cerebral perfusion appears to determine the pattern of cell death.

In the neonate, cells of *deep grey nuclei* are considered more mature. Manifesting a higher metabolic rate than those of the cerebral cortex, they may be more vulnerable to total anoxia. A specific pontosubicular pattern of neuronal necrosis has been found to be a specific consequence of episodes of hyperoxaemia in acidotic and hypoxic preterm infants (Skullerud and Westre, 1986). Association with any of the typical range of haemorrhagic lesions or PV leukomalacia has also been observed (Wigglesworth, 1987).

# SUBCORTICAL LEUKOMALACIA
# IN ASSOCIATION WITH LOCALIZED
# OR GENERALIZED CEREBRAL ATROPHY

Another form of leukomalacia recognizable in the neonate or infant is in a subcortical rather than periventricular location. It has been found particularly in association with victims of the sudden infant death syndrome or of congenital heart disease (Takashima et al., 1978).

Ultrasonography has furthermore established a relationship to eventual cerebral atrophy linked to a poor neurodevelopmental prognosis. It may represent encroachment of white matter undergoing anoxic/ischaemic pathology within the hypovascular subcortical zones *in the depths of the sulci*. Association with more generalized cerebral injury may be presumed, and the evidence is growing of it being more than an obscure element underlying cognitive deficit with or without cerebral palsy.

A lesion in this situation has been recognized in infant or child subjects of *the sudden infant death syndrome,* or of congenital heart anomalies (Takashima et al., 1978). An *hypovascular* subcortical region in the depths of the sulci has been postulated as the source. It may represent no more than a focal accentuation in this subcortical zone of a more typically widespread leukomalacia in the white matter associated with anoxic/ischaemic damage. Diagnosis of such a lesion by ultrasonography (Trounce and Levene, 1985) should therefore alert the physician to the possibility of more serious generalization of cerebral damage, more specifically including subsequent cerebral atrophy with a poor neurodevelopmental outlook.

# HYPOXANTHINE SECRETION IN HYPOXIC-ISCHAEMIC-INDUCED PERIVENTRICULAR LEUKOMALACIA (PVL)

There are also some important and challenging metabolic considerations in relation to PVL.

Hypoxanthine was postulated by Sangstad (1975 and 1988) as a measure of hypoxia, and with particular reference to foetal asphyxia (Thiringer, 1983). Assays of plasma hypoxanthine by high performance liquid chromatography have been developed as a marker of peripartum hypoxia and ischaemia. 116 infants at risk for PVL, which was detected within three days of birth by ultrasound, were studied by Russell and colleagues (1992). The median range gestation of 81 unaffected infants of 30 weeks (24-32) produced a plasma hypoxanthine of 7.8 $\mu$mol/l (24-48.9). The concentration in 7 infants with cavitating PVL and a median gestation of 28 weeks (26-30) reached 31.9 $\mu$mol/l (7.1-149).

That cavitating PVL was significantly dependent only on hypoxanthine when controlled for the effects of weight and gestation, supported peripartum hypoxia-ischaemia as one of the aetiological factors in cavitating PVL. The two groups with porencephaly, with or without PVL, had higher hypoxanthine concentrations than in the unaffected group but without significance, whereas in the group with PVL alone, the hypoxanthine was significantly higher at 31.9 $\mu$mol/l (p <0.005).

An increased concentration of hypoxanthine within two hours of birth, thought to indicate antenatal hypoxia, marked all three groups of parenchymal cavitation.

The relationship between early increases of plasma hypoxanthine and the emergence of PVL indirectly supports the hypothetical association of PVL with cerebral hypoxia-ischaemia. Increased hypoxanthine in cord blood and in its excretion has been found in asphyxiated babies with reduced "optimality score" - or abnormal neurological signs during the first week of life. Foetal cerebral oxygen uptake rapidly falls with falling arterial oxygen saturation especially when combined with acidaemia.

In term babies, increased concentrations of hypoxanthine are detectable for two hours after asphyxia, and in the preterm increased levels may persist for 24 hours after the hypoxic episode (Thiringer, 1983). About half of the babies who developed parenchymal cavitation showed birth asphyxia evidenced by increased hypoxanthine (>2SD from the mean:9.5 $\mu$mol/l). This would imply that the hypoxic-ischaemic insult occurring antenatally might be associated with subsequent parenchymal cavitation.

The degradation of hypoxanthine and xanthine to uric acid as the end-product of purine metabolism in man is catalysed by xanthine dehydrogenase. Co-factors are molybdenum, FAD and iron. Hypoxanthine is normally recycled by the salvage pathway for which xanthine is not an effective substrate in vivo. Indeed, there is an important role for hypoxanthine re-utilization in regulating the rate of purine synthesis.

# CONCURRENT FACTORS IN CEREBRAL ENERGY METABOLISM

In addition, one also begins to understand the underlying energy system by recognizing that the maintenance of the living state requires the rate of ATP synthesis of adenosine diphosphate to equal the rate of ATP breakdown. If stress of metabolism requires V (metabolic velocity) to approach Vmax, much higher quantities of the control chemical ADP are needed. A small additional load of metabolic stress would result in lack of control, with negative feedback control no longer possible. Metabolic needs of the brain are then no longer satisfied by its metabolic machinery, following which there is a rise of both ADP and inorganic phosphorus (Pi) which stimulates glycolysis. Lactate acidosis rises, ATP is depleted, and ADP by conversion to AMP monophosphate is lost. Finally there is excretion of hypoxanthine and uric acid. Insufficient ADP remains to allow resynthesis of ATP. Experimentally in rat brain, the loss of ATP in response to electric shock is accompanied by the production of *ammonia*, together with inosine and larger amounts of hypoxanthine. A possible correlation is suggested with the Krebs urea cycle and increased production of glutamate with its possible influence on cell death as postulated recently by Volpe (1993).

If the therapeutic technique adopted allows oxygen to reflow into previously ischaemic regions, free radicle damage may further impair capacity for recovery. When V and Vmax becomes equal, control is lost and life may be lost. This simplistic concept applies especially to the brain of the preterm where oxygen delivery may be jeopardised by many complications of the birth process.

To determine the V/Vmax for the newborn brain in a non-invasive, safe, and quantitative procedure, *Phosphorus Magnesium Resonance Spectroscopy (PMRS)* can now be exploited. This device can measure ATP directly in living tissues together with its back-up system - Phosphocreatinine (PCR) and creatinine kinase (CR).

In the cortical neurone, mitochondria in the cytoplasm comprise many places where ATP can be used at *synaptic junctions*, axons, etc., as well as in the cell body itself. Loss of ATP immobilizes the ion pumps, and allows effusion of potassium and entry of sodium and water. At the same time, *large amounts of neurotransmitters are released*, especially Glutamate, resulting in severe osmotic stress at the *neuronal membrane*. Osmotic forces would then tend to rupture the membrane leading to irreversible structural damage.

Direct measurements of several cerebral metabolites involved in oxidative metabolism are now also practicable via *Phosphorus Magnetic Resonance Spectroscopy*. As in part outlined above, serious disturbance of cellular energy metabolism follows acute hypoxic-ischaemic development during labour. The temporal sequence of patho-physiology must be studied in relation to concurrent disorder at a molecular level, especially in its culmination in late or secondary energy failure. *The end-points under increasing study are immediate and late neuronal necrosis.*

# OXYGEN-FREE RADICAL GENERATION
# AND
# POSSIBLE IMPLICATIONS FOR
# THERAPEUTIC INTERVENTION

Hypoxanthine is also a *free radical generator*. This had led to a reconsideration of *free-radical induced tissue damage*, and the role of free radical generation and hypoxia-ischaemia in the genesis of ischaemic disorders of the foetal or immature infant brain. The Oslo team of Rootwelt and colleagues (1992) have extended this perspective to the release of harmful oxygen free radicals during reoxygenation after severe hypoxia. The substrate hypoxanthine accumulates during hypoxia, and when xanthine oxidase catalyses its conversion to xanthine and on to uric acid, superoxide radicals and hydrogen peroxide and produced (Vettenranta and Reivio, 1990; Friedl and Smith, 1990). The release of xanthine oxidase to the systemic circulation during resuscitation from severe hypoxia

was experimentally studied in 19 hypoxaemic piglets but only confirmed in five of them.

Such ischaemic damage could therefore be secondary to the excessive release of free radicals via the xanthine oxidase-hypoxanthine reaction. Reduction of free radical release after perfusion/reoxygenation by prophylactic inhibition of xanthine oxidase might therefore limit the extent and intensity of tissue destruction. Such inhibition might be attainable by the application of Allopurinol and its major active metabolite, oxypurine. A promising advance has been confirmed experimentally that this approach can indeed *limit tissue damage* attributable to free radical activity (Martz et al., 1989; Palmer et al. 1990).

271

# References

Byrne P, Welch R, Johnson MA, Darrah J, Piper M. (1990) Serial magnetic resonance imaging in neonatal hypoxic-ischaemic encephalopathy. J Pediat 117: 694-700

Collaborative European Multicentre Study Group (1988) Surfactant replacement therapy for severe neonatal respiratory distress syndrome: an international randomised clinical trial. Pediatrics 82: 683-691

de Vries LS, Regev R, Pennock JM, Wigglesworth JS, Dubowitz LM. (1988) Ultrasound evolution and later outcome of infants with periventricular densities. Early Hum Dev 16: 225-233

Fitz C. (1989) Computed tomography: state of the art. In KE Pape, JS Wigglesworth (Eds) Perinatal Brain Lesions. Blackwell Scientific Publications, Boston, London. pp 25-53

Fitzhardinge PM, Flodmark O, Fitz CR, Ashby S. (1982) The prognostic value of computed tomography of the brain in asphyxiated premature infants. J Pediat 100: 476-481

Friedl HP, Smith DJ et al. (1990) Ischaemia reperfusion in humans. Appearance of xanthine oxidase activity. Am J Pathol 136: 491-495

Hagberg B, Hagberg O, Olow I, Von Vendt I. (1989) The changing panorama of CP in Sweden in the birth year period 1979-1981. Acta Paediat Scand 78: 283-290

Hirabayashi S, Kitahara T, Hishida T. (1980) Computed tomography in perinatal hypoxic and hypoglycaemic encephalopathy with emphasis on follow-up studies. J Comput Assist Tomogr 4: 451-456

Horbar JD, Soll RF, Schachinger H et al. (1990) A European multicentre randomised controlled trial of single dose surfactant therapy for idiopathic respiratory distress syndrome. Eur J Pediat 149: 416-423

Martz D, Rayes G, Schielke GP, Betz AL. (1989) Allopurinol and dimethylthioures reduce brain infarction following middle cerebral artery occlusion in rats. Stroke 20: 488-494

Miall-Allen VM, de Vries LS, Whitelaw AGL. (1987) Mean arterial blood pressure and neonatal cerebral lesions. Arch Dis Child 62: 1068-1069

Myers RE, Beard R, Adamson K. (1969) Brain swelling in the newborn rhesus monkey following prolonged partial asphyxia. Neurology 19: 1012-1018

O'Brien MJ, Ash JM, Gilday DL. (1979) Radionuclide brain-scanning in perinatal hypoxia/ischaemia. Dev Med Child Neurol 21: 161-173

Palmer C, Vannucc RC, Towfight J. (1990) Reduction of perinatal hypoxic-ischaemic brain damage with Allopurinol. Pediatr Res 27: 332-336

Perlman JM, McMenamin JB, Volpe JJ. (1983) Fluctuating cerebral blood flow velocity in the respiratory disress syndrome. Relation to the development of IVH. New Engl J Med 309: 204-209

Riikonen R, Raumavirta S, Sinivuori E, Seppala T. (1989) Changing pattern of cerebral palsy in the south-west region of Finland. Acta Paediat Scand 78: 581-587

Rootwelt T et al. (1992) Release of xanthine oxidase to the systemic circulation during resuscitation after severe hypoxaemia. Proc Annual Meeting, British Paediatric Association, Coventry

Russell GAB, Jeffers G, Cooke RWI. (1992) Plasma hypoxanthine a marker for hypoxic-ischaemic induced PVL. Arch Dis Child 67: 388-392

Sangstad OD. (1975) Hypoxanthine as a measurement of hypoxia. Pediatr Res 9: 158-161

Sangstad O. (1988) Hypoxanthine as an indicator of hypoxia: its role in health and disease through free radical production. Paediat Res 23: 143-149

Skullerud K, Westre B. (1986) Frequency of prognostic significance of germinal matrix haemorrhage, PVL and Pontosubicular necrosis in preterm neonates. Acta Neuropathol (Berlin) 70: 257-261

Takashima S, Armstrong DL, Becker LE. (1978) Subcortical leukomalacia. Arch Neurol 35: 470-472

Thiringer K. (1983) Cord plasma hypoxanthine as a measure of foetal asphyxia. Acta Paediatr Scand 72: 231-237

Trounce JQ, Levene MI. (1985) Diagnosis and outcome of subcortical cystic leukomalacia. Arch Dis Child 60: 1041-1044

Trounce JQ, Shaw DE, Levene MI, Rutter N. (1988) Clinical risk factors and periventricular leukomalacia. Arch Dis Child 63: 17-22

Vettenranta K, Reivio KO. (1990) Xanthine oxidase during human fetal development. Pediat Res 27: 286-288

Wigglesworth JS. (1987) Pathological analysis of haemorrhagic and ischaemic lesions in the preterm infant brain. In: Yabuuchi H, Watanabe K, Okada S (Eds) Neonatal Brain and Behavior. Nagoya, University of Nagoya Press. pp 35-43

# 11

# VULNERABILITY TO VASCULAR DAMAGE

Vulnerability to Vascular Damage

Potential for Prevention of Pneumothorax

Intraventricular Haemorrhage

Intraparenchymal Haemorrhage

Pathological Lesions as Delineated more Specifically by the Newer
Imaging Techniques

Periventricular Lesions
Focal Lesions
Infarction
Diffuse Lesions

Haemodynamic Factors and the "Lost Autoregulation Hypothesis"

**Periventricular Leukomalacia (PVL): Its Pathological Evolution and Association with Cerebral Palsy**

**Foetoscopy under Real-Time Ultrasound Control**

**References**

# 11

## VULNERABILITY TO VASCULAR DAMAGE

During the third trimester, progressive maturation of the cortex and white matter of the brain is accelerated. There is increasing elaboration, density and complexity of parallel neural interconnections and vascular supply, attended presumably by augmented and changing metabolic requirements. *31 p NMR Spectroscopy* has added a new tool to help clarify the accompanying metabolic changes in the newborn brain. Increasing vulnerability to different harmful influences accompanies those changes. So that despite many advances in the past decade, much remains to be learnt of the pathophysiological phenomena which may wreak havoc upon the immature brain.

Vulnerability to vascular damage is a risk of high priority, especially in preterm infants, and most of all in those under 1500g birth weight, or of less than 30 weeks gestation. Not unexpectedly, these suffer an extremely high incidence of periventricular and intra-ventricular haemorrhage of between 30-55% (Papile et al., 1978). The incidence of IVH, however, has declined in many major centres during the past few years. But the absolute number of infants with IVH and associated neurological sequelae remains high. Two dimensional cranial ultrasound has provided reliable detection of such periventricular haemorrhages, and we hope for an equally reliable prognostic role in predicting their neurodevelopmental outcome. It becomes vital, with prevention in mind, to localize the most frequent *sites of origin* of these early

preterm haemorrhages (Hambleton and Wigglesworth, 1976) particularly to include the subependymal/germinal matrix. It is crucial to realize that whether unilateral or bilateral, it usually first occurs in the region of the head of the caudate nucleus or caudothalamic notch. The region of the ganglionic eminence is also a frequent site. It is asserted that only occasional examples of such haemorrhage are encountered from then up to 38 weeks gestation (Ahman et al., 1980; Dolfin et al., 1983), most deriving from sites other than the subependymal matrix. But with gestation beyond 30 weeks there is also a vital and increasing proportion of bleeds originating from the *choroid plexus*, to the extent that Donat et al. (1978) postulated that by full term, nearly all intracranial haemorrhages are likely to be attributable to such choroid plexus bleeding. On the other hand, lesions of the basal ganglia are also believed to be commoner in the term infant (Fig 9).

An interesting localization of haemorrhage, again of possible patho-physiological bearing upon basal ganglia functions relevant to development of some manifestation of CP, is the entity of *thalamic haemorrhage* (Fig 9). Its recent recognition (Trounce et al., 1985) followed the application of ultrasonography to term infants even though they lacked evidence of perinatal asphyxia.

Related factors derived from a rise or fall in cerebral blood flow have also to be

# A horizontal section showing Thalamic and Putaminal Haemorrhages

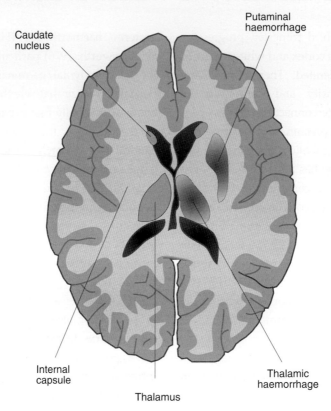

Putaminal haemorrhage

Caudate nucleus

Internal capsule

Thalamus

Thalamic haemorrhage

considered. Fluctuations in cerebral blood flow may play a part, as well as increases in venous pressure.

A broad gradation of the degree and extent of haemorrhage should of course have some bearing on its localization. I am indebted to Levene and his colleagues (1982) for the following simplified clinical grading which answers this requirement:

### Grade I: Small

Typically originates in the region of the germinal matrix, it shows no inferior or lateral extension beyond the lateral border of the lateral ventricle.

### Grade II: Moderate

Some downward extension into the basal nuclei on at least one side, or involvement of the caudate nucleus, extending to the region of the genu of the lateral ventricle posteriorly on parasagittal scans.

### Grade III: Large

Any degree of extension laterally or superolaterally into the cerebral parenchyma.

As identified by a Kranzbühler ADR real-time linear array machine, axial plane scans through the temporo-parietal region, and using a 5MHz transducer, an IVH would be visualized as echo density in the region of the lateral ventricle. On CT alone, ventricular "clots" can be seen clinging to the ventricular wall of the choroid plexus for three weeks or more. Transfontanelle scanning, using a 7MHz transducer, instead exposes germinal layer haemorrhage in the shape of dense subependymal echo densities in the region of the caudate nucleus.

Magnetic resonance imaging and its rapidly developing refinements, such as *Near Infrared Spectroscopy (NIRS)*, which permits non-invasive exploration of the cerebral circulation (Wyatt, 1992), promises to carry our understanding of the role of PVH in perinatal brain injury a stage further.

*The long-term sequelae* of each type of lesion will become clearer as they range from relatively limited haemorrhages in germinal layer matrix to the full extent and functional impact of intraparenchymal haemorrhage. Study of the correlationships between clinical patterns, findings of the new generation of ultrasound technology and magnetic resonance imaging, and the related neuropathology, should then become an integral part of perinatal/neonatal follow-up that will enable us to advance in our understanding of different entities of cerebral palsy. It is hoped thereby that future programmes of immediate or early management could become more rational and effective, depending upon our ability to prevent or even swiftly alleviate the underlying neuropathic lesions, or rather their anoxic/ischaemic or haemorrhagic causation.

Involved in this vital understanding of perinatal cerebral damage will be a combination of such longitudinal imaging studies in life, and a range of physiologic and neurological assessment methods practised by the neonatologist, as well as pathological exploration of the brains of infants who do not survive. It is also important that exploratory studies after cerebral damage extend to the possible compensatory modifications which can develop to support or strengthen alternative pathways subserving motor function.

It is expected that many of the *infarcted* areas observed early in preterm neonates will lead to functional deficits of the brain. Such "matured" infarcts in the brain of neonates with functional deficit are now readily detectable by magnetic resonance imaging, computerized tomography or ultrasound. Clinico-pathological correlationships between these and consequent dysfunction is by no means simple, especially because of the plasticity of the neonatal brain, hopefully compensatory, and because of the variety of regions that can be affected.

# POTENTIAL FOR PREVENTION OF PNEUMOTHORAX

Important preventive implications hinge upon the correlation between systemic hypotension associated with pneumothorax and IVH and its sequelae. The study of Mehrabani and colleagues (1991) was projected upon 67 very low birth-weight infants (<1500g at birth) of 32 weeks gestation, or suffering the respiratory distress syndrome and pneumothorax. 32 of the 36 infants with pneumothorax associated with hypotension (89%) incurred three or four examples of IVH which originates in the capillary network of the germinal layer. This compared with only 10% in infants with pneumothorax but normal blood pressure.

Pulmonary air leak or pneumothorax occurs in up to 35% of those being ventilated for the respiratory distress syndrome. The increased intrathoracic pressure is believed to bring about a fall in cardiac filling, cardiac output and systemic blood pressure. Cerebral infarction is seen as often the primary event with no IVH until after the systemic blood pressure rises to normal or above normal levels.

The work of Ahman, Lazzara and Dykes et al (1980) had indeed demonstrated a strikingly increased risk of IVH in infants. The risk was increased 2.5-fold compared to infants with alveolar rupture. In the work of Mehrabani et al (1991), 89% of 36 infants with pneumothorax developed Grade 3 or 4 IVH.

Whilst some instances of pneumothorax may be asymptomatic, others may be followed by severe circulatory disturbance including hypotension and hypoperfusion. When cardiac filling is inadequate in the presence of severe pneumothorax, leading to systemic hypotension, cerebral ischaemia could *specifically affect the arterial watershed zone* in the periventricular region.

When intrathoracic pressure is sufficient to compress the intrathoracic vessels severely, systemic hypotension results ("air block syndrome"). Cranial ultrasound scans were conducted in 17 infants of the hypotensive group before and 24 hours after their pneumothorax. Before the pneumothorax, 10 infants had normal cranial ultrasounds but 7 had Grade 1 or 2 IVH. When repeating cranial ultrasonography after the pneumothorax, all were abnormal. One had a Grade 1-2 IVH, and 16 had Grade 3 or 4 IVH.

In addition, infants with pneumothorax resulting in hypotension showed an increased incidence of cerebral ischaemia as expressed in periventricular leukomalacia with porencephaly and ventricular dilatation.

The sequence postulated is cerebral hypoperfusion or ischaemia precedes the severe IVH. Miall-Allen et al (1989) have recently shown that preterm infants developing hypotension in the first few days of life are likely to suffer cerebral parenchymal injury or severe IVH. It is suggested that since cerebral autoregulation had been lost, hypotension had led directly to cerebral hypoperfusion. The hypoperfusion accompanying systemic hypotension causes infarction of both the periventricular white matter and the germinal matrix. When the blood pressure and blood flow rise to normal values, the germinal matrix capillaries rupture followed by either germinal matrix or intraventricular haemorrhage.

*The prevention of moderate to severe hypotension* becomes the first challenge, and *the technical avoidance of pneumothorax during mechanical respiratory ventilation* becomes an important goal in the prevention of cerebral palsy as a sequel.

# INTRAVENTRICULAR HAEMORRHAGE

This most often results from extension of the initial subependymal haemorrhage. An important aspect in the extension of the intraventricular haemorrhage is the degree of its pathogenic spread throughout the ventricular system. The consequent distension of lateral ventricles, third ventricle, aqueduct and 4th ventricle is another sequel.

But any associated parenchymal extension, of course including parenchymal white matter, may occur either rapidly or be delayed for some days after the initial bleed. The latter may in part be associated with or the result of venous infarction, with the possibility of attendant obstruction of thalamo-striate vein branches.

Cytochemical markers can be exploited to detect and demarcate the contribution of proliferating astroglial cells and macrophages at the margins of such secondary parenchymal haemorrhage.

# INTRAPARENCHYMAL HAEMORRHAGE

These refer to any intrahemispheric haemorrhage other than those confined to the germinal matrix. Most occur in the periventricular region - especially anteriorly, and are either extensions anteriorly and laterally of a subependymal haemorrhage, or are part of a large primary haemorrhage into the periventricular region, including the subependymal area. An interesting experimental model of parenchymal haemorrhage was produced in the mouse by Yoshioka et al. (1989). When newborn mice were exposed to an hypoxic episode, only 34 survived, and in these cerebral parenchymal haemorrhage occurred. Cortical haemorrhage usually involved the parietal regions symmetrically. Neuronal destruction occurred in the deeper structures as well as in the cortex. The whole pattern of damage was comparable to parasagittal cerebral injury in humans. It was furthermore apparent that the cortical haemorrhage occurred as the cerebral blood flow recovered after the hypoxic event.

# PATHOLOGICAL LESIONS AS DELINEATED MORE SPECIFICALLY BY THE NEWER IMAGING TECHNIQUES

There are three broad categories of localization:

1. Periventricular
2. Focal
3. Infarction
4. Diffuse

## Periventricular Lesions

Early lesions are echogenic on ultrasound, and occupy characteristic sites *superolateral to the lateral ventricles*, ranging anywhere from the trigone to just anterior to the frontal horns.

Their localization is quite different from that involved in the typical *subependymal* haemorrhage. These lesions either slowly resolve over several weeks, or cavitation occurs with formation of cysts.

Periventricular leukomalacia is often associated, although mainly attributable to hypoxia-ischaemia. It was identified in 7.5% of 120 infants of birth-weight less than 1501g. Cavitation became apparent in 55% sometimes between the 5th and 73rd days. Residual ventriculomegaly is also likely to result.

## Focal Lesions

Focal abnormalities have been found in spastic CP which are predictable as regards their nature (atrophy, ischaemic areas, etc.) and their severity, with the more grossly handicapped children showing more extensive lesions (Kulakowski and Larroche, 1980; Pederson et al., 1982).

Echogenic areas are usually quite large. The cortex may be encroached upon, and the whole distribution of a major artery - often the middle cerebral - may be involved, although the focal bleed often arises from its most susceptible branch such as the recurrent artery of Heubner (Fig 10). Either gradual resolution or cavitation may occur, with a varying degree of dilatation of the adjacent ventricle being a common sequel.

282

# Thalamostriate arteries and Recurrent artery of Heubner

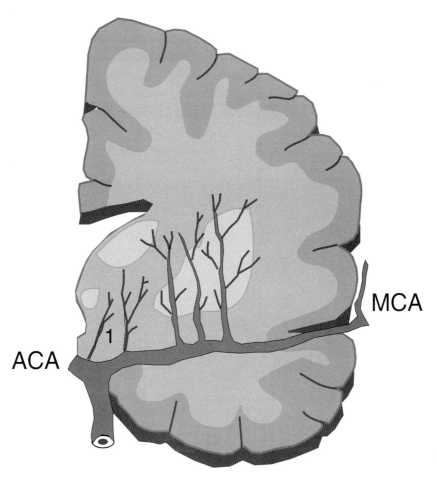

ACA

MCA

1

## Infarction

With the improved imaging and autopsy correlations it has been possible to distinguish between intraventricular and intraparenchymal areas of increased echogenicity. The former type of parenchymal lesion is thought to be due to an *area of venous infarction* in an area of parenchyma, the venous return to which has been compromised by distension of the ipsilateral *lateral ventricle* by a large intraventricular haemorrhage. Areas of venous infarction will form porencephalic cysts.

In their study of the application of Proton Magnetic Resonance Spectroscopy (II + MRS) to focal lesions (Rutherford, Dubowitz et al., 1993), four infants with *cerebral artery infarcts* showed no measurable signal *from the infarcted area* in terms of the

N-acetyl aspartate / choline ratio (as in earlier results of hypoxic-ischaemic encephalopathy) as well as decreased signals from the area around it. On an MRI rescanning at 4 months, glial tissue was demonstrated within the cerebral hemisphere but outside of the obvious infarct which may well precede the subependymal bleed. Conversely, a subsequent rise in systemic intracerebral blood pressure may lead to a spread of periventricular haemorrhage into infarcted tissue.

A more specific metabolic study (Tan et al., 1992) was focussed on the infarction which follows hypoxic-ischaemic injury in foetal sheep. This particular concentration was upon parasagittal cortical infarction and seizures in term neonates to which more detailed reference was made in relation to specific MRI findings making up a relatively specific clinicopathological entity (Fig 11). Brain lactate levels rose after the hypoxic-ischaemic insult, preceding the onset of epileptiform activity and the secondary cytotoxic oedema.

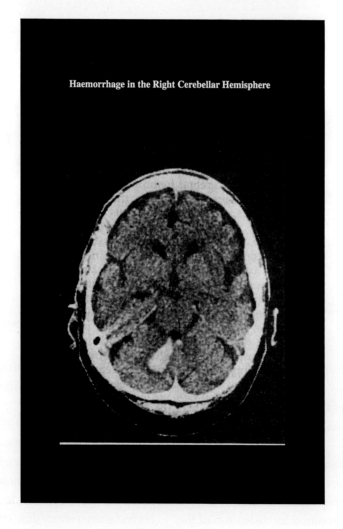

Haemorrhage in the Right Cerebellar Hemisphere

## Diffuse Lesions

These refer to widespread lesions even involving both hemispheres, or the thalamus and basal ganglia. Although the cerebral parenchyma remains echogenic, cystic areas of varying size appear. These may progress to diffuse *cystic encephalomalacia*. Ultrasound should prove to be useful in delineating the type, severity and evolution of the lesions listed, ultimately identifying those which appear most predictive of neurological deficit (Siegel et al., 1984).

# Cerebellar Haemorrhage

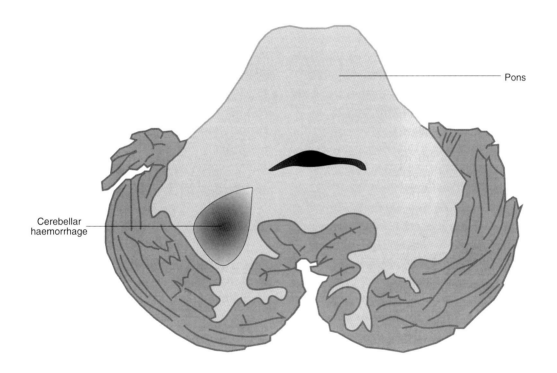

Pons

Cerebellar haemorrhage

# HAEMODYNAMIC FACTORS AND THE "LOST AUTOREGULATION HYPOTHESIS"

Further consideration is invited here of recent experimental studies of *haemodynamic* factors especially related to the *autoregulation of cerebral perfusion*, etc., which could be relevant to potential prevention and treatment. For example, as recently demonstrated in the newborn lamb (Szymonowicz et al., 1990), it is the choroid plexus which remains extremely vulnerable to haemorrhagic hypotension. *Vulnerability to hypotension, and lack of autoregulatory capacity* in the *white matter, caudate nucleus* and *choroid plexus* of the preterm lamb brain - which has also been successfully used as an experimental model for intraventricular haemorrhage - may well be the critical elements in the pathogenesis of both perinatal haemorrhage and ischaemic damage in the preterm neonates' brain.

Indeed Reynolds and colleagues had already shown in 1979 that a combination of asphyxia with intermittent increases in cerebral intravascular pressure was the most effective way to produce haemorrhages into the germinal layer.

The *preterm foetal lamb* has an extensive germinal layer overlying the head and body of the caudate nucleus similar to that of a 30 week gestation human infant, and the vascular supply to and from the germinal layer is similar to the basic pattern in the human preterm (Reynolds et al., 1979). At 125 days, the germinal layer is confined to small patches anterior to the head of the caudate nucleus and the brain resembles that of the term human infant.

In general there has been a growing appreciation of the probable role of haemodynamic factors in the pathogenesis of perinatal neurological disorder. Indeed the hypothesis incriminating *"failure of autoregulation"* of cerebral blood flow has been recognized as the probable key to understanding the development of hypoxic-ischaemic encephalopathy. Under "normal" conditions the unstressed newborn is capable of regulating vascular resistance to sustain constancy of cerebral perfusion despite relatively wide ranges of perfusion pressure. But this autoregulation of cerebral blood flow (CBF) *is lost in the stressed newborn* - exposing the brain to ischaemia even during moderate hypotension, and to an increased pressure gradient across the capillary wall during moderate hypertension with increased risk of intracranial haemorrhage.

In experiments partially occluding umbilical vessels, carbon dioxide was identified as a major determinant of the labile and fragile foetal mechanism of cerebral perfusion in utero, as it is after birth. A minor additional hypoxic insult such as accompanies normal birth suffices to abolish this protective mechanism. A sequence of events can be envisaged as potentially damaging... Firstly, defective auto-regulation, leading to hypotension, hence inducing ischaemic infarction. A subsequent rise in blood pressure would then evoke periventricular haemorrhage spreading into the infarcted tissues, with *perihaemorrhagic ischaemia* as a consequence. *Positron Emission Tomography (PET)* scanning by Volpe et al. (1983) demonstrated this very zone of intense ischaemia which surrounds intraparenchymal haemorrhage, ischaemia which may persist longterm.

Of possible value in either therapy or prevention was the significant correlationship to increased intracellular potassium concentrations demonstrable during this sequence of the first 2-3 days. The potassium concentration increases dramatically to about ten times - a level maintained for at least two weeks. Such intracellular potassium concentration (about 20-50 mcg) exerts a marked vasoconstrictor effect, which in itself could lead to peri-haemorrhagic ischaemia.

# PERIVENTRICULAR LEUKOMALACIA (PVL): ITS PATHOLOGICAL EVOLUTION AND ASSOCIATION WITH CEREBRAL PALSY

At least 7-15% of infants under 1500 g at birth ultimately reveal cavitating PVL (Trounce, Rutter and Levene, 1986). In a high proportion of these (47-80%), prospective studies (Graham, Levene and Trounce et al., 1987) especially in very low birth-weight infants, have shown that disturbances of tone and posture follow, with and without cognitive deficit.

The pathogenetic role of periventricular leukomalacia (PVL) was emphasised in the long term study of 399 preterm infants with gestation age less than 35 weeks by Kadoi (1992). Twenty-eight of these (7.0%) manifested "spastic CP" despite the absence of history of periventricular haemorrhage. Cystic periventricular leukomalacia was however evident in 14 on brain echography, and without cyst formation in an additional four, and indeed without any abnormality on neonatal brain echograms in tem. But on MRI cerebral lesions were definable in all these 28 infants whether periventricular high intensity areas on T2 weighted images, irregularity of ventricular wall, ventricular dilatation, decreased volume in periventricular white matter and thinning of the posterior body of corpus callosum, each compatible with the MR findings of PVL.

The Swedish team led by Hagberg (Krageloh-Mann, 1992) further substantiated this correlationship in the application of MRI to 38 children with bilateral spastic CP at the age of 5 years of more. Twenty-nine showed correlates of PVL. Especially was this defined in 20 of 21 preterms but it was also seen in 9 of 15 full terms without birth asphyxia, which does not therefore appear per se to be an essential antecedent to consider in either the pathogenesis or prevention of CP.

Likewise, Doran (1992) also demonstrated a strong predictive relationship between PVL and neuropathy, especially CP. His brief was to show how "carefully timed" intervention, with particular emphasis upon minimal handling, and the postnatal prevention of hypoxaemia, or of wide fluctuations in blood pressure, necessitating adequate ventilation and the continuous monitoring of oxygen saturation to help avoid and overcome hypoxaemic incidents.

Clarification of its evolution and distribution has been an excellent demonstration of the exploitation of high resolution ultrasonography to begin with, in monitoring the sequential advance of pathological lesions in the living infant. The ultrasound identification of parenchymal echodensities and echotranslucencies are being increasingly correlated with pathological findings at necropsy (Hill, Melson, Clark and Volpe, 1982; Leviton and Paneth, 1990). This is opening up a clearer understanding of the specifics of cerebral damage in cerebral palsy. Some preventable factors at play in its causation will be discussed later, bearing in mind also that antepartum haemorrhage and clinical perinatal asphyxia have also been clearly linked to subsequent development of PVL. Even hyperbilirubinaemia may also be involved in the pathogenesis of extensive (severe cystic) PVL in the preterm infant (Ikonen et al., 1992).

Its presumed site of origin mainly involves two locations. According to Shuman and Selednik (1980) the commonest presumptive site is the *optic radiation at the trigone of the lateral ventricle*. When it extends rostrally from the trigone, destruction of the *sublenticular portions* of the internal capsule follows. The second most common situation is in deep white matter near the foramen of Munro, especially at the juncture of corpus callosum, internal capsule, external capsule, and adjacent to the dorso-lateral angle of the lateral ventricle.

The pathological evolution of PVL could reflect a focal parenchymal venous infarction of the periventricular white matter, localized to the watershed between ventriculopetal and ventriculofugal vascular regions. Cavitation to the extent of porencephaly rather than PVL may be secondary to a contiguous large blood clot and release of vasoactive factors such as thromboxane, prostacyclin, or potassium (Edvinsson et al., 1986). Likewise, such infarction due to obstruction of veins of periventricular white matter by distension of the germinal matrix and ventricles after PVH could cause porencephaly and possibly PVL. Another hypothesis is that episodes of hypotension impair cerebral perfusion and oxygenation at the boundary zone between medullary artery branches entering the white matter from the cortex and the thalamostriate artery branches supplying the ependyma, and the immediate periventricular white matter. This phenomenon has been recently supported by evidence presented by Sinha and colleagues (1985) of a significant clinical association between clinical conditions causing hypotension and the development of PVL.

Areas of coagulative necrosis appear to mark its earliest stage. Infiltration of the necrotic tissue by lipid-laden macrophages then follows to produce the persistent "white spots". Oedema and astroglial proliferation are additional features. Where there is a limited area of damage, small foci of gliosis take over, often with ensuing focal calcification. But the more extensive lesions soon undergo central liquefaction with ensuing cystic changes.

This cystic phase is readily recognizable through real-time ultrasonography using a modern sector scanner, so that a fuller appreciation of the natural history of this condition becomes practicable. It is already clear, however, that most children with cystic PVL survive although in a neurodevelopmentally handicapped state, frequently manifested by varying degrees of spastic cerebral palsy.

Meanwhile, ultrasound and magnetic resonance imaging have revealed that typically the cysts cease to be visualized after two or three months. *On serial cranial ultrasonography*, parenchymal echodensities (of equivalent echodensity to the choroid plexus) seen in both coronal and parasaggital planes were regarded as pre-cavitating PVL (Russell, Jeffers and Cooke, 1992). Echodensities were visualised in three groups: (1) *Porencephaly*, widely communicating with the ventricle; (2) *Cavitating PVL-lucencies* 2-3 mm from the ventricular wall; and (3) *Porencephaly with associated PVL*, the lucencies within 2-3 mm of the porencephalic wall. Degrees of *ventricular dilatation* whether as a consequence thereof, or in some as yet unclear association, also tend to persist, as has been detailed in a separate chapter.

An excellent review of the outcome of cavitating PVL in 46 infants by Shortland et al. (1988) highlighted many of the features described above. Ultrasonic diagnostic outline was the basis of each case, providing a close correlation between the ultrasound findings and the later neurodevelopmental deficits. Its highest prevalence was in infants below 27 weeks gestation, appearing in 15% of very premature infants surviving for 14 days or more.

The cavities became definable 15 days after the onset of periventricular echodensities. In 24% of these, ventricular dilatation emerged. Of 27 infants still available for follow-up, 18 or 67% manifested significant neurodevelopmental handicap. Echolucent cavities appeared in these within anterior, middle or posterior cerebral zones or any combination thereof, cerebral palsy being closely correlatable to co-existence with them. Especially predictable of CP were the cavities within the occipital zone, and in addition the multifocal involvement of the brain, lesions larger than 1 cm in diameter and association with subcortical leukomalacia.

A magnetic resonance sequel of ominous significance, however, remains the appearance of severe impairment of myelination, especially encroaching upon the optic and auditory radiations. Residual scars demonstrated in the comprehensive studies at Hammersmith Hospital (Dubowitz LMS et al., 1985) also revealed persisting slit-like spaces flanked by scars of gliosis embodying groups of lipid-filled macrophages. Similar lesions had been previously described by neuropathologists as "white matter oedema" associated with perinatal asphyxia. The MRI visualization and monitoring of this and other pathological situations in which demyelination is a feature would certainly be a rewarding area for further research.

If crucial damage is in the area of periventricular leukomalacia, it might emerge either before or after birth, or before or after a subependymal or germinal layer bleed. A pathological extension of the leukomalacia would be the cystic changes, even porencephalic, which may not appear for one or two months. Within the basal ganglia themselves, spongiform changes may become grossly prominent.

289

# FOETOSCOPY UNDER
# REAL-TIME ULTRASOUND CONTROL

Amongst instrumental refinements of importance is that of foetoscopy under real-time ultrasound control. A sample of foetal blood could then be drawn under direct vision from a placental vein which for example opened the way to antenatal diagnosis of Duchenne muscular dystrophy. Foetal sexing would be done at around 14-16 weeks of gestation and if the foetus was male, the sample of blood would be taken at 18 to 20 weeks to demonstrate a significantly raised level of CPK (creatinine phosphokinase), optimal for the technique, and with time still to terminate pregnancy if the male proves to be presumptively affected.

## References

Ahman PA, Lazzara A, Dykes FD. (1980) Intraventricular haemorrhage in high risk preterm: Incidence and outcome. Ann Neurol 7: 118-124

Dolfin T et al. (1983) Incidence, severity and timing of subependymal and intraventricular haemorrhage in preterm infants as detected by serial real-time ultrasound. Pediatrics 71: 541-546

Donat JP, Okazaki H, Kleinberg F, Reagan JS. (1978) Intraventricular hemorrhage in full-term and premature infants. Mayo Clin Proc 53: 437-441

Doran L. (1992) Periventricular leukomalacia. Neonat Net 11: 7-13

Dubowitz LMS, Bydder GM, Muskin J. (1985) Developmental sequence of periventricular leukomalacia correlation of ultrasound, clinical and nuclear magnetic resonance function. Arch Dis Child 60: 349-355

Edvinsson L, Lou HC, Tvede K. (1986) On the pathogenesis of regimal cerebral ischaemia in intracranial hemorrhage: a causal influence of potassium. Pediatr Res 20: 478-480

Graham M, Levene MI, Trounce JQ, et al. (1987) Prediction of cerebral palsy in very low birth weight infants: prospective ultrasound study. Lancet 2: 593-595

Hambleton G, Wigglesworth JS. (1976) Origin of intraventricular haemorrhage in the preterm infant. Arch Dis Child 5: 651-659

Hill A, Melson GL, Clark HB, Volpe JJ. (1982) Hemorrhagic periventricular leukomalacia: diagnosis by real time ultrasound and correlation with autopsy findings. Pediatrics 69: 282-284

Ikonen RS, Janas MO, Koivikko MJ, Laippala P, Kuusinen EJ. (1992) Hyperbilirubinaemia, hypocarbia and periventricular leukomalacia leukamenia in preterm infants: relationship to cerebral palsy. Acta Paediat 81: 802-807

Kadoi N. (1992) Imaging evolution and incidence of periventricular leukomalacia in preterm infants. No To Hattatsu 24: 152-158

Krageloh-Mann I et al. (1992) Bilateral spastic cerebral palsy - pathogenetic aspects from MRI. Neuropaediat 23: 46-48

Kulakowski S, Larroche JC. (1980) Cranial computerized tomography in cerebral palsy. Neuropadiat 11: 339-353

Levene MI, Fawer CL, Lamont RF. (1982) Risk factors in the development of intraventricular haemorrhage in the preterm neonate. Arch Dis Child 57: 410-417

Leviton A, Paneth N. (1990) White matter damage in preterm newborn - an epidemiological perspective. Early Hum Dev 24: 1-22

Mehrabani D, Gowen CWJ, Korelman AE. (1991) Association of pneumothorax and hypotension with intraventricular haemorrhage. Arch Dis Child 66: 48-51

Miall-Allen VM, De Vries LS, Dubowitz LMS, Whitelaw AGL. (1989) Blood pressure fluctuation and IVH in the preterm of <31 weeks gestation. Pediatrics 83: 657-661

Papile LA, Burstein J, Burstein R, Koffler H. (1978) Incidence and evolution of subependymal and intraventricular haemorrhage: a study in infants with birthweights <1500 gms. J Pediat 92: 529-534

Pederson H, Taudorf K, Melchior JC. (1982) Computed tomography in spastic cerebral palsy. Neuroradiology 23: 275-278

Reynolds ML, Evans CAN, Reynolds EOR, Saunders NR, Durban GM, Wigglesworth JS. (1979) Intracranial haemorrhage in the pre-term sheep foetus. Early Human Dev 3: 163-186

Russell GAB, Jeffers G, Cooke RWI. (1992) Plasma hypoxanthine a marker for hypoxic-ischaemic induced PVL. Arch Dis Child 67: 388-392

Rutherford MA, Pennock JM, Murdoch-Eaton DM, Cowan FM, Dubowitz LM. (1992) Athetoid cerebral palsy with cysts in the putamen after hypoxic-ischaemic encephalopathy. Arch Dis Child 67: 846-858

Shortland D, Levene MI, Trouncer J, Ng Y, Graham M. (1988) The evolution and outcome of cavitating periventricular leukomalacia in infancy: a study of 46 cases. J Perinatal Med 16: 241-246

Shuman RM, Selednik LJ. (1980) Periventricular leukomalacia. Arch Neurol 37: 231-235

Siegel ML, Shakelford GP, Perlman JM, Fulling KH. (1984) Hypoxic-ischemic encephalopathy in term infants. Diagnosis and prognosis evaluated by ultrasound. Radiology 24: 418

Sinha SK, Davies JM, Sims DG, Chiswick ML. (1985) Relation between periventricular haemorrhage and ischaemic brain lesions diagnosed by ultrasound in very premature. Lancet 2: 1154-1156

Szymonowicz E, Walker AM, Yu YYH, Steward ML, Cannata J, Cussea. (1990) Regional cerebral blood flow after hemorrhagic hypotension in the preterm, near term and newborn. Pediat Res 28: 361-366

Trounce IQ, Fawer CL, Punt J, Dodd KL. (1985) Primary thalamic haemorrhage in the newborn: a new clinical entity. Lancet 1: 190-192

Trounce JQ, Rutter N, Levene MI. (1986) Periventricular leucomalacia and IVH in the preterm neonate. Arch Dis Child 61: 1196-1202

Volpe JJ, Herscovitch P, Perlman JM, Raichle MF. (1983) Positron emission tomography in the newborn: extensive impairment of regional cerebral blood flow with IVH and haemorrhagic intracerebral involvement. Pediatrics 72: 589-601

Wyatt JS. (1992) Understanding perinatal brain injury. In: Proceedings, Paediatrics into the 21st Century. p.19

Yoshicka H et al. (1989) New model of haemorrhagic hypoxic-ischaemic encephalopathy in newborn mice. Pediat Neurol 5: 1221-1225

291

# 12

# ADDITIONAL PREVENTIVE IMPLICATIONS:

# OTHER POSSIBLE ANTECEDENTS OF CEREBRAL PALSY

Additional Preventive Implications

Prevention of Preterm Delivery

Foetal Distress

Prevention Focussed on Hyaline Membrane Disease

The Negative Role of Maternal Drug Ingestion

Possible Role of Phenobarbitone

Pancuronium

Indomethacin

Ethamsylate

Vitamin E

Role of Other Direct or Conditioned Vitamin Deficiency

Coexistence of Major Coagulation Disorder including Disseminated
Intravascular Coagulation

Control of Hypotension

Control of Hydrocephalus

Conclusions

References

# 12

# ADDITIONAL PREVENTIVE
# IMPLICATIONS

Firstly we shall try to extract from all our preceding approaches an updating of preventive implications which are potentially most promising, or invite immediate application for this purpose. At the outset come the risk factors antecedent to germinal layer, intraventricular and periventricular haemorrhages, or their extension.

Follow up of preterm infants after periventricular haemorrhage of perinatal timing reveal neurodevelopmental sequelae especially when the cerebral parenchyma has been significantly encroached upon, or when ventricular dilatation has been significant. Refinement of diagnostic tools such as computed axial tomography, real-time ultrasound scanning and magnetic resonance imaging has begun the in vivo exposure of the extent of the problem and should allow more precise studies of antecedent events. With the advent of real-time sector scanners, a new era of intracranial sonographic evaluation was introduced to this preventive approach. What I believe to be practical comments have already been made disputing the glib claim that ultrasonography has virtually replaced computerized tomography (CT) as the primary diagnostic imaging modality in the preterm with suspected periventricular or intraventricular haemorrhage (IVH), or hydrocephalic sequelae. The relative roles of magnetic resonance imaging (MRI) or even positron emission tomography (PET)

have now to be appraised. Meanwhile, serial monitoring without risk of the preterm from birth, or even one day from the outset of foetal distress or imminent premature delivery, can become almost routine with either sonography or MRI.

Parenchymal damage probably most often reflects an haemorrhagic *infarction* of the brain that may arise in association with intraventricular bleeding, or primarily as a consequence of ischaemia with parallel or later bleeding into the hypoxic area as well as the adjacent ventricular system (Hill et al., 1982; Dolfin et al., 1983). The commonest site of haemorrhage in the preterm is the subependymal and periventricular area adjacent to the caudate nucleus. This has been variously ascribed to the presence of the germinal matrix, its abundant arterial supply, immaturity of the vascular rete and tenuous capillary integrity. But a primary preventive strategy should in the first place be aimed at reducing any increased tendency of the germinal matrix to bleed (germinal layer haemorrhage: GLH) and to prevent parenchymal lesions which would be secondary to consequent periventricular or intraventricular extension of the haemorrhage. Lesions primarily hypoxic and ischaemic could still have preceded, accompanied, or followed the haemorrhage or associated infarction.

Prevention here might be more successful if there was concentration upon

295

strategies to stabilize if not enhance cerebral perfusion. Indeed, an innovative approach to prevention could well concentrate predominantly upon techniques to stabilize otherwise rapid fluctuations in cerebral perfusion, as well as other haemodynamic factors. In this context, however, one should also focus upon modifications of therapy and management of gestation, with an objectively controlled assessment of changes in the incidence of cerebral palsy as a whole or of some of its associated components. Such attempts will be outlined, especially in relation to drug and vitamin prophylaxis focussing particularly where relevant on any potential for arresting or reducing the tendency to

specific intracerebral bleeds, or of their extension, or upon associated elements of hypoxic-ischaemic encephalopathy.

I have already dwelt briefly upon major factors in the aetiology of GLH/IVH and hypoxic-ischaemic encephalopathy and their preventive implications such as short gestation, intra-uterine growth retardation or "small for dates", foetal distress, hyaline membrane disease, and its attendant problems and complications such as pneumothorax. The relevant turn has come for the possible or established role of various micronutrients and potent pharmaceutical agents in the preventive campaign against CP.

# PREVENTION OF PRETERM DELIVERY

Preterm delivery is usually assumed to have reached an irreducible minimum in developed countries. But Finland and more recently France (Papiernik et al., 1985) have set an example. A programme of maternal education and early maternity leave ensured in high risk cases, has contradicted the previous popular bias with a substantial reduction in preterm delivery, hopefully with a presumptive reduction in the incidence of cerebral palsy as a secondary consequence yet to be realized. The greatest reduction was certainly effected in the lowest gestation group of preterm with a 50% fall in the births of infants weighing 1000 to 1500g, or of less than 32 weeks gestation. In other words, the group especially vulnerable to cerebral palsy.

Pharmacological applications to the prevention of preterm delivery and the

contribution of tocolysis have remained unconvincing. The prenatal use of steroids has more specific implications. First of all its effects in promoting foetal lung maturity (Collaborative Group of Antenatal Steroid Therapy, 1981). Although apparently effective in curbing hyaline membrane disease in a number of preterm infants, their overall impact on reduction of GLH/IVH is questioned. On the other hand, in a trial of combined Retrodrine and steroids involving infants of less than 28 weeks gestation, the incidence of hyaline membrane disease was more than halved (Kwong and Egan, 1986). There has been no evidence as yet of an accompanying fall in significant degrees of GLH and/or IVH which might well have been anticipated.

For a score of years, the pharmacological inhibition of uterine contractions using betaminetics had remained the mainstay of tocolytic therapy. *Magnesium sulphate* also had its advocates. It achieved tocolysis for more than 12 hours in 14 cases and for more than 7 days in 13 cases in the hands of Jirapinyo et al. (1990). But newer agents including Prostaglandin synthetase inhibitors, calcium channel blockers like Nifedipine and phosphodiesterase inhibitors are emerging to promise fresh hope of both safety and efficacy in prolongation of gestation. These are currently undergoing critical evaluation. A study of 102 women who received Nifedipine for the treatment of preterm labour (Murray et al., 1992) appeared to confirm that it was a well-tolerated and safe tocolytic agent in this population without deleterious uterine effects on the basis of foetal surveillance and neonatal outcome. In a comparison of the use of Ritodrine and Nifedipine in 42 women, 19 being randomized to the former group, 23 to the latter, they proved to be equally effective in the suppression of preterm labour, although there were fewer maternal and foetal complications in the Nifedipine group. Nor did it influence either the foetal or interoplacental circulation as evaluated by the Doppler technique (Mari et al., 1989).

Low dosage Aspirin is also having its day in reducing preterm birth. It appears to operate by reversing the functional balance between vascular prostacyclin and platelet derived thromboxane $A_2$ production. The outcome is an increased prostacyclin to thromboxane ratio. The conclusions reached were that effective reduction of preterm birth associated with intra-uterine foetal growth retardation and foetal growth retardation was a consistent result of the application of low dose Aspirin.

A fastidious appraisal of the effects of Magnesium on foetal haemodynamics was recently applied to 20 women presenting in preterm labour of between 23 and 35 weeks gestation. Pulse-wave Doppler measurements showed that there was a significant decrease in diastolic blood flow in the foetal middle cerebral ($p = 0.05$) whilst it increased significantly in the maternal uterine artery. The abberations in foetal haemodynamics were considered to indicate a physiological normalization process related to the stressed preterm infant and the preterm labour process itself.

The common usage of beta-adrenergic agonists to arrest premature labour delays delivery by 24 to 40 hours was challenged by a controlled trial (Canadian Preterm Labor Investigators Group, 1992). 708 women were assigned to receive the agonist Ritodrine (n=352) or placebo (n=356). Assessments were made via stratification to four categories of gestational age (20-23 weeks, 24-27 weeks, and 32-35 weeks). Amongst 771 infants born (including 63 pairs of twins), 23 deaths (6.1%) occurred in the *Ritodrine* group and 25 deaths (6.4%) in the placebo group. Meanwhile there was no difference between the groups in the extent of delay of delivery. Cerebral palsy occurred in only one infant in the Ritodrine group which showed as a group a slightly improved course on the Bayley Psychomotor Index at 18 months, whilst this affected five in the placebo group (p=0.09).

An illustration of combined therapy was that of Chimura (1992), in application to women suffering chorio-amnionitis with preterm PROM or threatened abortion in the 11th-34th week of pregnancy (n=9) and premature delivery, Imipenem/cilastin sodium (IPM/CS) was administered by intravenous drip infusion at daily dosages of 1-2 g concurrently with anti-ureteronics (Ritodrine HCl or Terbutaline sulfate). Response to IPM/CS was valued as good in all patients with threatened abortion and premature delivery. Latent periods were prolonged for more than seven days in 44.4%. The conclusion also reached was that treatment of preterm rupture of membranes before the 32nd week of pregnancy prolonged the latent period.

# FOETAL DISTRESS

Its amelioration, or control of associated factors, is likely to have significant prophylactic import. An association with germinal plate or intraventricular haemorrhage has been demonstrated in many studies. Following such distress or a prolonged labour, hypercapnia is often present, and may relate to the likelihood of subsequent GLH/IVH (Beverley and Chance, 1984). Since carbon dioxide exercises a vasodilator effect on the cerebral circulation, good physiological reasons exist for an aetiological role of hypercapnia at birth. An important claim was made by Lou and colleagues (1982) that hyperventilation in the immediate postnatal period afforded some protection against GLH/IVH.

# PREVENTION FOCUSSED ON HYALINE MEMBRANE DISEASE

In this context, the strong association of hyaline membrane disease with GLH/IVH points to a significant role for its prevention and management. Exogenous surfactants and modified mechanical ventilation to avoid pulmonary air leaks are promising innovations. Two trials of exogenous surfactant in preterm infants both report success in ameliorating the respiratory failure. This was attended by a reduction in smaller bleeds in the series of Hallman et al. (1985) who employed surfactant extracted from amniotic fluid. In the trial of Enhorning et al. (1985), using surfactant derived from corolung washings, the total numbers of infants with periventricular haemorrhage were halved. Equally significant effects in the prevention of GLH/IVH were achieved in a multicentre trial of artificial surfactant in the UK, as well as in the Belfast testing of porcine surfactant by McCord and team (1988).

# THE NEGATIVE ROLE OF
# MATERNAL DRUG INGESTION

A preventative approach in this context is also producing interesting results. A controlled study using prophylactic aspirin and dipyridamole by Wallenburg and colleagues (1986) showed improved outcome in infants born to mothers with a previous history of neonatal death due to maternal hypertension and related disorders. On the other hand, other reports have linked aspirin with a heightened incidence of neonatal bleeding; and of GLH/IVH in the preterm. So that it may be wiser to deny the use of aspirin especially during later pregnancy.

A curious observation under this heading is the result of a study by Cepeda et al. (1987) in which there was a significantly lower incidence of IVH in the progeny of drug-addicted mothers.

# POSSIBLE ROLE OF PHENOBARBITONE

A number of experimental studies of the value of phenobarbitone have been focused upon the prophylaxis of periventricular haemorrhage in very low birth-weight infants, predominantly applied in the immediate postnatal period. In that of Donn et al. (1981) 60 infants were randomized to phenobarbitone or "no treatment" groups. Two doses of 10 mg/kg intravenously were given 12 hours apart, followed by 2.5 mg/kg daily by any route for six days. The treated group showed a striking reduction in GLH/IVH from 46 to 13%. Such a beneficial effect was shown to persist in an extended trial by the same group (Goldstein et al., 1982). A trial by Morgan et al. (1982) in the following year, however, failed to confirm such an effect upon the incidence of GLH/IVH in a similar group of very low birth-weight infants. Nonetheless, there does appear to be a trend in most studies towards a reduction in major haemorrhage which could be of significant prophylactic value, possibly improved by modification of postnatal dosage.

Antenatal prophylaxis provides another approach of potential value. In the study of Shankaren et al. (1976) mothers in premature labour were randomized to receive 500 mg phenobarbitone intravenously, or no therapy. Cord blood levels were slightly higher at 9 $\mu$g/ml than maternal plasma levels at birth. A reduction in the incidence of IVH in premature infants of less than 30 weeks gestation following surfactant therapy was also claimed by Willinger et al. in 1987. The reduction in both mortality and severe IVH was significant, and suggests a method for coping with the adverse effects of labour on the very preterm foetus.

# PANCURONIUM

An alternative approach, the application of Pancuronium to this problem, and its induction of muscle relaxation, also appears promising. Using continuous wave Doppler examination of the anterior cerebral arteries, Perlman et al. (1985) have characterized haemodynamic factors and especially an unstable flow velocity pattern in infants who were at risk of later GLH/IVH. The use of Pancuronium abolished this pattern with immediate stabilization of blood flow velocity. Likewise Greenough et al. (1984) have also shown that Pancuronium reduces the high incidence of pneumothorax in ventilated preterm infants, and leads to fewer instances of GLH/IVH.

# INDOMETHACIN

Abnormally raised circulating levels of a number of prostaglandins characterizes the sick preterm infant, prostacyclin and thromboxane-A2 being particularly potent. Such high levels are also found immediately after birth. Especially prior to GLH/IVH. *A relatively low dosage of indomethacin*, a cyclo-oxygenase inhibitor drug, can rapidly suppress the raised concentrations of prostacyclin.

In the experimental animal, using a beagle puppy model, pretreatment with indomethacin has effected a reduction in IVH induced by hypotension and reperfusion. A parallel fall in the stable metabolite of prostacyclin could be measurable, alongside a more stable blood pressure. But even small doses of indomethacin carry the risk of increasing capillary bleeding time, although it has been shown by Maher et al. (1985) that this is not associated with any increased rate of extension in GLH/IVH. Curiously enough in extremely low birth-weight preterms of 900 g and below, prophylactic applications of indomethacin (Setzer et al., 1984) brought about significantly fewer haemorrhages, although no such effect was achieved in larger infants of 1250g birth-weight or more.

# ETHAMSYLATE

Pharmaceutical studies have suggested that Ethamsylate (diethyl ammonium 1,4-dihydrobenzene sulfonate), a water-soluble non-steroidal drug, hitherto empirically exploited for years as an "haemostatic" agent, altered platelet aggregation and increased platelet adhesiveness whilst raising capillary resistance. It has been used for decades to curb capillary bleeding in ear and buccal surgery. It has also reduced blood loss during transurethral resection of the prostate. Indeed it does reduce bleeding time, raise intrinsic thromboplastin release (Huguet et al., 1969) whilst presumptively maintaining capillary wall integrity by occlusion of endothelial lacunae. Significant reduction in the level of major metabolites of thromboxane-A2 and prostacyclin has been observed, as well as reduction of IVH in the beagle puppy model. Inhibition of prostaglandin and thromboxane synthesis has been accepted. It would appear logical that blocking production of prostacyclin, a potent vasodilator that is able to desegregate platelets, could prevent periventricular haemorrhage. Ethamsylate has thus been effectively exploited to prevent GLH/IVH in both human and animal studies, a vital consideration in lowering the frequency of subsequent neurological disorder.

In low birth-weight infants suffering the respiratory distress syndrome, ethamsylate did indeed reduce production of an immunoreactive prostacyclin metabolite (Rennie et al., 1986). A double-blind controlled trial has been undertaken involving initial intramuscular and intravenous administration of 12.5 mg/kg to 70 very low birth-weight infants within two hours of birth. It was then repeated 6-hourly for four days. The contemporary application of daily monitoring by scanning before entry, and on each day for the first week, was fully exploited. It produced a significant reduction in the incidence and severity of PVH (Morgan et al., 1981). This effect has been confirmed in a much larger study and controlled series (Cooke and Morgan, 1984). It was more obvious in those with extensive gradations of haemorrhage likely to produce subsequent neurological deficit. The lowered incidence

of GLH/IVH was most conspicuous at the GLH pole of the spectrum, although parenchymal haemorrhage was also reduced. Follow-up at one year of age confirmed lessened neurodevelopment sequelae including reduction in the number of ventriculo-peritoneal shunts inserted for hydrocephalus. A similar degree of effectiveness of ethamsylate in that prevention of PVH was effected in 330 infants of very low birth-weight without evidence of such haemorrhage on initial cranial ultrasound resulted in yet another multi-centre, placebo-controlled, double-blind study carried out in five centres from 1983 to 1986 by Benson et al. (1986). The dosage again was 12.5 mg/kg, the first dose being given intravenously or intramuscularly within an hour of delivery and was followed by 6-hourly doses intravenously for four days. The ethamsylate treated survivors had fewer total and fewer major haemorrhages than did the control survivors. Graded diminution in severity was also highly significant. In a group treated with both ethamsylate and Vitamin E, there were fewer haemorrhages than in those receiving vitamin E and placebo. Renal failure also occurred less frequently in the ethamsylate treated. The effect was most pronounced in those with more severe grades of haemorrhage which were more likely to lead to later neurological deficit.

In vitro, this agent has been shown to alter platelet aggregation, and block the synthesis of 6-keto-PGF1$_\alpha$ and thromboxane-B2. Inhibition of the synthesis of prostaglandin and thromboxane is apparent. Blocking in generation of prostacyclin, a vasodilator also able to desegregate platelets, is effective in preventing PVH. It has also been shown to reduce production of immunoreactive prostacyclin metabolite in low birth-weight infants manifesting the respiratory distress syndrome (Rennie et al., 1986).

It would appear that both the prevention and the outlook for PVL in very low birth-weight infants could be enhanced by ethamsylate, possibly even more so in conjunction with vitamin E and other advances in neonatal intensive care.

# VITAMIN E

*The prophylactic potential of Vitamin E is* still being pursued. Experimental evidence had long pointed to a protective role for Vitamin E in the immature central nervous system. Long ago, Pappenheimer et al. (1931) had demonstrated a nutritional encephalomalacia related to deficiency of Vitamin E, especially involving the cerebellum, which was marked by haemorrhage. A specific effect of Vitamin E deficiency, leading to swelling and fragmentation of the endothelial cells of the cerebral microcirculation was revealed on electron microscopy (Yu et al., 1974). Response to Vitamin E has been shown by Keeler et al. (1979) in the haemorrhagic necrosis involving the subependymal vasculature of the hamster which in my view bears analogy with areas of neuronal necrosis basic to the periventricular leukomalacia of the human preterm, and also advances to IVH. Subsequently, in the series of infants of less than 32 weeks subjected by Chiswick et al. (1982) to a double-blind controlled trial of 20 mg/kg intramuscularly of DL-alpha-tocopherol acetate in the first three days of life, intraventricular but not germinal layer haemorrhage occurred significantly more often in the control group. In a larger randomized controlled trial in 226 infants of

32 weeks gestation or less (Chiswick et al., 1983), these findings were reinforced very significantly. Giving three intramuscular doses of 20 mg/kg of alpha-tocopherol acetate at 24 hour intervals as soon as possible after birth, periventricular haemorrhage occurred in 6.5% of the newborn infants, whereas it emerged in 40% of untreated controls. Intramuscular free tocopherol combined with oral tocopherol for five days, as used by Speer et al. (1984) in the apparently effective prophylaxis of retinopathy, at the same time demonstrated a convincing reduction in both the incidence and severity of germinal layer and intraventricular haemorrhage, particularly in infants of less than 1000g birth-weight.

Plasma Vitamin E assay was established to be low in infants of 32 weeks or less. When 231 such infants were subjected to Vitamin E supplementation, significant elevation of plasma Vitamin E was confirmed, attended moreover by a lessened prevalence of periventricular and intraventricular haemorrhage in the treated group. Given promptly on the first day of life, a vital effect of Vitamin E appeared to be to rapidly *curtail the extension of subependymal haemorrhage within 24 hours of its occurrence,* rather than preventing the original bleed. As a *free radical scavenger*, it would appear to trap the free radicals stemming from ischaemic tissue damage in the subependymal region, thus curbing its progress, or the extent of periventricular haemorrhage on re-perfusion.

In beagle pups, as an experimental model, another free radical scavenger, *superoxide dismutase*, appeared to provide *protection against periventricular haemorrhage* in pups exposed to hypovolaemic hypotension and volume re-expansion.

## ROLE OF OTHER DIRECT OR CONDITIONED VITAMIN DEFICIENCY

The recent vindication of an important role for folic acid and its metabolites in the embryogenesis of the nervous system (Smithells et al., 1981) revives other empirical considerations in the field of prevention. However, no specific relationship of folate to the causation of cerebral palsy has been identified. An MRC trial lasting eight years in 33 centres in seven countries involved 1817 women who had had a previous pregnancy in which the foetus had a neural tube defect. 4 mg daily of folic acid was given to the trial group until the 12th week of pregnancy. Of 1195 pregnancies, 27 resulted in a foetus with neural tube defect, including anencephaly, spina bifida or encephalocele. Only seven of these were in those who had partaken of folic acid, implying a protective effect of 72%. No such protective effect could be demonstrated for other vitamins administered in this trial.

A crucial issue has been resolved, with a firm basis for significantly reducing what was formerly the commonest source of disability in children in the UK. To reduce the incidence still further, the timing of the introduction of 5.0 mg daily of folic acid at the time of conception, or even before, requires fuller study. After all, this was a bold empirical trial, as were initially the experimental trials of Vitamin E in the prevention of both retinopathy and cerebral bleeding. Similar large-scale trials of supplementation, with other selected vitamins, whether in conjunction with Vitamin E or not, may well be justified for the prophylaxis of neuropathology in cerebral palsy.

## COEXISTENCE OF MAJOR COAGULATION DISORDER INCLUDING DISSEMINATED INTRAVASCULAR COAGULATION

Whilst not initiating GLH/IVH, *disseminated intravascular coagulation* may provide its widespread extension. It can be overcome by 10-15 ml/kg of fresh frozen plasma given over a few hours, but its efficacy in preventing extension of the bleed has not yet been established.

# CONTROL OF HYPOTENSION

At the onset of cerebral haemorrhage, or even just preceding it in the neonate, a fall in blood pressure and haematocrit, most likely to be neurogenic or the response to vasodilatory prostamoid, is often observed. Correction of the hypotension and the anaemia would be urgent in the light of the dangers of ischaemic cerebral damage. An infusion of 10-20 ml/kg of whole blood, or partially packed cells, usually suffices. Where the myocardium is also under threat, 5 to 7 $\mu$g/kg/min of dopamine via a central catheter should reinforce this effect.

# CONTROL OF HYDROCEPHALUS

Hydrocephalus in this context is definable as a progressive distension of the ventricular system stemming from raised intracranial pressure. This complication develops in as many as 50% of the survivors of germinal plate haemorrhage with or without intraventricular extension (Burstein et al., 1979). According to Flodmark and colleagues (1981), whilst 52% of preterm infants display ventriculomegaly, progressive hydrocephalus of a degree necessitating a diversionary shunt develops in only 16%. The prognostic indices of the degree of haemorrhage has pointed significance. Grade I or small germinal layer haemorrhage has no increased risk of developing progressive hydrocephalus (Conlon, 1981). Grade II increases the risk to 25%, Grade II to 75%, and Grade IV, unequivocally, to 100%. He also observed the greater tolerance of premature neonates - without leading to hydrocephalus - than term neonates, attributing this to a greater release of fibrinolysin to lyse blood clots before intractable adhesions emerge.

Routine monitoring of ventricular size after GLH/IVH should permit early detection of such progressive ventricular dilatation. Such ventriculomegaly does not necessarily imply advance to progressive hydrocephalus. Control with diuretics or removal of cerebral spinal fluid, or even invasive intervention at the outset of symptoms including convulsions, apnoeic episodes or vomiting, may nevertheless be warranted to achieve relief of symptoms for several weeks, in preparation for serial surgical drainage of bloody cerebral spinal fluid, limiting the occlusive process as soon as indicated (Kreuser et al., 1985). The insertion of an implanted reservoir to allow for daily aspiration of cerebral spinal fluid may avert some disadvantages of daily LP or external ventricular drainage (Marlin, 1980).

In infants with significant cerebral parenchymal loss even when associated with ventriculomegaly, microcephaly may be the end result of the head's failure to grow. When this is the case, or the head size remains normal in the presence of ventriculomegaly, a cerebral atrophic process can be presumed.

Obviously computed tomographic scanning demarcates the ventricular size more accurately than serial measurements of head circumference. But it is not so useful as ultrasound in indicating particulate matter or other characteristics of the cerebral spinal fluid within the ventricular system. Monitoring of intracranial pressure over a 12-24 hour period helps to clarify this issue, having in mind that the normal intracranial pressure between 33 and 35 weeks is always <8mm of mercury (Hoffman, 1989). He attained continuous monitoring thereof by placing a pressure sensor to the anterior fontanelle. This will often allow diagnosis of progressive hydrocephalus even before abnormal increases in head circumference. At the same time one should remain alert to the natural course of events: that as intracranial pressure mounts, the fontanelle bulges and sutures spread apart... whereupon the intracranial pressure falls, a cycle which repeats itself in the typical situation.

Measurement of cerebral spinal fluid dynamics using radionucleotide flow studies typically confirms that there is a disturbance of cerebral spinal fluid flow. Injection of technetium into the lumbar subarachnoid space helps to demonstrate a communicating hydrocephalus amenable to lumboperitoneal shunting. This should be undertaken whenever there is unequivocal evidence of progressive hydrocephalus.

# CONCLUSIONS

Preventive studies have focussed on preventing the specific cerebro-vascular bleeding phenomena, with unfortunately sparse emphasis upon probably interrelated hypoxic-ischaemic factors. Follow-up studies of preterm who have suffered PVH in the neonatal period, have certainly confirmed their association with neurodevelopmental sequelae, especially after involvement of brain parenchyma or following significant ventricular dilatation. Most follow-up series establish that the poorest outcome mainly follows parenchymal lesions. Preventive approaches have focused on *the prevention* of these haemorrhages, or of *their extension*.

Whilst extension of a small GLH through an intraventricular stage towards parenchymatous involvement is usually assumed, the parenchymal lesion may be the first manifestation to be identified. Probably, it may stem from an haemorrhagic infarction secondary to intraventricular bleeding or primarily in association with ischaemia with later bleeding into the damaged area and adjacent ventricular system. A preventive strategy would focus on damping down the tendency of the germinal matrix capillaries to bleed, and preventing parenchymal lesions secondary to IVH. Primarily ischaemic infarctions could still arise. These lesions might be prevented by increasing cerebral perfusion, but perhaps only at the cost of evoking more GLH/IVH.

The overall evidence in the majority of cases, however, indicates that GLH/IVH in preterm infants is the outcome of an unstable cerebral circulation induced by respiratory disorders and its complications. Prolonged capillary bleeding time is an associated factor and may contribute to the extension of haemorrhage.

Some preventive strategies have been cited. A reduction in preterm deliveries as a social disease through health education, maternal protection and specific therapy during the third trimester whether with Nifedipine, Indomethacin, etc., or low aspirin dosage is one important pathway. Advances in the prevention and management of respiratory distress with surfactants is another. Improved stabilization of affected infants, possibly through the use of capillary stabilizers such as Ethamsylate and Vitamin E may add to the armamentarium available to markedly reduce the clinical problems stemming from GLH/IVH, possibly including cerebral palsy. It remains to be proven whether this can also lead to a parallel reduction in the incidence of ischaemic brain damage and its sequelae, again including cerebral palsy.

It may also be reasonably expected that current research with excitatory neurotransmitters may lead to specific therapy which could limit the progression of neurone injury towards irreversible loss and such permanent brain damage as characterizes cerebral palsy.

## References

Benson JWT, Drayton MR, Hayward J et al. (1986) Multicentre trial of ethamsylate for prevention of PVH in very low birth weight infants. Lancet 2: 1297-1299

Beverley DW, Chance D. (1984) Cord blood gases, birth asphyxia, and intraventricular haemorrhage. Arch Dis Child 59: 384-386

Burstein J, Papile I, Burstein R. (1979) IVH and hydrocephalus in premature newborns: a prospective study with CT. Am J Roentgenol 132: 631-635

Canadian Preterm Labor Investigators Group (1992) Treatment of preterm labor with the beta-adrenergic agonist Ritodrine. New Engl J Med 327: 308-312

Cepeda EE et al. (1987) Reduced frequency of intraventricular haemorrhage in the infants of drug-addicted mothers. Acta Paediat Scand 76: 16

Chimura T. (1992) Clinical studies of Imipenem/Cilastatin sodium in the early therapy of preterm premature rupture of the membrane or threatened abortion and premature delivery. Jap J Antibiotics 45: 1023-1028

Chiswick ML, Wynn J, Toner N. (1982) Vitamin E and IVH in the newborn. Ann NY Acad Sci 393: 109-118

Chiswick ML, Johnson M, Woodhall C. (1983) Protective effect of Vitamin E against IVH in premature babies. Br Med J 287: 81-84

Collaborative Group of Antenatal Steroid Therapy. (1981) Effect of antenatal dexamethasone in the prevention of respiratory disress syndrome. Am J Obstet Gynecol 141: 276-286

Conlon RA Jr. (1981) Outcome of intraventricular haemorrhage in the neonate based on CT scan and/or post mortem grading. In: Am Soc Pediat Neurosurg Concepts, Vol 1, pp 148-173. New York, S Karger

Cooke RWI, Morgan MEL. (1984) Prophylactic ethamsylate for periventricular haemorrhage. Arch Dis Child 59: 82-83

Dolfin T et al. (1983) Incidence, severity and timing of subependymal and intraventricular haemorrhage in preterm infants as detected by serial real-time ultrasound. Pediatrics 71: 541-546

Donn SM, Roloff DW, Goldstein GH. (1981) Prevention of intraventricular haemorrhage in preterm infants by phenobarbitone: a controlled trial. Lancet 1: 215-217

Enhorning G, Shennan A, Possmayer F, Dunn M, Chen CP, Milligan T. (1985) Prevention of neonatal respiratory distress by tracheal instillation of surfactants. Pediatrics 76: 145-153

Flodmark D, Scott G, Harwood-Nash DC. (1981) Clinical significance of ventriculomegaly in children after perinatal asphyxia. J Comput Assist Tomogr 5: 663-673

Goldstein G, Donn S, Roloff D. (1982) Further observations on the use of phenobarbital to prevent neonatal intracranial haemorrhage. In: J Lucey (Ed) Second Special Ross Conference on Perinatal Intracranial Haemorrhage. Columbus, Ross Labs. pp 810-815

Greenough A, Wood S, Morley CJ, Davis JA. (1984) Pancuronium prevents pneumothorax in ventilated premature babies. Lancet 1: 1-3

Hallman A, Merritt A, Jarvenfaa F, et al. (1985) Exogenous human surfactant for treatment of severe respiratory distress. J Pediat 106: 963-965

Hill A, Melson GL, Clark HB, Volpe JJ. (1982) Hemorrhagic periventricular leukomalacia: diagnosis by real time ultrasound and correlation with autopsy findings. Pediatrics 69: 282-284

Hoffman HJ. (1989) Diagnosis and management of posthaemorrhagic hydrocephalus in the premature infant. In: KE Pape and JS Wiggleworth (Eds) Perinatal Brain Lesions. Oxford, Blackwell Scientific Publications. pp 219-229

Huguet G, Thomas J, Raynaud C. (1969) Action of cyclonamine, a haemostatic drug, on capillary permeability and resistance. Therapie 24: 429-450

Jirapinyo M et al. (1990) Prospective study on premature labour with magnesium sulphate. Asia-Oceania J Obstet Gynaecol 16: 91-96

Keeler RF, Young S. (1979) Role of Vitamin E in etiology of spontaneous haemorrhage necrosis of the central nervous system of fetal hamsters. Teratology 20: 127-132

Lou HC, Phibbs RH, Wilson SL, Gregory GA. (1982) Hyperventilation at birth may prevent early periventricular haemorrhage. Lancet 1: 1407

Kreusser KL, Tarby TJ, Kovnar F. (1985) Serial lumbar punctures for at least temporary amelioration of neonatal post-haemorrhage hydrocephalus. Pediatrics 75: 719-724

Kwong MS, Egan EA. (1986) Reduced incidence of hyaline membrane disease in extremely premature infants following delay in delivery in mothers with preterm labour. Use of ritodrine and betamethasone. Pediatrics 78: 767-774

McCord FB, Curstedt T, Halliday HL, McClure G, Reid MMc, Robertson B. (1988) Surfactant treatment and incidence of IV haemorrhage in severe respiratory distress syndrome. Arch Dis Child 63: 10-16

Maher P, Lane B, Ballard R, Piecuch R, Clyman RI. (1985) Does indomethacin cause extension of intracranial haemorrhages: a preliminary study. Pediatrics 75: 491-499

Mari G et al. (1989) Doppler assessment of the fetal and uteroplacental circulation during Nifedipine therapy for preterm labor. Am J Obstet Gynecol 161: 1514-1518

Marlin AE. (1980) Protection of the cortical mantle in premature infants with posthaemorrhagic hydrocephalus. Neurosurg 7: 464-471

Morgan MEI, Benson JWT, Cooke RWI. (1981) Ethamsylate reduces the incidence of periventricular haemorrhage in very low birth weight babies. Lancet 2: 830-831

Morgan MEI, Massey RF, Cooke RWI. (1982) Does phenobarbitone prevent PVH in very low birth weight infants. A controlled trial. Pediatrics 70: 186-189

Murray C et al. (1992) Nifedipine for the treatment of preterm labor: a historic prospective study. Am J Obstet Gynecol 167: 52-56

Papiernik E, Bouger J, Dreyfus J et al. (1985) Prevention of preterm births: a perinatal study in Haguenau, France. Pediatrics 76: 154-158

Pappenheimer AM, Goettsch M. (1931) A cerebellar disorder in chicks of nutritional origin. J Exp Med 53: 11-26

Perlman JM, Goodman S, Kreusser KL, Volpe JJ. (1985) Reduction in intraventricular hemorrhage by elimination of fluctuating cerebral blood flow velocity in preterm infants with Respiratory Distress Syndrome. New Engl J Med 312: 1353-1357

Rennie JM et al (1986) Ethamsylate in the reduction in immunoreactive prostacyclin metabolite in low birth weight infants. Early Human Dev 14: 239

Setzer ES, Morse BM, Goldberg RN, Smith M, Bancalari E. (1984) Prophylactic indomethacin and intraventricular haemorrhage in the premature. Pediat Res 18: 345

Shankaren S et al. (1976) Antenatal phenobarbitone for the prevention of intracranial hemorrhage. Am J Obstet Gynecol 154: 53-57

Smithells RW, Sheppard S, Schorah CJ, Seller MJ, Nevin NC, Harris R, Reid AP, Fielding DW. (1981) Parent prevention of neural tube defects by periconceptional vitamin supplementation. Arch Dis Child 56: 911-918

Speer ME, Blifield C, Rudolph AJ. (1984) IVH and Vitamin E in very low birthweight infants: evidence for efficacy of early intramuscular Vitamin E. Pediatrics 74: 1107-1112

Wallenburg HCS, Dekker GA, Makovitz JW, Rotmaus P. (1986) Low dose aspirin prevents pregnancy induced hypertension and pre-eclampsia in angiotensin-sensitive primigravidae. Lancet 1: 1-3

Willinger SM et al. (1987) Reduction of intraventricular hemorrhage in premature infants of less than 30 weeks during surfactant therapy. Pediat Res 21: 381a

Yu WA, Yu MC, Young PA. (1974) Ultrastructural changes in the cerebrovascular endothelium induced by a diet high in linoleic acid and deficient in Vitamin E. Exp Mol Pathol 21: 289-299

# 13

# NEUROPATHOGENESIS OF CEREBRAL DYSFUNCTION AND FUNCTIONAL RECOVERY

# 13

# POSSIBILITIES OF FUNCTIONAL REORGANISATION AFTER PRETERM CEREBRAL DAMAGE

The brain of the preterm, particularly if less than 34 weeks, is thus at major risk of haemorrhagic or ischaemic lesions, or a combination of both. Basically, nevertheless, in the event of limited damage being incurred, its developmental status can still be regarded as an appropriate setting for *functional reorganisation*.

Bearing in mind the evidence already raised elsewhere of other pathogenic implications relating to the *striatum* and *subthalamic nucleus* and especially to the *caudate nucleus*, the contributory role of the *degree of maturation* of basal ganglia in structure and function at the time of pathological impact may even be a crucial primary factor. In that context, we may recall that both the *structural and functional maturation* of basal ganglia nuclei, thalamic, subthalamic, globus pallidus and caudate/putamen (striatum) is arrived at much earlier than that of the cerebral cortex.

First of all, therefore, one must try to relate to *the possibilities of functional reorganisation* after *preterm* cerebral damage. Re-establishment of function may be dependent upon several such possibilities. A particular function or set of functions may be reassigned to *an adjacent area* of the *same* cerebral hemisphere. As previously mentioned, reassignment of function to the *opposite* hemisphere is another possibility, as

is almost total failure of such compensatory modifications of function. After *unilateral* lesions of cortex and related white matter, however, there is experimental and other evidence of a potentially better chance of structural recovery. Intrinsic to it is an extensive development of cross innervation, a critical factor being the preservation of ipsilateral target cell groups at basal ganglia level, or more specifically at thalamic level.

The *nature* and *extent* of underlying cerebral damage is critical to the restoration of valid function. In turn it is a vital determinant of the *critical* mass of *residual* healthy cerebral cortex, or other area, which remains to permit significant redevelopment of function.

An extensive pathological sequel such as *cystic periventricular leukomalacia* tends to spread diffusely through periventricular zones. According to the boundaries of such spread there are likely to be levels of interruption of potential routes of interconnection between cortex and other target areas. Precise localization could determine whether the breach in communications is disproportionate to the volume of brain destroyed, which is in keeping with the frequent clinical experience of discrepancy between size of lesion and the extent of neurological impairment.

Where there has been a particularly large intraventricular haemorrhage, parenchymatous extension into white matter is likely to have been sufficient to interfere with maturation and integrity of the long tracts of the CNS. Resultant defects in a survivor would include hemiplegia or spastic diplegia and tetraplegia. To those immediate consequences there could be additive effects stemming from what may be *secondary* pathology, predominantly the *cystic leukomalacia* already emphasized. Any concomitant cerebellar lesions would add ataxic elements. The laterality, extent and degree of such a combination of effects could then be expressed clinico-pathologically in the extent, degree and character of the cerebral palsy, whether one of its more specific or discrete entities or a more or less mixed pattern.

# EXPERIMENTAL NEURONAL "RESCUE": NEUROPROTECTION

## Induction of Insulin-Like Growth Factor 1 in Neuroprotection

Impressive neuronal protective effects for insulin-like growth factor 1 (IGF-1) have been demonstrated experimentally by Peter Gluckman and colleagues in the Research Centre for Developmental Medicine and Biology, Auckland, New Zealand. Using in situ hybridisation, it was induced in astrocytes in the area of neuronal death within 72 hours of unilateral hypoxic-ischaemic injury in 21 rats. The infarction rate was simultaneously reduced ($p < 0.01$) from 87% to 16%. Behavioural testing also revealed protection of somatosensory function. IGF-1 used prior to hypoxic-ischaemic injury was not neuroprotective suggesting that it operates through some active mechanism, possibly apoptosis initiated by the hypoxia-ischaemia. It therefore appears that hypoxia-ischaemia activates endogenous IGF-1 production. The implications of this finding could be important therapeutically, since such therapy may be potentially valuable in neuronal "rescue".

## GM$_1$ Ganglioside

A different neuroprotective effect was illustrated in the use of GM$_1$ ganglioside after hypoxic-ischaemic injury to the brain of foetal sheep subjected to three 10 minute episodes of reversible central ischaemia. The GM$_1$ was given as 30 mg/kg through the umbilical vein.

The course of GM$_1$ led to improved recovery of the primary cytotoxic oedema within the parasagittal cortex, as well as "markedly reduced histologic damage" ($p < 0.001$) especially within the striatum, hippocampus and cortex. The results implied stabilised membrane function and enhanced neuronal outcome following subsequent hypoxic-ischaemic insults with the exciting promise of possible therapeutic value during repeated prenatal hypoxia-ischaemia.

# EARLY PREDICTION OF NEURODEVELOPMENTAL OUTCOME

Efforts to identify predictable parameters and related factors in at risk infants, and to improve their precise definition, are crucial steps in both the primary and secondary prevention of cerebral palsy. These include the possible management or control of phenomena that correlate strongly with the development of cerebral palsy (de Vries et al., 1985), such as germinal matrix, ventricular and parenchymatous haemorrhage or cystic periventricular leukomalacia (PVL). *All infants with an ultrasound diagnosis of cystic PVL, for instance, appear to go on to develop cerebral palsy.* Major ultrasound abnormalities (Grade IIb-III, cystic PVL) assessed together with developed NI latency show no better sensitivity as predictors for cerebral palsy. Nevertheless, in *specificity* and positive predictive value, both reached 100%. This has assumed especially dread importance in the light of estimates of steadily increasing survival of low birth weight infants alongside increasing numbers of the premature infants amongst them who develop cerebral palsy.

In the study of a cohort of 126 premature infants with and without abnormalities on cranial ultrasound (de Vries et al., 1992), 14 of the 25 infants who incurred cerebral palsy following large haemorrhages as well as cystic PVL, showed a normal NI latency. Only in some of them was the parenchymatous involvement in periventricular white matter zone possibly without effects upon the somatosensory tracts. On the other hand, 11 of the 19 infants demonstrating persistent delay of NI latency were to manifest cerebral palsy. Other techniques being tested for such predictive outcome in full term infants with postasphyxial encephalopathy (Gibson et al., 1992), including somatosensory evoked potentials of the posterior tibial and the medial nerve, have shown promising although inconclusive results.

## The Place of PVL and the Status of Myelination in this Prediction

**PVL**

Whilst PVL is demonstrable in the early postnatal period by ultrasound imaging (US) of the brain through the anterior fontanelle, only MRI achieves *optimal* differentiation of brain tissue, and of its abnormalities. It is especially valuable after fontanelle closure in following the evolution

313

of PVL. A follow-up was performed after 1 year of 95 full-term and term infants with cystic or non-cystic leukomalacia (Cioni et al., 1992). In 32 of these, a serious neurological outcome came to be exposed. This was mainly CP, sometimes associated with mental retardation and/or cerebral visual impairment. The main categories included *cystic lesions, enlarged ventricles* with irregular outlines, *delayed myelination, high intensity areas in the long tract images* within the white matter, and *cortical atrophy*. Their conclusion was chastening: that clinical outcome cannot be predicted by neuro-imaging alone. A more comprehensive approach is warranted, including *longitudinal, functional and neurophysiological testing*.

## Process and Stage of Myelination

Cranial ultrasound had detected periventricular and intraventricular haemorrhage and periventricular leukomalacia in 33 preterm infants of less than 32 weeks gestation. MRI at 44 weeks post-menstrual age was performed with especial focus upon the *process and stage of myelination*. The neurodevelopmental outcome was then appraised at 3 years of age in 31 children. A significant correlationship was found between the ultrasound findings, neurodevelopmental outcome, and stage of myelination... The detection of periventricular leukomalacia with ultrasound was calculated as showing the best predictive factor for neurodevelopmental outcome, so that the MRI assessment at 44 weeks proved to be unnecessary.

## References

Cioni L et al. (1992) Neuroimaging and functional outcome of PVL. Behav Brain Res 49: 7-19 ·

de Vries LS, Dubowitz LMS, Dubowitz V, et al. (1985) Predictive value of cranial ultrasound: a reappraisal. Lancet II: 137-140

de Vries LS, Eken P, Pierrat Y, Daniels H, Cassaer P. (1992) Prediction of neurodevelopmental outcome in the preterm infant: short latency somatosensory evoked potentials compared with cranial ultrasound. Arch Dis Child 67: 1177-1181

de Vries LS, Eken P, Dubowitz LMS. (1992) The spectrum of leucomalacia using cranial ultrasound. Behav Brain Res 49: 1-6

Gibson NA, Graham M, Levene MI. (1992) Somatosensory evoked potentials and outcome in perinatal asphyxia. Arch Dis Child 67: 393-398

Gluckman PD, Williams EB, Guan J. (19  ) Neuronal rescue after hypoxic-ischaemic injury (HI) using insulin-like growth factor 1.

# 14

# IMPLICATIONS OF NEURONAL "PLASTICITY" OR REGENERATIVE EXPERIMENTATION IN CEREBRAL PALSY

Implications of Neuronal "Plasticity"

Remodelling and Emergence or Restoration of Function after CNS Damage

Functional Outcome after Cerebral Lesions: Dependence upon Environmental Enrichment

Neutralization of Myelin and Oligodendrocyte Intubation of Neurite Outgrowth

Experimental Induction of Neuronal Generation

The Future Potential of Stereotactic Neurosurgery and Transplantation

**Experimental Cerebral Transplantation**

**Cochlear Implantation**

**References**

# 14

# IMPLICATIONS OF NEURONAL "PLASTICITY"

*Plasticity* in the development of the nervous system reflects proliferative or maturational changes following upon or associated with those which are predominantly regressive or degenerative. Its role in neonatal or postnatal recovery from perinatal cerebral damage is of critical importance.

Experimental studies after CNS injury have long demonstrated some degree of recovery or sparing of function, or even an element of neural regeneration which offers some promise for future habilitation after perinatal cerebral damage. That recovery tends to be more complete in *younger* animals is especially relevant to cerebral palsy. Recent evidence from work with children suggests that new pathways are indeed laid (or their regression *offset*) after early injury to the motor system (Carr et al., 1991; Cohen et al., 1991; Farmer et al., 1991).

Firstly, one may visualize the normal complex evolution of the basic neural pathways as a programmed development. Chemotactic (Sperry, 1963) and physical influences are conceived as guiding to their final target the growth cones at the tips of sprouting axons. That axons may follow a predetermined innervative pathway in response mainly to chemical cues despite destruction or other deviations, was illustrated by Landmesser (1981) who showed that chick lumbosacral motor neurones can reach their appropriate target muscles even if an aberrant course is induced from entry.

Experimentally, one instance worthy of mention is simply the anatomical and functional result of resection of areas of dorso-lateral prefrontal cortex. Normal acquisition of functions subserved by these areas is important whilst anatomically there is initially abnormal ectopic gyral formation, but eventual bilateral macroscopic symmetry. A point of probable relevance to cerebral palsy is the preservation of the *thalamic* neurones which normally project to the excised portion of cerebral cortex.

Even more promising physiologically, however, is the "massive" ipsilateral *sprouting* of pyramidal tract fibres 1-3 mm above experimental lesions (Kalil and Reh, 1979). Even more striking, however, is that true *crossing* of most of the fibres followed, and served to re-innervate sites which had been deprived by the initial lesion.

Occasional clinical experiences indicate that the compensatory mechanism after a serious cerebral lesion must include a structural modification with partial redirection of neural pathways subserving motor functions included in the regenerative phenomenon.

*Regulated cell death* appears to be an essential morphogenetic and even normal antecedent to the precise formation of an organ or of any specific neural structure (Janowsky and Finlay, 1986). The morphogenetic death of considerable numbers of neurones has already been shown to precede the formation of ventral horns at the nonlimb levels of the mouse spinal cord (Flanagan and Harris, 1969). Even between 5 and 10 days of postnatal age in the mouse and hamster (Heuman and Leuba, 1983), considerable numbers of neurones are thereby lost from the most recently generated outer layer of the neocortex. At the medial cingulate cortical level (Finlay and Slattery, 1983) the loss approaches 100%. Similar cell losses varying from 20 to 70% characterize the amygdala, midbrain tectum, central grey matter, auditory relay nuclei, Purkinje and granule cell layers of the cerebellum (Janowsky and Finlay, 1986); and also *the thalamus and caudate nuclei* in which we are especially interested in this context because of their possible relevance to cerebral palsy.

The establishment of connections - and of integrated function - appears to parallel, or immediately precede, the outset of these cell losses. In the mouse neocortex, it is maximal soon after the completion of migration of cells to the cortical cell plate (Finlay and Slattery, 1983). Jacobson (1978) extrapolates this to about 30 to 34 weeks in the human foetus, when there is a marked increase in connectivity within the brain, reflected also by augmented dendritic spines or neuronal axons (Purpura, 1975). The timing in the cerebellum would be soon after term.

The purpose of these cell losses are probably two-fold. Firstly, that they are part of an overall *population-matching* process whereby cells are restricted to those capable of involvement in making efficient connection with target structures. Elimination *during development of errors in connectivity*, is another process. So the relationships between developing neurones and their ultimate target cells are worthy of careful exploration (Wigglesworth, 1989).

Most of the cells that die have already made peripheral connections, although cell death also follows failure to make appropriate connections. Oppenheim (1981) has demonstrated a relationship between natural cell death and the number and distribution of *acetylcholine receptors*, apart from evidence of critical physiological factors in the regulation of the number and distribution of receptors.

*Reduction of connectivity* is also an important phenomenon. At the outset of muscle activity, axon collaterals retract - followed by reduction in axon number - until a later reduction in polyneural innervation is reached with a one-to-one ratio between axons and muscle fibres. *Functional competition between axons* is reflected by the delay or inhibition of depressed polyneural innervation produced by partial denervation of individual limb muscles in the newborn rat. It may well be of practical significance to early habilitative techniques that electrical stimulation, or resultant "functional" muscle hypertrophy (Oppenheim, 1981), can hasten such loss of polyneural innervation. It is retained in the "staggerer mouse" (Crepel et al., 1980) which lacks either granule cells or synaptic contacts between climbing fibres and cerebellar Purkinje cells, an aspect which may be relevant to atactic cerebral palsy.

*Influences promoting cell proliferation* are no less important. Increasing the quantity of target tissue and thus diminishing the rate of cell death is the expression of one such group of influences which may not necessarily induce any improvement in CNS function. Exploitation of an *enriched environment* is another approach (Rosenzweig et al., 1962), to which we shall again refer.

*Sensory input is another vital influence* upon cell proliferation in specific pathways. In the monkey, monocular occlusion from birth leads to impaired development of those ocular dominance columns in the visual cortex which are related to the occluded eye (Hubel et al., 1977). Conversely, this was accompanied by compensatory widening or hypertrophy of the dominance columns of the visual cortex related to the non-occluded eye.

# REMODELLING AND EMERGENCE OR RESTORATION OF FUNCTION AFTER CNS DAMAGE

It was an important finding of Goldman and Galkin (1978) that resections of dorso-lateral prefrontal cortex in foetal Rhesus monkeys of less than 119 days postconceptual age, were followed by recovery of the functions subserved by the related cortical areas. Underlying this, there is preservation of thalamic neurones normally projecting from the relevant excised section of cortex, whilst abnormal arrangements of corticostriatal, callosal and corticothalamic projections are attended by a marked increase in crossed projections to the opposite hemisphere.

*Another aspect of reserve for recovery* was expressed in the *persistence* of the corticospinal neurones that normally disappeared after ablation of corticospinal neurones in the infant rat cortex (D'Amato and Hicks, 1978). A study of considerable topical interest was on the effect of irradiation of the foetal rat on day 12, which produced death of 50 to 75% of primitive cells in the dorsal pallidum of cerebral hemispheres, optic vesicles, diencephalon and dorsal midbrain, etc. *72 hours later there was almost complete recovery.* Subsequent normal motor performance was revealed on follow-up, although ocular maldevelopment remained in three of the ten animals.

*Sprouting is a vital structural change* that can follow damage to newborn as distinct from adult motor cortex. Massive ipsilateral sprouting of the pyramidal tract arises 1-3 mm above the section of the left pyramidal tract just above the decussation (Kalil and Reh, 1979). *The actual crossing of fibres to reinnervate sites deprived by the initial lesion* is

319

a striking regenerative phenomenon, the application of which is more than worthy of continuing intensive study.

Sparing of function is less marked after *early* subcortical lesions. Experimental involvement in the Rhesus monkey of the antedorsal sector of the *caudate* nucleus, or of the dorsomedial nucleus of the thalamus produces equally severe dysfunctions in infants or adults (Goldman and Galkin, 1974).

After left hemispherectomy in the Sturge-Weber syndrome, some language deficit did ensue *but the right cerebral hemisphere appears able to take over some development of language function*, albeit less efficiently than the left hemisphere (Dennis, 1981). This transfer of function reflected two basic "recovery" or "compensatory" mechanisms. One is recognized as *Substitution* where the destroyed function is replaced by a substituted behaviour performed by an intact system. The second is *Functional Reorganization* referring to a compensatory take-over phenomenon first studied as long ago as 1938 by Kennara.

Children with *congenital agenesis of the corpus callosum*, or surgical section thereof at under 10 years, can still fulfil *tasks dependent upon interhemispherical connection* (or bilateral cortical representation) despite this being a function of the intact corpus callosum. Possible *bilateral representation of functions* such as speech and language that are normally lateralized, may account for the compensatory mechanism. It has been assumed (Dennis, 1976) that sensory input has access to both hemispheres through simultaneous use of crossed and uncrossed

projections resulting from absence of callosal suppression.

Nuclei of basal ganglia, thalamus, midbrain and brainstem mature both structurally and functionally in the mammalian brain, especially that of the human brain, at a far younger age than does the cortex. Preterm stages of less than 30 weeks, although so vulnerable to haemorrhagic and ischaemic incidents, are believed to reflect a favourable developmental setting for functional reorganization of much of the CNS. After *unilateral lesions of the cortex and related white matter without involving thalamus or caudate nucleus*, a good structural recovery is linked to development of cross-innervation, and the preservation of ipsilateral target cell groups at thalamic or basal ganglia levels.

After total destruction of an area of infant *brain before establishment of the function it is to subserve*, three possibilities of functional reorganization arise: function may be reassigned to the opposite hemisphere, it may be assigned to an adjacent area of the same hemisphere, or it will not develop... Thus despite left hemispherectomy, normal language development may still emerge. Or after unilateral or bilateral *prenatal* cortical lesions, cortical functions may be transferred either to the opposite hemisphere or to adjacent areas of the same hemisphere. The degree of recovery of function appears to depend upon the *site, extent and timing* of destruction of mature cerebral regions *such as the thalamus and caudate nuclei*. But it is very difficult to delineate the precise size and location of the underlying cerebral destruction by imaging near the time of the event. By diffuse spread through the periventricular region, however, a cystic degree of periventricular leukomalacia tends to pose a problem of extensive interruption of routes of connection between the cortex and other target areas to an extent disproportionate to the volume or size of the brain lesion.

# FUNCTIONAL OUTCOME AFTER CEREBRAL LESIONS: DEPENDENCE UPON ENVIRONMENTAL ENRICHMENT

Recovery of function is certainly not a passive phenomenon. It has been convincingly demonstrated in the monkey (Goldman and Lewis, 1978) that after frontocortical (motor) resections at 50 days, some form of developmental or training stimulation is essential to effect the functional reorganization required to restore the ability to perform spatial tasks, as assessed at 2 years. Such a favourable outcome of *environmental enrichment* embodying non-specific stimuli, has also been shown in rats subjected to brain damage at the post-weaning stage (Will et al., 1976). These functional results of brain lesions have also been reinforced by laboratory parameters in brain tissue such as *enhanced RNA-DNA ratios* (Ferehmin, Eberovic and Caputto, 1970).

In the same way, differences in outcome of cerebral lesions in the human preterm may be influenced by variations *in the range, intensity or specificity of external stimulation*. Particular difficulties in achieving a broadly favourable outcome to adequate or appropriate stimulation may be the consequence of co-existing damage to cerebral areas subserving *visual* or *auditory*

pathways. Other factors which will determine this outcome to a greater or lesser extent include the precise timing, site or extent of the lesions.

Specific trophic influences may be engendered from damaged or destroyed neurones as a result of experience, or external stimulation, and these may constitute a balanced physiological basis underlying behavioural recovery from early brain damage. *Nerve growth factor*, and a range of neurotransmitters, are probably included. Loss of these trophic influences may evoke *depression of postsynaptic cellular metabolism*, and external stimulation may therefore operate by reversing this depression. This may well be especially difficult in socially disadvantaged situations, or where appropriate or adequate stimulation after damage to brain tissue subserving visual or auditory pathways is unlikely. Functional reorganization, however, also appears to be paralleled by *structural reorganization* in terms of fundamental axon sprouting, which presumably equally hinges more or less equally upon environmentally-based trophic stimuli.

Outcome will, of course, be affected either favourably or unfavourably by the underlying structural reorganization after cerebral damage or ischaemia. This may be basically defined in terms of neuronal axon sprouting and its degree and direction, quite apart from the trophic stimuli referred to as derived from the environment. Such influences may operate via rises in the cell population of the developing brain. But increasing the quantity of target brain tissue, with decreases in the rate of cell death, may not necessarily lead to improvement in central nervous system function. In earlier experimental studies applied to young rats housed in groups in spacious cages with a variety of toys and other objects to stimulate exploratory activity - being changed frequently to offer a continuous challenge - the cerebral cortex became heavier and thicker than that of rats reared under standard laboratory conditions (Rosenzweig, Kresh and Bennett, 1962). Underlying such increases in cortical mass were increases in glial cell number, together with enlargement of neuronal cell bodies and augmented elaboration of dendritic branches and spines. Biochemically an increase of RNA content and enhanced metabolic activity were associated (Ferehmin et al., 1970).

# NEUTRALIZATION OF MYELIN AND OLIGODENDROCYTE INTUBATION OF NEURITE OUTGROWTH

Recently, an inhibitory substrate effect of CNS myelin and oligodendrocytes has been discovered to be directly involved in the limited neurite regeneration of which the CNS is capable (Schwab et al., 1991). These inhibitory components of myelin were characterized as two proteins of 35 and 250 kD molecular weight. To neutralize these inhibitory effects, a specific monoclonal antibody was generated. When these specific myelin components are thereby neutralized, regeneration is significantly enhanced within several different lesions of CNS pathways, including the cholinergic septo-hippocampal pathway and the optic nerve. The application of such specific monoclonal antibodies, during or as soon as is practicable after the basic cerebral damage, *may help in the promotion of early regeneration.*

# EXPERIMENTAL INDUCTION OF NEURONAL GENERATION

It is reassuring to end this academic review of the implications of cerebral neuronal "plasticity" in the restoration of function after cerebral damage with an exciting note of promise. The dogma has long been accepted that regeneration of neurones can never occur except in the earliest stages of neurodevelopment. But the radical, even revolutionary, finding from Alberta has shown that neurones can be generated. Samuel Weiss and Brent Reynolds have demonstrated transmutation of stem cells in the cerebral environment of mice, into astrocytes and in particular neurones, in response to the injection of *epithelial growth factor* (1992). The stem cells gradually modified in shape to assume the full anatomical shape and immunogenic characteristics of astrocytes and neurones. If these cells exist in the human brain, it may be possible to trigger the production of neurones and then transplant them back into the same person, or to stimulate their production within the brain itself. Whilst early estimates of its therapeutic implications may be deferred for a decade or more, one hopes that its application to overcome highly localized damage to basal ganglia components, such as that in the substantia nigra in Parkinson's disease or even that of the striatum, which was the experimental source of this neuronal generation. This would be so specifically relevant in Huntington's chorea or attained much earlier in the choreo-athetoid form of cerebral palsy that can derive from anoxic/ischaemic damage in the preterm in that localization.

# THE FUTURE POTENTIAL OF STEREOTACTIC NEUROSURGERY AND TRANSPLANTATION

Not only have the new techniques of neuro-imaging enhanced our interpretation of the nature and localization of particular congenital brain defects and prenatal damage, including hypoxic/ischaemic, they have in parallel facilitated advances in stereotactic neurosurgery. Such highly sophisticated procedures depend upon the precise positioning of an electrode carrier, a radio frequency probe or a needle directly into discrete regions of the brain for biopsies, stimulation, destruction or ablation. The future role of such an approach becomes realistic, with particular relevance to the alleviation or elimination of such involuntary movement disorder, as choreo-athetosis stemming from lesions of basal ganglia constituents or of their inter-communicating functions in their cortical-hypocampal, collicular, cerebellar loops, or in overcoming intractable epilepsy which in this context is so frequent a complication.

Stereotactic surgery including stereotactic thalamotomy has been vainly applied to the relief of spasticity. On the other hand, stereotactic dendatomy has its advocates in cerebral palsy, including some of its subjects with athetosis. It is believed to be also useful in dystonia (Gornall et al., 1975).

# EXPERIMENTAL CEREBRAL TRANSPLANTATION

Technological advance in this area also holds out promise for brain tissue transplants. The experimental rat studies of Donald Stein and his colleagues at the Clark University of Worcester, Massachusetts, have already produced challenging results. Limited frontocortical ablation in 21 rats was followed in 8 by implantation of pin-head sized laps from the frontal cortex of normal rat embryos. Although the treated rats did not learn as rapidly as normal, their rate of learning was significantly faster than the remaining untreated brain-damaged rats.

After neural or cerebral transplantation the new axons sprouting would lack the ability to function in the transmission of neurological stimuli without the supervention of membranes of myelinogenesis. The formation of myelin or myelin-like membranes is an intrinsic property of oligodendrocytes. Concurrent transplantation, or side by side placement of oligodendrocyte cultures, would seem rational in the light of studies of their transplantation (Seil, 1989) although the prompt response of pre-existing or residual oligodendroglia may suffice. Oligo-dendrocytes from all three sources which he used, although especially from dissociated oligodendrocyte cultures, migrated into the host explants to form myelin around appropriate host axons.

It is hoped that the clinical results of transplantation experiments in the adult monkey may one day be truly meaningful for the child victim of cerebral palsy. One promising extension is the reversal of a Parkinsonian syndrome, and its characteristically continuous tremor induced with MPTP (1-methyl-4 phenyl-1,2,3-6 tetrahydro pyridine), by experimental transplantation elsewhere of foetal dopamine neurones of the substantia nigra. Extension of neurites was defined, attended presumptively by integration with the host brain. Comparable neuritic outgrowth, both axonal and dendritic, appears to be directed by a terminally expanded specialized organelle - the *growth* cone. This is responsive to, and can align actively towards a *nerve growth factor* or kindred as yet undefined substance from nerve or muscle media. *Neuronal cell adhesion molecules (NCAM)* and their antigens have been identified with a role in such *alignment processes* and antibodies against one of them have been shown to disrupt fascination of the retinofugal protection of chicks. Indeed, it would be characteristic of the young neurone to move along a glial fibre as in embryonic neural migration, with the neuronal-glial interaction probably derived from a selective *molecular* affinity between surfaces of neurones and glial cells. We can be forgiven a conviction that the manifestations of Parkinson's disease in the human adult may one day be finally overcome if not at least significantly modified by appropriate neurological transplantation. Another reassuring aspect of such transplants is that the brain shows less tendency to reject such new tissue than do other parts of the body.

Some forms of blindness may also become a suitable substrate for such creative tissue manipulation. Indeed a great deal of experimental regenerative study in the CNS has been focused upon a progenitor cell of the rat optic nerve: the oligodendrocyte-type-2 astrocyte (0-2A). In vitro, this cell can be induced to generate oligodendrocytes or type-2 astrocytes (Noble, 1992). Astrocytes of a different glial line modulate differentiation of 0-2A progenitor cells via secretion of one of an extraordinary array of newly-defined growth factors: PDGF or platelet derived growth factor. The ciliary neurotropic factor, for example, has been shown to hasten the growth and differentiation of oligodendrocytes. Cooperative interaction of growth factors, in this instance, included the addition of basic fibroblast growth factor (6FGF), which can together induce continuous self-renewal of the growth of the 0-2A progenitors, so-called conditional immortalization of these precursor cells. This process has been successfully exploited (Noble, 1992) in the repair of demyelinating lesions involving myelin regeneration and the "remyelination of axons" essential for remodelling axons within the pathological area. The recent demonstration of differentiation of the mouse brain stem cell into neurones and astrocytes, also heralds a new understanding of neural regeneration.

A variety of cell types has also been effected in the presence of Gamma-interferon, using a novel strain of transgenic mice. This new experimental tool should facilitate developmental biological studies moving towards neuronal and axonal regeneration, and delicate techniques of intrusive plasticity of the central nervous system which could one day help in the otherwise irreparable cerebral damage underlying cerebral palsy.

# COCHLEAR IMPLANTATION

For some profoundly deaf children with sensory or cochlear hearing loss but intact cochlear nerve, implantation of a cochlear device may now provide a valid answer (House, 1986). In the UK alone, the prevalence of severe sensorineural hearing loss ranges between one and two per thousand (Taylor, 1985), but only during the past decade has implantation of a device such as the Nucleus or Ineroid multi-channel unit achieved widespread clinical application. More than 800 children have already been so served by a multi-channel implant which is significantly more beneficial than the single-channel type.

It is, in essence, a highly sophisticated hearing aid or microphone which is implanted so as to bypass the inner ear hair cell system and directly stimulate the ganglion cells of the 8th nerve. It is connected to an externally-worn speech process, filtering speech and extracting dormant information data which are transmitted to the receiver/electrode package in the implanted part.

In the FDA trials, 64% of those implanted were deafened at or before 24 months of age, being considered pre-linguistic, with 43% being congenitally deaf (Staller et al., 1991). Preliminary evaluation includes general medical and otological assessment, as well as computed tomography, an important check in examples of deafness due to meningitis, or to labyrinthine ossificans which constitutes a contra-indication. It also extends beyond hearing to include spoken language and other communication skills, In the pre-verbal stage, video analysis of the child with a known adult may be used both before and after implantation. The post-operative rehabilitation process is a protracted one and preliminary study of the management programme evolved by the Nottingham team is essential (Gibbin, 1992), at present the major paediatric implant centre within the UK. Implantation is warranted solely for the proportion of children with sensorineural hearing loss who have not been helped by suitable conventional amplification coupled with appropriate habilitation. This technique should lend itself to severe sensorineural deafness associated with cerebral palsy which has not responded to the conventional amplification approach.

## References

Carr LJ et al. (1991) Evidence of bilateral innervation of homologous motor neurone pols in man. J Physiol 446: 567

Cohen et al. (1991) Reorganisation in motor pathways following a large congenital hemispheric lesion in man: different ipsilateral motor representation areas for ipsi- and contralateral muscles. J Physiol 438: 33

Crepel F, Delhaye-Bouchaud N, Guastavino JM, Sampaio I. (1980) Multiple innervation of cerebellar Purkynge cells by climbing fibres in staggerer mutant mouse. Nature 283: 483-484

D'Amato CJ, Hicks SP. (1978) Normal development and post-traumatic plasticity of corticospinal neurons in rats. Exp Neurol 60: 551-569

Dennis M. (1976) Impaired sensory and motor differentiation with corpus callosum agenesis. Neuropsychologist 14: 455-469

Dennis M. (1981) Language in a congenitally acallosal brain. Brain Lang 12: 33-53

Farmer SF et al. (1991) Plasticity of central motor pathways in children with hemiplegic cerebral palsy. Neurology 41: 1505-1510

Ferehmin PA, Eberovic VA, Caputto R. (1970) Studies of brain weight and RNA content after short periods of exposure to environmental complexity. Brain Res 20: 49-57

Finlay BL, Slattery M. (1983) Local differences in the amount of early cell death in neocortex predict adult local specialization. Science 219: 1349-1351

Flanagan A, Harris E. (1969) Differentiation and degeneration in the motor horn of the foetal mouse. J Morphol 129: 281-306

Gibbin KP (1992) Paediatric cochlear implantation. Arch Dis Child 67: 669-671

Goldman PS, Galkin TW. (1974) Prenatal removal of frontal association cortex in foetal Rhesus monkey: anatomic and functional consequences alternative to developmental plasticity heterology of CNS in infants and adults. In: Plasticity and Recovery of Function in the CNS. Eds. Stein et al. New York, Academic Press. pp 149-174

Goldman PS, Galkin TW. (1978) Prenatal removal of frontal association cortex in foetal Rhesus monkey: anatomical and functional consequences. Brain Res 152: 451-485

Goldman PS, Lewis ME. (1978) Developmental biology of brain damage and experience. In: Neuronal Plasticity. Ed. Cotman CKI. New York, Raven Press. pp 291-310

Gornall P, Hitchcock AHS, Kirkland IS. (1975) Stereotaxic neurosurgery in the management of cerebral palsy. Dev Med Child Neurol. 17: 279-286

Heuman D, Leuba G. (1983) Neuronal death in the development and aging of the cerebral cortx of the mouse. Neuropathol Appl Neurobiol 9: 297-311

House WE. (1986) Cochlear implants: present and future. Otolaryngol Clin N Am 19: 217-218

Hubel DH, Wiesel TN, Le Vay S. (1977) Plasticity of ocular dominance columns in monkey striate cortex. Philos. Trans R Soc London(Biol) 278: 377-409

Jacobson M. (1978) Developmental Neurobiology, 2nd Ed. New York, Plenum Press. p 66

Janowsky IS, Finlay BL. (1986) The outcome of perinatal brain damage: the role of normal neuron loss and axon retraction. Dev Med Child Neurol 28: 375-389

Kalil K, Reh T. (1979) Regrowth of several axons in neonatal central nervous system. Science 205: 1159-1161

Kennara MA. (1938) Reorganisation of motor function in the cerebral cortex of monkeys deprived of motor and premotor areas in infancy. J Neurophysiol 1: 477-496

Landmesser L. (1981) Pathway selection by embryonic neurons. In: Studies in Developmental Neurobiology. Ed. Cowan WM. New York, Oxford University Press. pp 53-73

Noble M. (1992) Development, repair and neoplasia in the central nervous system. Proc Paediatrics in the 21st Century. Institute of Child Health, London. p.36

Oppenheim RW. (1981) Neuronal cell death and some related regressive phenomena during neurogenesis. In: Studies in Developmental Neurobiology. Ed. Cowan WM. New York, Oxford University Press. pp 74-133

Purpura DP. (1975) Dendritic differentiation in human dendritic cerebral cortex: normal and aberrant developmental patterns. Adv Neurol 12: 91-134

Rosenzweig MR, Kresh D, Bennett EL. (1962) Effects of environmental complexity and training on brain chemistry and anatomy. J Comp Physiol Psychol 55: 429-437

Schwab ME, Schnell L, Cadelli D. (1991) CNS myelin associated inhibitors of neurite outgrowth, and their role in regeneration 1011 glial control of neuronal development and regeneration. 14th Meeting European Neuroscience Assoc Abstr. Oxford University Press. pp 1011, 1013

Seil FJ. (1989) Tissue culture models of myelination after oligodendrocyte transplantation. J Neural Transplant 1: 44-57

Sperry RW. (1963) Chemoaffinity in the orderly growth of nerve fibre patterns and connections. Proc Natl Acad Sci USA 50: 703-710

Staller SJ, Dowell RC, Beiter AL, Brimacombe JA. (1991) Perceptual abilities of children with the nucleus 22 channel cochlear implant. Ear Hear 12: suppl.

Taylor VE. (1985) Aetiology of bilateral sensori-neural hearing loss in young children. J Laryngol Otol: suppl. 10

Weiss S, Reynolds B. (1992) Generation of neurones and astrocytes from isolated cells of adult mammalian central nervous system.

Wigglesworth JS. (1989) Current problems in brain pathology in the perinatal period. In: Perinatal Brain Lesions, Eds. KE Pape, JS Wigglesworth. Blackwell Scientific Publications, Boston, Oxford, London. p. 1

Will BE, Rosenzweig MR, Bennett EL. (1976) Effects of differential environments on recovery from neonatal brain lesions measured by problem-solving scores and brain dimensions. Physiol Behav 16: 603-611

# 15

# THE IMMATURE LOCOMOTIVE PATTERN OF THE CP CHILD AND ADAPTATION FOR WALKING AND PROGNOSIS FOR ULTIMATE WALKING

# 15

# CONCEPT OF IMMATURE EVOLUTION
# OF THE LOCOMOTIVE PATTERN
# IN THE CP CHILD

In the human species, at least early in ontogeny, the influence of a provisional localization within the spinal cord of *locomotor generating circuits* has been indicated by the stepping movements of the foetus even from the first half of pregnancy. An alternative perspective would envisage them as an expression of the nervous system's capacity to generate rhythmical motor patterns, influenced, even modified, by afferents from the sole of the foot touching the surface. Prechtl has drawn attention to another centrally generated pattern with rhythmical characteristics in the side to side movement in the rooting response of the hungry young or preterm infant. The same interpretation would apply to the anencephalic infant (AndreThomas and Autgaerden, 1966), or to the normal infant during his first two months of life. Both the reflexive stepping and spontaneous kicking, which are presumed to represent the same stereotyped movement patterns, appear to be the forerunners of mature locomotion according to Thelen and associates (1981). In other words, they can also both be envisaged as a basic component of future locomotion, or as a probable muscle synergism later incorporated into erect locomotion.

One explanation of the earlier dominance of a spinal locomotor generating complex, or its initial autonomy from corticospinal control, may relate to the earlier maturation of myelinogenesis of the spinal roots relative to the control tracts of the cord. For instance, roots of segments C8 to T1 are myelinated first, and finally those of the lumbar segment.

In the same context, fibres of the striato-acoustic system attain myelination before birth. With foetal reflexive stepping in mind, this could reflect a link between *the basal ganglia system* - the striatum in particular - *and the spinal locomotor system*. It may in any case be presumed that such a correlationship would not come to be strengthened and reinforced until corticospinal control fully matures.

After those first two months or so, reflexive stepping tends to disappear or becomes difficult to elicit over the next eight to nine months. Spontaneous kicking persists, however, with locomotion reappearing solely as "supported walking" after those first eight to nine months. Implicit in what is called "support" at that stage, is that effected by parent or experimenter standing in front of the child with hands under the child's arms or holding the child's hands. The child may also walk voluntarily or bear body weight on one leg.

Although *independent* walking is the next stage in most children by 11.3 to 12 months, the *more gradual maturation* of gait, betokened by several so-called *plantigrade* components (Saunders et al., 1953) evolves to eventually attain a *"mature gait"* between the second and fourth years (Fig 13). Firstly, comes the prominent *heel strike*, with *knee flexion* following during the supported phase, then asynchronous joint movements and specific patterns of muscle activation.

The earlier exhibition of the innate capacity of the spinal cord to autonomously generate locomotion, as in the rat or cat, is either lost or depressed in human ontogeny. Attention must therefore be focused on supraspinal control, and upon concepts of its pathophysiology in cerebral palsy. Although the principal focus had previously been on the role of the sensorimotor cortex and related higher brain centres, or the remodelling of supraspinal centres (Forrsberg, 1985) or transcortical pathways related to them (Dietz, 1987), more specific disorders in other directions have also been invoked. Of especial relevance in this context, these have included disturbance of higher cerebral functioning influenced by cognition and motivation (Zelazo, 1983). Interference with basic circuitry governing pattern-generation has also been suggested by Berger et al. (1984), whilst Mycklebust et al. (1986) have pointed to the possibility of failed maturation of spinal reflexes and/or the descending tracts which control them. Another pathogenic source should be added in terms of potentially failed maturation of *myelogenesis* of these pathways (Fig 15), bearing in mind that this process normally proceeds from the 32nd week of gestation at least beyond the end of the first year of life.

*The basic circuitry* that could be so affected by neural damage or incomplete myelinization, includes neural loops interconnecting the basal ganglia system with somatosensory cortex and related subcortical areas, but also functional maturation of the map linking cerebellar and vestibular nuclei on the one hand, and both locus ceruleus and the superior colliculi on the other.

In what way could such factors associated with failed maturation of corticospinal circuits, and/or interrelated myelin processing, account for the pathophysiology of cerebral palsy, of spastic diplegia for example, within the first year of life. Failed maturation of ultimate locomotion is a fundamental issue. Could there be a more direct pre- or perinatal impact upon *interneural spinal levels* affecting what in earlier stages of ontogeny appears to have been the autonomous spinal source of locomotion?

Our discussion was introduced by the hypothesis of at least a *provisional* localization of such autonomous locomotor generating circuits within the spinal cord of the human foetus. Furthermore, that the reflexive stepping and spontaneous kicking of the foetus reflected its operation prenatally, then extending into a short postnatal phase, but was to be the forerunner of ultimate mature locomotion in the normal child once corticospinal controlling mechanisms are functionally interconnected in parallel with the completion of myelination (Thelan et al., 1981). If this does not eventuate, as in the cerebral palsied infant, what alternative mechanisms can take over? And is it true

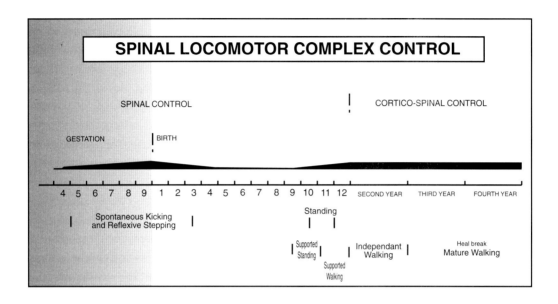

that facilitatory activation initially derives from the reticular activating centre in the brain stem, or is there loss of forebrain control of the inhibitory reticular formation which inhibits extensor neurones, and excites flexor neurons?

In the diagram above (Fig 13), an hypothetical course has been mapped out to illustrate the probable evolution of normal maturation of locomotor generating circuits. Firstly, spontaneous foetal kicking and reflexive stepping emerge from the fifth month of gestation. Whatever metabolic and other factors of ongoing foetal maturation or pathophysiology may depress or intensify these movements, they persist beyond birth until about two months of age. These movements appear to represent uninhibited activation of autonomous locomotor generation independently of

corticospinal regulation, such as we have mentioned as having been revealed in the lamprey, cat and rat. The stepping and spontaneous kicking then disappear, or become difficult to elicit, until the next stage towards independent locomotion is attained. This is marked by supported walking from 8 to 9 months or age. Flat feet are sustained until independent walking takes over from 11.3 to 12 to 13 months. Although stability is gradually achieved, presumably with progressive and parallel maturation of myelinogenesis as well as of corticospinal control, the immature pattern of locomotion continues in the normal toddler until the normal gait pattern asserts itself between 2 and 4 years of age.

When exploiting instrumented gait studies it has become possible to more precisely analyse the supported gait of cerebral palsied infants and children in the second year of life, and compare it with that of:

(a) normal infants during the supported phase: from 8 to approx 12 months;

(b) normal infants on attaining independent walking from approx 11.5 months to 14 months; and

(c) children who have achieved a mature or plantigrade gait from 2 to 4 years of age.

Firstly, it appears that the locomotor patterns of infants with cerebral palsy are comparable to normal infants during their supported phase of walking, but not beyond. They do not lose this pattern whilst retaining some of these infantile characteristics as they grow. In other words, they cannot evolve the transformation to plantigrade gait without intact corticospinal or sensorimotor cortical influence. And these corticospinal projections exercise direct control of, and integration with, pre-existing interneural circuitry within the spinal cord, or its ontogenic neural remodelling.

Thus, *foot control leads immediately to ankle flexion* during that crucial phase of supported locomotion in both normal and cerebral palsied children. Reflexive stepping in the foetus and neonate mirrors the same pattern due to "placement", or surface contact of the forepart of the foot. To reiterate the background neurophysiology, therefore, this appears to reflect relatively autonomous activation of spinal interneural complexes.

*Brisk ankle extension* then follows this foot contact in normal independent walkers,

being considered the mature plantigrade sequel of a heel strike first evoking passive plantar flexion torque. Cerebral palsied children neither develop heel strike, nor such ankle extension, following foot contact. The ankle continues to flex until the end of the supported phase, when it extends to flex again during the swing phase.

Whether the child suffers cerebral palsy or is normal, the knees proceed to flex during the beginning of this swing phase, extending for ground contact at the end of swing. Bending of the knee during mid to late stance - as the body "passes over" the knee - is another characteristic plantigrade feature which Saunders and colleagues long ago claimed (1953) as serving to curb vertical body oscillation during walking. In the excellent contemporary studies of Leonard, Hirschfield and Forssberg (1991) such smooth flexion-extension wave forms were never observed, with only one very mild hemiplegic achieving anything comparable. Likewise, *in movement about the hip joint*, cerebral palsied children could not achieve the smoother stable wave-form during stance characterizing normal independent walkers.

In the cerebral palsied infant and child, however, *the flat-footed and immature pattern of gait* which appears to represent and solely reflect spinal control, persists indefinitely. *Instrumented gait analysis* has permitted a clarification of these stages of independent walking in the normal child, as well as their pattern of impairment in the child suffering cerebral palsy. What such analysis appears in essence to have vindicated, in confirmation of meticulous clinical observation, is that the gait or locomotor antecedents of the cerebral palsied infant and child closely resemble, or is identical with, that of the normal infant and child from early in pregnancy until 2 months of age or so, and thence during the initiation of supported walking *albeit delayed in the cerebral palsied child*. The locomotor pattern of this initial phase introducing supported walking, persists in the CP child.

A more or less limited degree or residue of corticospinal or pyramidal control and maturation accounting for the hypertonus, exaggerated stretch reflexes and babinski, nevertheless obtains whether initiated pre- or postnatally according to the timing of cerebral damage. In the choreo-athetoid or extrapyramidal clinical picture, predominant damage may be largely concentrated upon the striatum and/or related basal ganglia elements leaving the intervening internal capsule and pyramidal tracts relatively free.

Involvement of pathways connecting the cerebellum, colliculi and even vestibular elements could also be expressed in an ataxic pattern or in its more intense equivalent of dysequilibrium.

Basically, however, if the continuity of corticospinal or pyramidal tracts and connections is interrupted as the result of ependymal or periventricular haemorrhage or infarction, and/or ischaemic/anoxic pathology and its sequel, periventricular leukomalacia, the otherwise provisional spinal locomotor generative activity persists with varying degrees of autonomy.

Reducing all this to a practical attainment of independent mobility although solely through a pattern of "immature" gait differing from the normal but practicable for that particular entity of cerebral palsy. Indeed, subsequent adaptation of gait is a gradual illustration of Petö's axiom "that what the baby does not learn in maturation, he must now learn as a skill". There is a shift towards a conscious learning situation also eventually involving language and cortical concepts, so that the original system of Conductive Education started with the two to three-year-old. From then on, the child is learning how he, be he spastic, athetoid or ataxic, can manage to function effectively. This is not based on pursuing normal development but on spontaneous and contrived sequences leading to valid function whilst at the same time overcoming his main problems, his abnormal motor patterns, his lack of symmetry and normal asymmetry, but the ability to retain midline orientation while fixing with one hand and moving the other. In Ester Cotton's words, in order to achieve this, Petö avoided rotation but used *pivoting* and turning so that the child can sustain his newly acquired straight arms and legs and midline orientation.

The immature walking pattern practicable for the cerebral palsied child is therefore a reasonable and pragmatic stage to work for *rather than copying the complicated rotation in normal walking* which is almost unattainable in CP and also destroys the external rotation of the lower limb. Symmetry is the dominant need to be continually stressed in the life of the cerebral palsied child.

# PROGNOSIS FOR ULTIMATE WALKING OR "AMBULATION"

The above discussion helps to eliminate some well-worn myths and to clarify the nature of the ultimate walking in cerebral palsy. It is therefore not normal "mature" walking but a modified gait illustrated, for example, by the absence of mature heel strike. Various authorities have retreated to the term "ambulation" rather than walking. Nevertheless, "independent walking" recently earned a somewhat limited definition by Campos et al., (1994) as the ability to stand and "ambulate" indoors or outdoors without "needing sticks, crutches or walkers" with the possibility of using orthosis for ankle support.

A number of recent long-term clinical studies focus especially upon this issue of the anticipated prognosis for walking in the CP child, correlated with earlier functional motor capacities. For instance, Molnar (1979) demonstrated a significant correlationship between the ability to sit unsupported when appropriately positioned, and ambulation. He also concluded with undue pessimism, in my view, since there is no reference to the possible potentiality in response to the long-term Petö approach, that the chances of a child attaining independent ambulation diminish after the age of 4 to 5 years and that it is unlikely after 8 years.

According to the results of the study of 50 CP children categorized as spastic diplegia by Badell-Ribera (1985) "sitting and crawling" at 1½ to 2½ years was predictive of subsequent ambulation *in all cases*.

In the prospective study by Watt and colleagues of the ambulatory potential of 14 neonatal survivors of intensive care later diagnosed as CP, a positive relationship appears to have been established between sitting at 2 years of age and "ambulation" at 8.

But more helpful neurodevelopmental criteria appear to have been firmly established by the recent, very thorough, prospective analysis of 270 examples of spasticity by the team of Campos et al., (1994). The age of attainment of gross motor milestones was thus offered as an alternative method for prediction of locomotor prognosis. Achievement by 9 months of *head balance* (Bayley, 1969) as outlined in Chapter 3, apparently proved to be an important index of a good motor prognosis, whereas if deferred until beyond 20 months, the prognosis for walking was poor. *Sitting by 24 months* can also serve as an indicator of favourable outcome in vindication of the previous conclusions by Molnar (1979) and of Watt and colleagues in 1989. They finally added crawling. An additional milestone was added, however, in the shape of crawling by 30 months as a valid predictor for good "locomotor" prognosis. A broad practical perspective of the whole issue is bravely addressed by a true veteran in the field, Ester Cotton, in Chapter 11 of the accompanying volume.

# References

AndreThomas A, Autgaerden S. (1966) Locomotion from pre to postnatal life. Clinics Dev Med 24: SIMP with Heinnemann

Baddell-Ribera A. (1985) Cerebral palsy: postural locomotor prognosis in spastic diplegia. Arch Phys Med Rehab 66: 614-619

Bayley N. (1969) Manual for the Bayley Scale of Infant Development. Psychological Corporation, New York

Berger W, Altenmueller E, Dietz V. (1984) Normal and impaired development of children's gait. Human Neurobiol 3: 163-170

Campos A, Paz A et al. (1994) Walking prognosis in cerebral palsy: a 22 year retrospective study. Dev Med Child Neurol 36: 130-134

Dietz V. (1987) Role of peripheral afferent and spinal reflexes in normal and impaired human locomotion. Revue Neurologique 143: 241-254

Forssberg H. (1985) Ontogeny of human locomotor control. 1: Infant stepping, supported locomotion and transition to independent locomotion. Exp Brain Res 57: 480-493

Leonard CT, Hirschfield H, Forssberg H. (1991) The development of independent walking in children with cerebral palsy. Dev Med Child Neurol 33: 567-577

Molnar GE. (1979) Cerebral palsy: prognosis and how to judge it. Pedaitr Ann 8: 596-606

Mycklebust BM, Gottlieb GL, Agarwal BC. (1986) Stretch reflexes of the normal infant. Dev Med Child Neurol 28: 440-449

Saunders JB de CM, Inman VT, Eberhart HD. (1953) The major determinants in normal and pathological gait. J Bone Joint Surg 35A: 543-558

Thelen E, Bradshaw G, Ward JA. (1981) Spontaneous kicking in month-old infants: manifestation of a human central locomotor program. Behavioural Neural Biol 32: 45-53

Watt et al. (1989) Early prognosis for ambulation of neonatal intensive care survivors with cerebral palsy. Dev Med Child Neurol 31: 766-773

Zelazo PR. (1983) The development of walking. J Motor Behaviour 15: 99-137

# 16

# THE ROLE OF MYELINOGENESIS IN THE MATURATION OF MOTOR FUNCTION AND ULTIMATE WALKING

Role of Myelinogenesis in Maturation of Motor Function

Delays or Deficits in Myelination

References

# 16

# ROLE OF MYELINOGENESIS IN MATURATION OF MOTOR FUNCTION

When mature, the motor axons of lower motor neurones are large myelinated fibres (6 to 20 $\mu$u in diameter). They comprise two distinct fibre types, nearly half being *alpha motor fibres* innervating *extrafusal* muscle fibres. The remainder are *gamma motor fibres* of smaller calibres originating in smaller anterior horn cells, which innervate the muscle spindles (*intrafusal* muscle fibres). Only for a few microns at their terminal ramification, on a neuro muscular end-plate, is the motor axon unmyelinated.

Myelin itself is a multilamellar membrane investing and wound around axons in both the central and peripheral nervous system (Fig 14). Lipid layers alternate with protein layers, both developing from the all-surface plasma membranes of the Schwann cell in the peripheral nervous system, and from oligodendroglia within the brain. It is produced at an enormous velocity, illustrated by the myelin synthesis of each oligodendrocyte in the rat, amounting to over three times its own weight *per day*.

## Myelin Formation
### Multi-layered protein-lipid membrane

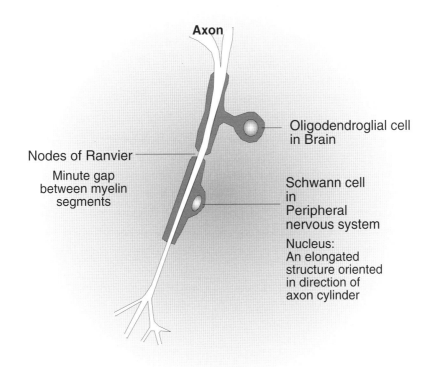

Axon

Oligodendroglial cell in Brain

Nodes of Ranvier

Minute gap between myelin segments

Schwann cell in Peripheral nervous system

Nucleus: An elongated structure oriented in direction of axon cylinder

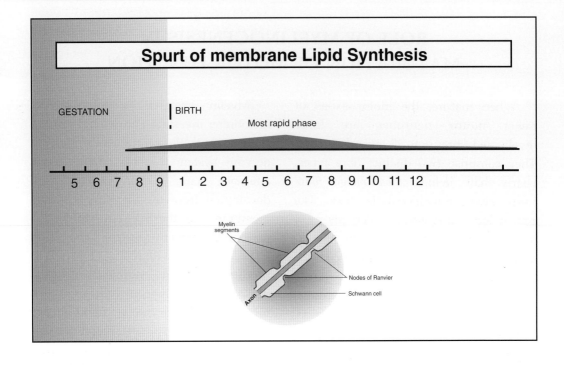

Such a *spurt* of membrane lipid synthesis illustrated in Fig 15, and maximal for plasmalogens, begins at 32 weeks of gestation. And within the human central nervous system, *in the forebrain*, an explosive proliferation of axons, dendrites and dendritic spines parallels this spurt of myelinogenesis at 32 weeks which is even precisely identifiable in clear EEG changes. Like all membranes, myelin is rich in phospholipids, but three main biological groups are involved:

1. Phospholipids and cholesterol - general membrane lipids;

2. Gangliosides as neuronal lipids - enriched in synaptic membranes; and

3. Plasmalogens - as membrane lipids relatively enriched in myelin. These are end products of phospholipid biosynthesis and account for one fifth of all phospholipids in the human body.

Sphingolipids which represent about 30% of the myelin lipids are implicated in various hereditary neurological disorders. Of all parameters studied, only those referable to myelination especially plasmalogens, and particularly in the forebrain, are affected by *undernutrition*. And this is to a degree directly proportional to the duration of the nutritional insult, although with significantly less impact upon the cerebellum. Indeed in relation to Galactolipids - only the cerebrum is affected.

The timetables for myelination and the development of complex motor functions are thus roughly parallel. The most rapid phase is between 30 weeks prenatally, and 6 months postnatally. When myelination of the pyramidal tract is believed to be almost complete, at the end of the first year and beginning of the second, independent walking is normally considered a "spontaneous" achievement.

The spinal roots achieve myelination earlier than the central tracts of the cord which is in keeping with the sequence of maturation discussed, and the initial autonomy from corticospinal control of the spinal locomotor generating complex. The anterior roots of segments C8 to T1 become myelinated first, and finally those of the lumbar segment. Growth of the intrinsic axons appears to be in parallel, bearing in mind that increase in axon diameter stimulates myelination.

That the fibres of the striato-acoustic system also attain myelination before birth (Myersberg and Post, 1979) may, with "reflexive stepping" in mind, reflect a link between the basal ganglia system - the striatum in particular - and the spinal locomotor system. It is probable that this correlationship is strengthened and reinforced until corticospinal control fully matures.

Motor roots are myelinated by the end of the first month which may allow for the earliest stage of motor control when the infant is suspended vertically to induce "placing" and reflexive stepping. But the myelination of the pyramidal tract and of the striatum is largely complete by the end of the first year, so that supported walking may be accomplished by 8-10 months, standing alone by 10-11 months, and independent walking by 11.3-13 months.

The benefits of myelination include lower energy requirements for nerve conduction, rapid conduction and marked reduction of space required, together with a much reduced flow of sodium ions. The most reliable functional assessments of myelin maturation derive from motor and sensory conduction velocity studies. Completion of its maturation is finally acceptable in normal children between two and five years of age. Conductive velocities in infancy, less than half those in older children, correlate closely with the "incomplete" stage of maturation.

The circumstantial and indeed experimental evidence nonetheless supports a critical role for myelinogenesis in the maturation of the motor control system, cortical, subcortical and basal gangliar,, and inevitably in the ultimate maturation of walking and gait modification. It is logical to assume that rapid transmission of neural impulses from both central and peripheral receptors is essential for such modification. *The organisation of myelin along axons permits the propagation of action potentials* in a highly characteristic "*saltatory conductive*" manner. If myelin is lacking, as in multiple sclerosis, or in experimental demyelinating forms, or distorted by sulfatide accumulation as in the segmental demyelination of metachromatic leukodystrophy (Russell and Yatziv, 1985), the entire axonal membrane must depolarize and then repolarize. Control of the conductive system would be slow and the energy requirement high.

Experimental studies of such demyelination in monkeys focused upon allergic encephalomyelitis as a model for multiple sclerosis. An equivalent state was found moreover to be reproduced by repeated injections of cerebral tissue.

# DELAYS OR DEFICITS IN MYELINATION

MRI clearly demonstrates the process of normal myelination which begins just before the neonatal period and close to the 32nd week of gestation. Myelination is generated peripherally by the Schwann cells, centrally by oligodendroglia, and proceeds along sensory tracts before the motor tracts, whilst that of the internal capsule precedes the great commissures and lateral cerebral hemispheres (Valk and van der Knaap, 1989). The T1 of unmyelinated white matter gradually decreases so that by 3 to 6 months it is equal to that of grey matter. The "edge enhancement" appearance of the cortex is then lost.

Evidence of focal or diffuse delayed myelination on CT or MRI is also frequent in many metabolic defects, especially in mitochondrial cytopathies and peroxismal disorders. Methionine deficiency also plays a role in the pathogenesis of demyelination. Is there a specific metabolic basis for the demyelination and neuronal necrosis that complicates immune diseases?

Delays are difficult to recognise before about 6 months since myelin is still relatively sparse. Delays or deficits are most conspicuous therefore from 6 to 24 months of age, by which time myelination is complete or approaches completion. Delays or deficits such as have been claimed in prenatal rubella, post-haemorrhagic hydrocephalus, ischaemic-hypoxic encephalopathy and in cystic periventricular leukomalacia, may only be precisely definable in the absence of myelination of named tracts or commissures where these are present in the control (Lily Dubowitz and Bydder, 1990).

Damage or abnormality of myelin formation and/or maturation must therefore be taken into consideration in researches into the pathogenesis of cerebral palsy and its associated disorders of hearing, vision, and cognitive and behavioural function. MRI is thus increasingly identifying delayed myelination as a factor in the pathogenesis of CP. In all nine cases studied by Byrne and colleagues (1990), this delay was already detectable at 8 months, which they considered was the earliest time at which the MRI findings correlated with the subsequent neurological outcome.

Various groups of myelin disorders of progressive character, and therefore non-CP, are also potent in seriously impairing or even preventing the ultimate attainment of erect posture and walking.

Myelinoclastic or disorders of myelin destruction or necrosis of *abnormally formed* myelin comprise the first such group, whereas demyelination strictly refers to destruction of normally formed myelin. Leukodystrophies or degenerative disorder of white matter including myelin make up a second group. *Segmental demyelination*, is the product of a disease or metabolic process involving the Schwann cell, as in metachromatic leukodystrophy or in the category with deficiency of the multiple arylsulfatases (Russell and Yatziv, 1985) Severe disease of this kind may be associated with secondary axonal destruction and Wallerian degeneration. A more transitory and recurrent process of repetitive demyelination and remyelination is even found in certain genetic disorders of peripheral nerves.

## References

Byrne P, Welch R, Johnson MA, Darrah J, Piper M. (1990) Serial magnetic resonance imaging in neonatal hypoxic-ischaemic encephalopathy. J Pediat 117: 694-700

Dubowitz LMS, Bydder GM. (1990) Magnetic resonance imaging of the brain in neonates. Sem Perinatol 14: 212-223

Myersburg HA, Post RM. (1979) An holistic developmental view of neural and psychological processes: a neurobiol-psycho analytical integration. Br J Psychiat 115: 139-155

Russell A, Yatziv S. (1985) A metabolic basis for idiopathic torsion dystonia: a new variant of metachromatic leukodystrophy. World Pediat Child Care 1: 25-29

Valk J, Van der Knaap MS. (1989) Magentic Resonance Imaging of Myelin, Myelination and Myelin Disorders. Springer Verlag: Berlin, Germany

# 17

# HYPOTHETICAL EARLY POTENTIAL NEUROHABILITATION

# 17

# HYPOTHETICAL EARLY POTENTIAL NEUROHABILITATION

We have already discussed the diagnostic implications in the premature or early neonate of the newer techniques of neuro-imaging, including MRI and PEP. Notes have been added for their further exploitation in measuring intracerebral metabolic changes, or even more recently in appraising changes in blood flow or neuronal activity in specific cortical areas related to speech, hearing, vision or even tongue movement. Their *localizing* evidence indicative of gradations of intracerebral or intracerebellar haemorrhage, or of ischaemic or ultimate cystic damage as in periventricular leukomalacia can be related firstly to their timing and secondly to the ultimate clinical manifestation of the different entities of cerebral palsy. More fundamental morphological defects of cerebral and/or cerebellar neuronal migration and maturation such as lissencephaly, inevitably to be expressed in CP, can likewise be recognized in early CT-scanning or MRI.

Although such accurate diagnostic definition is now feasible, can the eventual clinical manifestation of CP be reliably predicted thereby, and within days or at most weeks postnatally, rather than after 6 to 15 months according to severity as is expected even in the best of Western hands. Farenc Katona's programming of what he describes as damaged behaviour patterns in the brain involving reliance on impaired movement and sensory behaviour as evidence of relevant brain injury is certainly not enough. *If it were truly practicable to identify the causal cerebral damage within days or weeks of birth, could early postnatal activation of normal movement and postural control* lead to effective neurohabilitation so as to avert any manifestation of CP. As yet there is inadequate neuro-biological evidence in support of Katona's presumption that such early activation of genetically-coded movement and postural coordination is practicable, and that whatever is achieved in that direction can ensure the normal growth and even realignment of axonal tracts (Chapter 14). To be effective for neurogenic function this must also include restoration of active myelinogenesis where it has been interrupted.

Elementary sensori-motor patterns gradually disappear when the infant begins to sit and crawl, yet spontaneous movement still follows a pattern established by the elementary codes. But when the elementary codes is missing or has been disrupted because of brain damage in utero or at birth, the development course will be abnormal so that abnormality in spontaneous movement will gradually emerge. It is as if the infant is not "aware of his legs" or has an indefinable or abnormal awareness of them, recalling Oliver Sack's brilliant monograph on the phantom limb, "A leg to stand on".

It is emphasized for instance that the complex coordination movements encompassed in sitting and crawling come naturally to the newborn, and furthermore that the right impetus or "stimulus contingent" which can be effected by a slight incline of the crawling surface aided by gravity can trigger off this activation. Abnormality or even absence of these movements can be another parameter of damage to the underlying cerebral programming.

Diagnostically, the analysis is postulated as solely defining weakness or paralysis of limbs or groups of muscles rather than disorders of tone, movement or balance which are the classical clinical expressions of CP.

Katona's claim is that the restoration of correct movement patterns lays the foundations of the infant's eventual movement ability and posture. By his sequence of training he aims to prevent the development of abnormal motor patterns, or to correct the "defaults" by giving normal spontaneous development a platform from which to evolve.

The early postnatal adaptation or testing includes the child "Sitting on our Posture" and entails a baby, 2-3 weeks old or somewhat older, sitting erect supported only by the thighs, gripped at mid-thigh, the head held upright unaided with the baby ostensibly enjoying a reflection of himself in the mirror, they are induced to spontaneously creep down along a surface which is gently sloped for this purpose. He also places the infant in hypothetically specific positions aimed at triggering "primitive areas" of the brain and/or initiating reflex movements presaging the human characteristics of "locomotion" and verticalization. In the cardinal exercise, the baby is induced to spontaneously creep down an inclined ramp, sloped to assist gravity to propel the infant down the ramp. The spontaneous movements of hands and arms resemble swimming and disturbance of such movement, or unilateral impairment, are considered indicative of underlying brain dysfunction heralding development of an ultimate clinical pattern of cerebral palsy.

His team also focuses upon more specifically localized abnormality involving coordination of sucking, swallowing and breathing, which they attempt to objectively evaluate in the first weeks of life. Developing specialized stimulatory techniques of electrotherapy, including small electrodes to stimulate muscles responsible for swallowing, they report sustained coordination achieved within a couple of weeks.

A weakness inherent in his claim to unequivocally predict the evolution to ultimate CP in those first few weeks of life rather than awaiting 5 to 15 months for conventional diagnosis. He believes that such diagnosis can be confirmed by comprehensive computerization of brain, nerve and muscle scans, and then that the outcome of his early infantile intervention represents 45% of "cures" of cerebral palsy by the end of 2 years. Little or no allowance is made for the many false positives that may thereby be concealed. The need for complex controlled study is inescapable, with at least statistically adequate exclusion from this specific approach of an appropriate proportion of the neonates diagnosed in this way. In any case, deferring this particular approach in an appropriate group for 9 to 12 months could well demonstrate how many of his diagnostic predictions can be substantiated. Such an extension of his studies could at least promise more conviction one way or another than the long-term expectation suggested by Bax (1990) of a significant fall in the prevalence of CP below 2 per 1000 live births.

My postulate envisages the potential incorporation or addition of infantile swimming under water to Katona's technique. Despite flaws in his claims for precise diagnostic definition, Katona's concept embodies an important and logical rationale. That natural and spontaneous movements of the neonate and infant can not only prevent axonal and even neuronal degeneration, by preserving the integrity and survival of axons subserved by the neurons so damaged intracerebrally, but can also activate the ongoing function and growth of the corresponding cortico-spinal communication. If we accept this concept, and can confirm it in the experimental animal, then the cultivation of movement from the neonatal phase onwards would be warranted. His diagnostic interpretation of predictive cerebral damage could be coupled with that of one or more authoritative experts engaged in the same research area such as Victor and Lily Dubowitz.

My suggestion is that the activation of movement be reinforced by adoption of a technique of infantile swimming, or rather swimming under water such as strongly advocated and practised by the Swedish paediatrician Bo Bille. His team has adapted an effective technique of breath-holding under water by his handicapped infants and prides itself on valuable habilitation through the use of this early swimming approach.

The emphasis of Michael Crawford (1992) that babies are born *knowing how to swim*, although losing this ability after about 6 months, supports the concept of a spinal locomotor centre in control during this phase. I have postulated an analogous concept to explain the phase of reflexive stepping beginning in the 5th or 6th month of gestation and continuing to be manifest in the early postnatal life of a normal infant. Likewise, this reactivity or ability ends after about 2 months with supported standing and walking beginning only when early cortico-spinal connections mature or are myelinated after 8 to 10 months or thereabouts.

The extraordinary Russian male midwife, Igor Charkovsky, has also exploited this adaptability, and what is claimed as a natural affinity for water of the neonate and infant, in his controversial *birth under water* technique and subsequent cultivation of infant swimming; especially in remarkable unison with dolphins. This recalls theories of our descent from sea mammals rather than primates and the related postulate that "voluntary breath control" enabled our ancestors to swim under water, an ability still confined to humans and aquatic mammals such as seals and dolphins, which is of especial interest in relation to Charkovsky's initiative.

## References

Bax M. (1990) Motor delay and cerebral palsy. Dev Med Child Neurol 32: 283-284

Crawford, Michael (1992) Personal communication. Institute of Brain Surgery. Proc Br Assoc Sci Festival, Southampton University

# SECTION III:

## SIMULATION OF CEREBRAL PALSY ENTITIES BY PROGRESSIVE NEUROMETABOLIC AND NEURODEGENERATIVE DISORDER

# GENERAL INTRODUCTION

The symptomatology of different categories of the *non-progressive* disorder of cerebral palsy is *simulated* at some stage in the natural history of many genetically-determined metabolic encephalopathies underlying *progressive* forms of childhood neurological disability. In the main, the consistent difference lies in their *progressivity*, however gradual, linked to other overt clinical criteria, apart from specifically distinctive and pathognomonic biological evidence of the fundamental disorder. A similar simulation applies, however, to various so-called degenerative disorders which instead manifest developmental regression. Whatever the category of cerebral palsy, a metabolic or degenerative basis or certain specific entities of unknown aetiology would become suspect once it becomes clear that the cerebral dysfunction is progressive and is combined with other neuropathic manifestations.

The functional correlations between these clinical expressions and any identifiable molecular or biological defect whether involving enzyme, mitochrondrium, peroxisome, metal or other co-factors, or GABA dysfunction or other primary or secondary disturbances in cerebral neurotransmitters, are not fully understood. Although some of the proposed hypotheses touched upon in subsequent individual descriptions are based upon *in vitro* experimentation, it goes without saying that this never adequately reproduces conditions as they exist *in vivo*.

This rapidly growing range of inborn metabolic and molecular disease overlaps all the specialities of paediatrics in their co-existing simulation of cerebral palsy. Differences in their many attributes to be emphasized whenever relevant in our subsequent analyses include (1) their clinical course and rate of evolution, and (2) their more rapid progressivity or developmental regression than many categorised as degenerative. The initial hypotonia, or even "simple" spastic paraplegia becomes modified by varying degrees and duration of ataxia, athetosis, myoclonus or even rigidity, and peripheral neuropathy.

This can never belittle the importance of such neuro-metabolic and "degenerative" situations in the differential diagnosis of the classical entities of cerebral palsy. No less challenging is the potential patho-physiological significance of such biochemical, metabolic or "degenerative" influences whether primarily in the foetus, or primarily within the pregnant mother as are expressed in their cardinal neurological manifestation, or directly and indirectly in the impaired growth differentiation and other pathology of cerebral and cerebellar tissues. It is our fervent hope that study of these interrelationships must eventually help add to our knowledge and understanding of more or less specific aspects of the clinico-pathological concept and causation of the cerebral palsies. Especially would this apply to the small proportion of cerebral palsy per se, in the region of 10%, with an apparently genetically-determined basis.

Many more of the analogous progressive disorders, which at some stage embody symptoms and signs of cerebral palsy are themselves the outcome of single gene mutations.

Judgement as to whether even a spastic paraparesis, let alone a somewhat equivocal hypotonia, is either static and stable or truly progressive may have to be reserved for a long period. One form of *spastic diplegia* known in a few families to become maximally manifest at somewhat different infantile or pre-school age phases, can nonetheless be described as *non-progressive*. If there is evident worsening during early or late childhood, or new movement abnormalities emerge, such as dystonia, there should be a reconsideration of the basic diagnosis of cerebral palsy of obscure origin. This would be aimed at identification of a previously unsuspected metabolic or other genetic disorder. One example demonstrating such a sequence is *Pelizaeus Merzbacher* disease and other types of Sudanophilic disorder with leukodystrophy, or in rare instances of familial spastic paralysis (as described by Poser et al., 1957) or linked to dementia as described by McKusick (1956) and others. Likewise, the *Strumpell-Lorain familial paraplegia*, an inherited neuronal atrophy of either autosomal dominant or recessive type, wherein the underlying bi-pyramidal syndrome clinically emerges in later childhood, is marked by progression, albeit exceedingly slow over years.

*Inborn metabolic errors* or molecular biological pathology may thus be given initial clinical expression in different developmental age phases from the foetus onwards. In other words, the realization has come about that enzymatic factors, including metallo-enzymes and those of intermediary metabolism, including that of essential or nutritional co-factors, also have specific developmental phases during the evolution of life.

The *progressive clinical expression* of these disorders in terms of aberration of movement, posture and tone can thus be divided into relevant age phases. *Neuropathological* sub-division could also focus on those with a major impact on:

(1) *grey matter* (the poliodystrophies), a presumption favoured by convulsions, myoclonic jerks and spike abnormalities in the EEG, the relationship to the underlying component of the metabolic disorder still to be clarified by computerised fractional analysis etc.; or upon

(2) *white* matter, compatible with long-tract disorders such as spastic weakness, hemianopia, optic atrophy, polyneuropathy and slow-wave or other abnormality in the EEG.

A common early pattern of symptoms and signs comprise *a core syndrome* which embodies:

*Combinations of initial hypotonia*, with delay in the acquisition of:
- head control
- sitting posture
- eye-hand coordination

and later hypertonic or spastic weakness with apparent pyramidal involvement also reflected in hyperactivity of deep tendon reflexes, positive Babinski responses and clonus.

In addition: disinterest in the environment associated with perceptual delays, and hyperirritability together with persistent inexplicable crying, or difficulty in swallowing adding to overall malnutrition and failure to thrive.

More specific clinical findings associated with this core syndrome, and those that parallel psychomotor regression, will usually determine the initial steps in the differential diagnosis. For instance, the hyperaceusis and the amblyopia with cherry-red macular spots would indicate either Tay Sachs or GM$_2$ gangliosidoses, whereas significant *hepatosplenomegaly* linked to the cherry-red *macular* spots, would add up to the infantile Niemann-Pick. Comparable macular spots linked to a pattern of dysmorphic facies including oedema and gingival hypertrophy, as well as co-existing hepatosplenomegaly, distinguish GM$_1$ gangliosidosis. *Infantile Gaucher* would be supported by the additional signs of ophthalmoplegia and head retraction apart from splenomegaly, whilst early optic atrophy and blindness, tonic extensor spasms and progressive megaloencephaly especially characterize the syndrome of Canavan-Van Bogaert-Bertrand. Early head enlargement is also a characteristic of Alexander's leukodystrophy with Rosenthal fibre formation, whilst to the presentation of Leigh's encephalomyelopathy is added episodic respiratory disorder and ocular palsies but without any significant hepatosplenomegaly. Hepatomegaly, together with the characteristic craniofacial dysmorphism including of eyes and ears, and supraorbital ridge and mid-face hypoplasia marks the Zellweger syndrome.

Many of these "progressive" disorders are recessively inherited so that a history of consanguinity or of stillbirth or neonatal death would be supportive. With a possible background of ornithine transcarbamylase deficiency (Russell, 1972), its X-linkage is to be kept in mind so that a history of *male* - neonatal or early infantile - deaths on the maternal side would be particularly suspect. A convulsing male subject of this disorder may, in any case, rapidly lapse into coma. The introduction of increased protein or of amino acids like leucine in the first few days may precipitate such clinical symptoms. Likewise, in galactosaemia or fructose intolerance, a change of feeds to include the offending galactose or fructose sources, may bring this about.

Even a pathognomonic odour of skin or of sweat, especially accentuated when the infant's temperature is raised in an incubator, may point directly to the diagnosis in isovaleric acidaemia, glutaric aciduria Type II, or maple syrup urine disease.

### References

McKusick V. (1956) Hereditable Disorders of Connective Tissue. Mosby, St. Louis

Poser CM, De Wolf A, Van Bogaert L. (1957) Atypical cerebellar degeneration associated witih leukodystrophy. J Neuropathol Exp Neurol 16: 209-237

# 18

# PROGRESSIVE AND METABOLIC SOURCES OF INITIAL AND/OR PERSISTENT HYPOTONIA

## SOMETIMES ASSOCIATED WITH DISORDERS OF MOVEMENT AND BALANCE

## *ALTERNATIVELY ENTITLED PROGRESSIVE* DISORDERS WITH *HYPOTONIC* COMPONENT SIMULATING HYPOTONIC CEREBRAL PALSY

**Metabolic Sources of Neuromuscular Hypotonia**

**Initial Hypotonia: Acute or Persistent**

Acute Infective Sources: Acute Encephalitis or Encephalopathy
Hypotonia in Congenital and Metabolic Myopathies
1. Associated with specific underlying biochemical abnormality.
2. Associated with specific structural and enzymological abnormality.
3. Congenital muscle dystrophy.

## Initial Hypotonia: Acute or Persistent continued

Spinal Muscular Atrophy
    Werdnig-Hoffman Syndrome
    Intermediate forms
    Later onset of a relatively mild form, or the Kugelberg-Welander syndrome
Benign Congenital Hypotonia
Myasthenia Gravis
    Congenital Open-mouth or Lockjaw as the end product of foetal myasthenia
Dystrophia Myotonica or Steinert's Syndrome
Dermatomyositis
Riley-Day (Familial Dysautonomia)
Pontocerebellar Hyperplasia
Demyelinating and Axonal Neuropathies
Central Positive Myelinolysis (CPM)
Formimino Glutamic Aciduria (FIGLU: McKusick 22910)
    Impaired Remethylation of Homocysteine by 5-methyl-tetrahydrofolate
Methylmalonic Acidaemias and Combined Homocysteinuria and Methylmalonic
    Aciduria (McKusick 27740 and 27741)


## Hypotonia: Initial and Transitory

Syndromes of Chromosomal or Cytogenetic Anomaly
    XXXXY syndrome
    Down's syndrome
    Prader-Willi syndrome
    Tetrasomy 12 or Pallister-Killian syndrome
    5p or Cri-du-chat syndrome
    4p syndrome: Partial deletion of short arm of 4 (Wolf-Hirschhorn syndrome)
    9p Monosomy syndrome
    18p syndrome
    Trisomy 13 syndrome
    Trisomy 20 syndrome
Miscellaneous Disorders of Unknown Aetiology
    Hypermobility of Joints
    Camptomelic Dysplasia

# Initial Hypotonia followed by Spasticity or Accompanied by Intermittent Hypertonic Reactions and/or Ataxia

Hyperammonaemia/Urea Cycle Defects and Intermittent Extensor Hypertonicity and Transitory Ataxia
HHH Syndrome
Lysinuric Protein Intolerance
Non-Ketotic Hyperglycinaemia
Lysosomal Enzyme Disorders
Tay-Sachs (Early Infantile GM$_2$-Gangliosidosis) Disease
Sandhoff's Disease (GM$_2$-Gangliosidosis, type 2)
Congenital Amaurotic Idiocy
Early Infantile GM$_1$-Gangliosidosis (type 1)
Infantile Niemann-Pick Disease
Infantile Neuronic Ceroid Lipofuscidosis or Polyunsaturated Fatty Acid Lipidosis
Lowe's Syndrome (Oculo-Cerebro-Renal Syndrome)
3-Hydroxy-3 Methylglutaric Aciduria
Multiple AcylCoA Dehydrogenase Deficiency (MADD) or Glutaric Aciduria Type II
3-Methyl Glutaconic Aciduria
3-Ketothiolase Deficiency
Dihydrolipoyl Dehydrogenase Deficiency
α-Thalassaemia: X-linked Mental Retardation Syndrome
Metachromatic Leukodystrophy
Mucolipidosis: Type IV

# Peroxisomal Disorders

Glycogenosis Type II (Pompe's disease)
Zellweger's Disease (Cerebro-hepato-renal transport defect)
Mevalonic Aciduria

# Initial Hypotonia followed by Choreo-athetosis

Purine Disorders
    Lesch-Nyhan or Congenital Hyperuricaemia
Other Disorders of Purine Metabolism
    Phosphoribosylpyrophosphate (PRPS) Syndrome
    Combined Xanthine Oxidase/Sulphite Oxidase (XOD/SO) Deficiency
    Defects of enzymes involved in re-utilization of ATP degradation

## Initial Hypotonia followed by Choreo-athetosis continued

Mitochondrial Myopathy
    Defects of Mitochondrial Oxidation
        *Acyl-CoA Dehydrogenase Deficiency*
        *Enoyl CoA Hydratase (Erotonase) Deficiency*
    Defects of Mitochondrial Respiratory Chain Complexes
Infantile Refsum (Phytanic Acid Storage Disease)

## Other Miscellaneous Rare Metabolic Abnormalities with Clinical Expression in Initial Hypotonia and Other Disorders of Movement, Posture and Balance

Aspartyl Glucosaminuria
Menkes' Kinky Hair Syndrome
Spongy Degeneration of Nervous System White Matter:
    (Canavan-Van Bogaert-Bertrand disease)
Neurobiological Disorder: Peroxisomal Defect of Neuronal Migration)
    *Sudanophilic Leukodystrophy with Deficient Hepatocellular and Renal Peroxisomes*
        *(Zellweger's cerebro-hepato-renal syndrome)*
Neurobiological Disorder of Uncertain or Unknown Aetiology
    *Meckel-Gruber syndrome*
    *Cerebro-Oculo-Facial (COFS) [Neurogenic arthrogryposis]*
    *Neu-Laxova syndrome*

## Disorders with Conspicuous Cardinal Features other than Hypotonia

Coffin-Siris Syndrome
Generalized Gangliosidosis Type I
Miller-Dieker Syndrome (Lissencephaly Syndrome)
X-linked Hypophosphataemic or Vitamin D Resistant Rickets
Rieger Syndrome
Stickler Syndrome or Hereditary Arthero Ophthalmopathy
Thanatophoric Dysplasia Syndrome
William's Syndrome
Foetal Aminopterin Syndrome
Hyperthermia-induced Spectrum of Defects
Fabry Syndrome
Shprintzen Syndrome (Velo-Cardio-Facial)
Osteogenesis Imperfecta Syndrome Type I
Pena-Shokier II Syndrome (COFS Syndrome: Centro-Oculo-Facial Skeletal)
Langer-Giedion Syndrome
Marfan Syndrome

# 18

## METABOLIC SOURCES OF
## NEUROMUSCULAR HYPOTONIA

Hypotonia is a common element of many metabolic syndromes which will be outlined subsequently. The infantile "failure to thrive" syndromes associated with deepening hypotonia and the clinical "surrender" pattern of a pithed frog, are also attended by a resistance to feeding, vomiting, "obstipation" and abdominal distention. Outstanding examples of this include infantile hypercalcaemia, renal tubular acidosis, nephrogenic diabetes insipidus and infantile hypoaldosteronism (Russell et al., 1963). In each of these, the deep reflexes are noticeably brisk. The specific differential diagnostic features of other infantile situations especially marked by hypotonia are to be outlined later in this section, such as Lowe's syndrome, Pompe's glycogenosis, and hypothyroidism. Hereditary metabolic encephalopathies are of clearly progressive character, being especially emphasized. For example, non-ketotic hyperglycinaemia is included as well as Lowe's syndrome and Zellweger syndrome, both of which are recognizable by characteristic ocular, visceral and skeletal features. *Atonic cerebral palsy* nonetheless remains a serious basis to be considered in the non-progressive presentation of a floppy baby. An aside of interest at this point is that tone normally diminishes from birth until the second to sixth month, gradually increasing again in later childhood.

Infants with severe chronic illness predictably manifest a degree of gross motor hypotension (Markestad and Fitzhardinge, 1981) which is difficult to differentiate from hypotonia directly stemming from neuropathic sources in the first year of life. The effects of gradual improvement in general health will clarify this diagnostic issue. Basic disorders other than neuro-muscular which may underlie hypotonia and delayed motor milestones, involve the central nervous system and include forms of general retardation, both intellectual and motor. But one must also exclude even connective tissue disorder, or as already mentioned, the Prader-Willi and Down's syndromes, and finally even truly idiopathic "benign" hypotonia.

A special group of syndromes that present in infancy with muscle weakness and hypotonia in association with lactic acidaemia include Fakahara's disease, mitochondrial encephalopathy, and the Kearns-Sayre syndrome (Rowland, 1983). They also share hepatomegaly and growth failure. Add episodes of hypoglycaemia and the presenting features are comparable to those of a deficiency of another gluconeogenic enzyme: fructose 1,6,diphosphatase. An essential key to muscle weakness and hypotonia in their case may have fundamental significance as their biochemical source in many other progressive disorders of tone and power encompasses a lack of mitochondrial PEPCK (Phospho enol pyruvate carboxykinase) activity in muscle where it could play an essential role in regulating the pool size of 4-carbon intermediates. Rowland's group also included a death in the neonatal period in overwhelming acidosis due to severe muscle deficiency of cytochrome oxidase.

Specific structural brain damage has also been related to pyruvate dehydrogenase E3 deficiency such as that confined mainly to the brain stem described by Robinson (1983), or to the cerebral cystic lesion identified by Reynolds and Blass (1970).

# INITIAL HYPOTONIA: ACUTE OR PERSISTENT

## Acute Infective Sources:
## Acute Encephalitis or Encephalopathy

Inflammation of the brain of infective source, or encephalopathies, when no infective basis can be defined for analogous neurological symptomatology (e.g. Reye's syndrome or Leigh's syndrome). The child with concurrent or recent mumps, measles, chicken-pox or pertussis, etc. will be at increased risk for the supervention of encephalitis. Indeed its neurological manifestation may sometimes precede that of other clinical expression of the underlying infection. This typically includes CSF pleocytosis, or suggestive EEG patterns. Children who are immunologically compromised by, for example, lymphoma, leukaemia or AIDS, etc., are at increased risk, especially from infections wherein cell-mediated immunity is crucial, eg chicken-pox, cytomegalovirus and fungi.

The encephalitis may be localized or involve multiple areas of the brain, with diagnostic references reflecting this involvement, eg acute cerebellar ataxia, meningo encephalitis or the exceptionally lengthy compound, meningo encephalo myelo radiculitis.

Only about 25% of encephalitis have established causes, although the seasonal pattern of disease, for example, in the USA indicates that the majority of the remainder reflect entero-virus infection, ranging from mild aseptic meningitis to severe encephalitis ending in death or significant sequelae, or those due to arboviruses due to infection by an arthropod virus, and herpes viruses (1-2, and varicella zoster) cytomegalovirus or Epstein-Barr.

Non-viral infections may include a whole series of agents, from Rickettsiae, mycoplasma and bacterial to fungal, protozoal or metazoal.

Neurological damage and its expression results from direct invasion and destruction of neural tissue leading to nervous tissue reaction to corresponding antigens which probably induces demyelinization together with vascular and perivascular destruction.

Clinical manifestations of acute encephalitis may range from a sudden lapse into coma, or high fever and convulsions interspersed with bizarre movements and hallucinations. More commonly, the onset is typical of an acute systemic illness eith fever and headache, or in infants, screaming spells accompanying nausea and vomiting or abdominal distress. The nuchal rigidity may not be an unquivocal as in meningitis. Specific or complication expressions may include acute transverse myelin or Guillain-Barre, or acute cerebellar ataxia. The latter is characterized by the abrupt onset of truncal ataxia with varying severity of disturbed gait. Tremor of the head and neck when upright, spreads to the extremities when moved against gravity. The illness and symptoms may continue for a week to several months.

*Acute encephalitis or encephalopathy* must therefore be considered as a source for hypotonia which may be interrupted by jitteriness and repetitive stereotyped movement. In hypoxic-ischaemic encephalopathy *in the neonate*, the rapid loss of consciousness is usually preceded by a short prodrome of lethargy, disinclination to feed and pyrexia. Seizures may mark the onset and multifocal myoclonic jerks especially typify an hypoxic or metabolic source. Pallor marked by petechiae and ecchymosis is common with ocular chemosis and subhyaloid haemorrhage to be watched for especially if there is co-existing or primary cavernous thrombosis or subarachnoid haemorrhage.

The commonest aetiology in such an infant is infection, whether bacterial, viral, fungal or protozoal (including malaria). More recently specific viruses, eg varicella, have been identified swiftly by using the technique of polymerase chain reaction, although careful specimen collection of faeces, urine, throat swab, as well as paired serum titres, is still crucial. Alpha-interferon and specific IgG subsets in the CSF are also helpful diagnostically. E coli, listeria monocytogens and "septic shock" associated with Group B Streptococcus constitute many of these infections, with an especial initial impact from meningitis, when neck stiffness may be the cardinal sign, although possibly attended by local foci such as otitis media and a background of palatal sinus, thrombosis, with or without epiglottitis of probably influenzal basis. More general signs such as anterior and/or posterior cervical lymphadenopathy and hepato-splenomegaly are likely to be associated. One can anticipate neurological sequelae in 50-60%. Of vascular causes, apart from haemorrhage, subdural, subarachnoid and intraventricular forms already discussed, the "near miss" sudden infant death syndrome should take first place although thrombosis, embolism, and vasculitis can be responsible.

Cytomegalovirus is the commonest of the viral or TORCH group, infecting the infant *transplacentally*, and later via the birth canal, such as herpetic involvement for which acyclovir is relatively effective. Their impact earlier, in the third or fourth month of gestation, can effect neuronal migrational disorders, as described elsewhere.

HIV has introduced another threatening source, since its perinatally acquisition accounts for most of such childhood infection. Transmission is estimated as 25-35%, leading to encephalopathy in at least 13%.

The chronically sick preterm, or the immunologically embarrassed neonate suffering immunity disorders such as that of the Di George syndrome is especially vulnerable to viral and/or fungal infection and associated encephalopathy. The commonest pathogen is candida, with the most effective therapy for disseminated fungal infection being intravenous amphotericin B and/or ketoconazole.

## Hypotonia in Congenital and Metabolic Myopathies

These present either as the "floppy infant syndrome" combining muscle weakness and profound hypotonia of "central" nervous origin or related to more remote sources in early infancy, or with poor tone and proximal muscle weakness in later infancy and childhood. The important distinction is from weakness linked to involvement of the lower motor neurone or muscle itself. The basic syndrome of generalized hypotonia in the neonate or infant is attended by feebleness of voluntary movements and depressed or absent deep tendon reflexes manifest at birth or during early infancy. It was at one time encompassed by the classical term amyotonia congenita. In due course it was recognized that a congenital myopathic basis or that of a lesion of the anterior horn cell of the cord (infantile spinal muscle atrophy or Werdnig-Hoffman) accounted for most such cases. Congenital myopathies are so heterogeneous a group of disorders, although they all share in common a varying degree of muscular weakness from birth or from early infancy, in association with the conspicuous hypotonia.

Assessment of different aspects of tone still lacks objective measurement. It is still customarily assessed by gauging the resistance to passive movement, testing the range and flexibility of movement especially flexion/extension at the elbows, supination and pronation of forearms or in abduction of hips and extension of knees. This is related to extensibility, involving slow movement of joints through their full range. Other facets of tone emphasized by AndreThomas et al. (1960) include the *consistency* of a muscle tested subjectively by palpation, by wobbling the muscle laterally with a finger, if not by shaking the limbs. When the proximal part of a limb is shaken, the amplitude of the flapping movement is appraised as an expression of *passivity*. Another aspect is *recoil* when a muscle is at full stretch. Tone can also be appraised simply by observing posture in supine or prone, at rest and against gravity. The infant lies supine with hips abducted and flexed, the knees flexed, and arms flexed or extended. At the same time, in hypotonia the joints tend to show enhanced mobility. A condition of abnormal joint mobility or hyperextensibility may be associated, although not infrequently it is an isolated phenomenon so that we have addressed this dilemma is a separate section. *On traction* of the arms to raise the infant, there is complete head-lag, and *on ventral suspension*, head, arms and legs hang limply - the so-called "rag-doll" or "U-position". If hyperextension of the head derives from hypertonus, or following upon face and brow presentation, the head provisionally remains extended even when the child is prone. Unlike muscle dystrophy, the weakness is non-progressive, or only slowly progressive. Detailed histochemical and electron microscopical studies of muscle (Dubowitz, 1985) offer precise differentiation from CP, in addition to electro-diagnostic investigation as a screening test aimed at clarifying a myopathic, neurogenic or normal pattern of muscle activity. Differentiation is essential firstly between spinal muscular atrophy and congenital muscular dystrophy, and subsequently in the identification of forms of congenital myopathy associated with specific structural abnormality of muscle.

It is definable in three main groups:

1. *Associated with underlying biochemical abnormality specifically diagnosable on analyses of muscle biopsy material.* These include skeletal muscle glycogenosis (GSD) affecting muscle, Types II and III (acid maltase and debranching enzyme deficiency) presenting in infancy as a "floppy baby syndrome". This is linked to hepatomegaly and cardiac involvement, including a characteristically short PR interval on ECG. Another milder form of GSD Type II appears much later in childhood as the *juvenile* type, showing predominantly skeletal muscle involvement simulating muscle dystrophy.

2. *Associated with specific co-existing enzymological as well as structural abnormality, both identifiable in muscle biopsy material*, such as:
   (a) the absence of enzymatic activity in the core of muscle (*Central core disease*); or

(b) the rod-like structures arising from the Z-line material of muscle fibres in *Nemaline myopathy*; or

(c) *Centronuclear or Myotubular myopathy* with the nuclei centrally placed: this form, also usually progressive, being marked by *ptosis* as well as *symmetrical weakness of limbs*. The abnormal cell resembling a myotube is found in foetal muscle between 12 and 20 weeks of gestation; or

(d) longitudinal fibre disproportion embodying disproportion in the size and number of biochemical fibre type; and

(e) mitochondrial myopathies incorporating various mitochondrial anomalies.

3. *Congenital muscle* dystrophy makes up the third broad group of congenital myopathies. In these infants there is a combination of *hypotonia with weakness*, multiple *contractures* and a *myopathic EMG*. Biopsy findings are very similar to those in Duchenne muscle dystrophy. Although it tends to be non-progressive (Donner et al., 1975) and akin diagnostically to CP, it is also distinguished by its good prognosis for recovery.

In the congenital form of *myotonic* dystrophy, however, the sole anomaly may be a tendency of the Type I fibres to atrophy so that the diagnosis is often more readily confirmed by clinical and electro-diagnostic appraisal of the mother, who herself demonstrates the dominantly inherited condition.

# Spinal Muscular Atrophy (SMA)

Where the infantile hypotonia is *associated with prominent muscle weakness*, several conditions warrant careful exclusion:

## Werdnig-Hoffman Syndrome

The prevalence of some form of SMA is almost as frequent as that of Duchenne muscle dystrophy. The spinal muscular atrophies with predominantly *proximal* muscle involvement can be subdivided according to age of onset correlatable with the degree of clinical severity. The *earlier* form is an hereditary disorder characterized by degeneration and loss of the anterior motor neurons of spinal cord and brain stem which is expressed in even more profound hypotonia in association with the primary paralysis of limbs, etc., and absent reflexes.

The earliest manifestation may already be identified *in utero* with decreased or even cessation of foetal movement, or there may be sudden paralysis equally abruptly within the first two to three relatively normal months of life. A history of poor sucking and swallowing may nevertheless have anticipated this. A preceding infection may appear to precipitate the overall illness.

The *proximal* muscles are more severely affected, and the lower limbs more than the upper. *This paralysis is superimposed upon profound hypotonia*, with the infant in the characteristic frog-like or "surrender" posture with limbs spreadeagled, totally unable to raise the legs against gravity. The hips are abducted and flexed, and arms internally rotated in a jug-handle position with elbows flexed and forearms pronated. Whilst mild contractures are often associated, that documented with arthrogryposis multiplex probably represents a distinctive clinical entity.

Facial expression, however, is alert, and the infant can smile and make his wants known. But as well as inability to control the head, the trunk muscles are also severely affected. *Fasciculation of the tongue* - expressed in small furrow-like depressions rapidly appearing and disappearing - are diagnostic, but its careful differentiation is still necessary in infancy from tongue tremor. Eventual bulbar paralysis with accumulation of secretions associated with a persisting difficulty in swallowing, is almost invariable. Respiration is almost entirely diaphragmatic. All reflexes are diminished or absent, but there is neither sphincter disturbance nor obvious sensory impairments.

## Intermediate Form

In an intermediate or autosomal recessive form, the child is less severely affected. Indeed the condition is intermediate in severity between infantile Werdnig-Hoffman and the juvenile or Kugelberg-Welander syndrome, and more closely resembling muscular dystrophy. It is also distinguishable by *fasciculation* of the tongue and occasionally of skeletal muscle, and a characteristically coarse *tremor* of the outstretched hands. They differ especially in the later onset. Early motor development is indeed relatively normal, with unaided sitting actually achieved by 8 to 9 months. Beyond this, there is no further motor progress, but they survive longer, even into their late teens. They also differ clinically in *eversion of the feet* so that they are flat-footed rather than toe-stepping as in muscle dystrophy. Legs are again more affected than arms by a symmetrical weakness, but the deep reflexes, although often absent, may still remain unaffected.

### Later Onset of a Relatively Mild Form, or the Kugelberg-Welander Syndrome

In this relatively mild late and autosomally recessive form, the weakness remains static, sometimes increasing the difficulties of differentiation from cerebral palsy. A pattern of very slow progression is also occasional. In all proximal muscles, the interference pattern of activity is reduced, the motor units being of higher amplitude, longer duration and more polyphasic to the extent of producing the so-called giant units.

A form described in an inbred Japanese community in the Ryukyuan islands is a possible variant (Kondo et al., 1970), to which *pes cavus* and *scoliosis* is also added. A variant of juvenile proximal SMA likely to present diagnostic difficulties in differentiation from CP is that documented by Spiro et al. (1967) in association with microcephaly and severe learning difficulty.

## Benign Congenital Hypotonia

In this entity, first named by Walton (1957), *hypotonia and flaccidity*, coupled with a degree of symmetrical muscle weakness, is already manifest at birth, or during the infant's first year. In another group, onset is consistently between 2 and 12 months. Deep reflexes of normal strength are elicitable. Whilst the hypotonic evidence is most marked in the legs, both the trunk and arms are also often involved. There is accompanying delay in motor development, and diminished muscular activity. Gradual improvement is characteristic and often complete, although there may be mild residual disability. Reiteration should be forgiven to ensure clinical awareness of the simulation of mild hypotonia in infants with marked joint *extensibility*, sufficient to also encourage faulty interpretation of delayed motor development.

Congenital hypotonia of this type may be associated with *the Robin sequence* of anomalies (Herrman and Opitz, 1974), comprising a principal triad of micrognathia, cleft palate and glossoptosis. Whether there is oligohydramnios, or already established prenatal neurogenic hypotonia, *prenatal lack* of mandibular exercise probably accounts for the micrognathia. A phenocopy of this anomaly was produced by Poswillo (1966) in rats by puncturing the amniotic sac *prior to palatal closure*, with resulting failure of palatal closure attributable to prenatal pressure of the undescended tongue upon the palate.

In accordance with Walton's initial description, this benign category has been confined to those with "widespread congenital muscle hypotonia of undetermined aetiology which eventually recovers completely" (Walton, 1956). The "benign" term should therefore be reserved for those in whom hypotonia can be demonstrated at or shortly after birth, but with active limb movements and tendon reflexes, and without delay in motor development. Their improvement with gradual restoration of tone stretches over months although several years duration is more likely. Concurrently serum enzyme assays, EMG and muscle have remained normal throughout.

For example there was analogous recovery from hypotonia in seventeen of Walton's original series of 109 infants initially diagnosed from 1930 to 1954. This recovery was complete in eight, although remaining incomplete in nine. Those showing incomplete recovery presumably embrace examples of the metabolic myopathies which have subsequently been unearthed.

Of especial importance in this context was Lundberg's review in 1979 of 78 children with a history of delayed development of gross motor functions such as sitting and walking but without defect of manipulative functions or other neuropathic signs. In 65 of these children manifesting delay in walking beyond 27 months, infantile hypotonia has been significant in 72%. Half had been "bottom shufflers". She also demonstrated as a classical sign amongst these late walkers, "sitting on air" with a posture of hip flexion and knee extension.

## Myasthenia Gravis

This is characterized more specifically by muscular weakness enhanced by progressive fatiguability. It rarely presents in childhood, when it may first emerge in the guise of a *relapsing* and *remittent* weakness.

In the flaccidity and hypotonia associated with *myasthenia* of *congenital or early infantile onset*, the tendon reflexes gradually diminish, and tremor may involve fingers, hands and arms. The "floppy infant" is one guise, and may be its clinical expression in the progeny of an affected mother. Bilateral ptosis, like the muscular weakness elsewhere which increases in the latter part of the day - or after repetitive activity - as the most conspicuous element of the facial weakness, is characteristic. So is rapid fatiguability and weakness of oropharyngeal musculature in feeding. But when emerging soon after birth difficulties in sucking, swallowing and handling secretions predominate, as well as a feeble cry. Accumulated secretions may bring on respiratory difficulties which could especially highlight bulbar paresis in congenital myasthenia. In the older child, sudden strabismus, diplopia, or ptosis again, may first manifest. Other early signs may include weakness in the lower extremities, also sometimes sudden in onset, when it may be represented as "episodic weakness" in the congenital form. Dysarthria and external ophthalmoplegia are also later manifestations. All may be swiftly overcome diagnostically in response to Tensilon (physostigmine derivative: 1mg I.V.).

**Congenital Open-mouth or Lockjaw as the product of foetal myasthenia** (Russell and Shapiro, 1994)

*Congenital myasthenia* is usually defined as an autosomal recessive disorder dating from birth with ptosis and external ophthalmoplegia on muscle fatigue as dominant features. Any involvement of facial and skeletal musculature is initially very mild, although a decremental response on electromyography may still be detectable. Progressive skeletal muscle weakness may be its ultimate clinical expression (Fenichel, 1983).

There is a good response in early childhood to anticholinesterase agents such as the Tensilon Physostigmine derivative, and ACh antibodies are assumed to be absent in male cases. In Vincent et al's five examples (1981) the findings indicated a defect in acetylcholine receptor. A partial response to anticholinesterase agents was possibly augmented by treatment with 3,4-diaminopyridine. A different postsynaptic defect was suggested in two of these cases,

including one studied by Lecky et al. (1986) who hypothesized a defect in the structure of the AChR macromolecule.

When of sufficient *prenatal* potency it may also lead to a "fixed open-mouth syndrome" postnatally, as described by Russell and Shapiro (1994) in two pairs of siblings who exemplify the considerable prenatal impact of congenital myasthenia on mandibular growth. Foetal impairment of growth, with obtuse angulation of the mandible consequent upon diminished prenatal pull of the masseters and related musculature upon the maturing foetal mandible, is presumably the direct explanation of the subsequent failure of jaw closure.

The infant eventually exhibiting the *choreo-athetoid* category of cerebral palsy may also manifest first with hypotonia and defective postural reactions. The irregular choreo-athetoid movements only gradually emerge towards the end of the second year of life.

## Dystrophia Myotonica or Steinert's Syndrome

The primary abnormality in this progressive genetically-determined disorder is within muscle itself, although other clinical features indicate multi-system involvement. Its onset may be in infancy or late childhood, but may be already evident at birth. so that poor sucking and swallowing would be the earliest manifestations, although *generalized hypotonia and weakness* are the usual presenting features. This muscle weakness is generalized, extending to facial,

sternomastoid, and limb muscles. On the other hand, asymmetry of this involvement may occur, and distal muscles are more affected than proximal.

In the *Steinert's Syndrome* of myotonic dystrophy, manifold anomalies in association with *myotonia* and *hypotonia* in infancy are encountered as a product of a single mutant, autosomal dominant, gene. The myotonia may be so mild that it is elicitable only on careful testing. Associated anomalies such as cataract ("myotonic dust" on slit lamp microscopy), cardiac conduction defects with arrhythmias, and testicular atrophy, appear much later.

Although the syndrome does not usually appear until after 8 years of age, subjects have commonly been initially hypotonic and "floppy", with developmental delay and apparent mental defect, sometimes linked to microcephaly, already manifest during infancy (Pruzanski, 1966). Occasionally clinodactyly, talipes, and kyphoscoliosis co-exist, as well as ocular features such as ptosis and ophthalmo-plegia; blepharitis and keratitis sicca may also emerge early. Likewise for the muscle wasting and weakness, which most often involves the facial and temporal muscles to produce the expressionless "myopathic facies", also marked by a triangular-shaped mouth. Dysphagia is also distinctively associated. A highly sensitive *early* index of localized impact of such muscle dysfunction is the radiological demonstration of partial pharyngeal retention of radiopaque material after swallowing.

The *myotonus* (or difficulty in relaxing a contracted muscle) may be elicitable by inability to release a grasp, or a furrow of sustained contraction of an inter-rib segment of muscle after percussion, for example of the pectoralis major. *Delayed opening of the eyes after crying*, and a *protracted grasp-reflex* may also draw attention to the possibility of an underlying myotonic syndrome. This may be suspected on finding facial weakness in mother or father, with subclinical evidence such as inability to completely close the eyes, the sluggish release of a hand grasp, or the characteristic myotonic discharge on EMG in either or both mother and child to confirm the diagnosis. The earliest clinical feature may however prove to be prenatal, in the form of *hydramnios*.

Myotonia is also the dominant clinical feature of myotonia congenita which is benign and without muscle weakness. Quinine, procainamide or steroids may solely alleviate the myotonia.

## Dermatomyositis

Although uncommon in the under-fives, it is important to consider this diagnosis in any child manifesting generalized weakness, especially when intermittent or associated with overall undue fatiguability. *The differentiation of weakness from hypotonia* is always a critical diagnostic issue. Gradually progressive weight loss, mainly due to muscle wasting, and the characteristic violaceous colouring and skin desquamation above the eyelids becomes conspicuous. The natural history is one of relapses and remissions which may be induced by steroids.

The EMG shows a mixed picture of fibrillation potentials *at rest* - indicative of denervated fibres - and of myopathic potential on activity.

# Riley-Day Syndrome (Familial Dysautonomia)

Another progressive autosomal recessive disorder without known metabolic basis or specific aetiology which is characterized at the outset by *hypotonia* and hyporeflexia in the neonate, also expressed initially in difficulties in feeding and failure to thrive. Developmental delay persists from the first year and is punctuated by episodic fevers and incidents of apnoea and breath-holding usually provoked by oesophageal regurgitation linked to dysphagia. Undue apprehensiveness is a marked characteristic, as is striking sinus tachycardia, excessive drooling, transitory spreading erythematous blotchiness on face, neck and extremities, and paroxysmal hypertension which it induces.

Other multifocal neurological features include insensitivity to pain, sensorineural deafness, sparse tear production, and sometimes mild ptosis in association with impairment of taste in the early neonate (Russell and Perlman, 1992). The causative absence of fungiform papillae is definable from the first few days of life, especially during elucidation of the difficulties in feeding and swallowing. Other pathognomonic criteria include the absence of a weal and flare reaction to intradermal histamine, and the miosis of the pupil following installation of methacholine.

Histology of the dorsal root ganglia could help to account for the absence of response to deep pain in terms of its extensive neuronal loss and proliferation of nodules of Nogeotte. Predominantly sensory peripheral nerves show loss of small diameter myelinated and unmyelinated axons. Both dorsolateral tracts and dorsal columns show equally severe loss of neurones, with some loss from the intermediate lateral grey columns.

# Pontocerebellar Hypoplasia (Dubowitz and Davies, 1991)

Hypotonia and floppiness from birth is associated with hyporeflexia and muscle weakness affecting proximal muscles more than distal. The co-existing fasciculation of the tongue would initially point to Werdnig-Hoffman or infantile spinal muscular atrophy manifesting at birth. Narrowing of the thoracic cage with subcostal recession, including that of the intercostal musculature associated with poor function, would oppose that diagnosis, as would the absence of that bright and alert expression typical of Werdnig-Hoffman. This neurobiological defect of cerebellar and pontine hypoplasia can be clearly defined by cranial ultrasonography and confirmed on magnetic resonance imaging. Loss of anterior horn cells comparable to that in SMA has been identified at autopsy.

# Demyelinating and Axonal Neuropathies

This differential diagnosis from CP is, of course, particularly difficult in infants and young children. *Peripheral weakness* and *absence of reflexes* are predominant, so that the fundamental differentiation of weakness from hypotonia, likewise with hyporeflexia, necessitates very careful assessment of tone and exclusion of the peripheral neuropathies.

*Demyelination, or myelinoclastic disorder* implies normal myelin which is attacked by exogenous agents to be broken down into its component, lipids, etc. In *dysmyelination* or leukodystrophy, there is abnormal formation of myelin owing to a genetically-determined error of metabolism.

*Segmental demyelination* would be the expected and natural consequence of Schwann cell or axonal pathology, i.e. of neuronal segments. It may be confined to the peripheral nervous system, or is part of a more widespread disorder involving the CNS. It occurs, for example, in the globoid cell type or metachromatic variants of leukodystrophy already mentioned. These can be distinguished from other progressive degenerative disorders of the CNS by virtue of the accompanying slow motor nerve conduction velocities. Analogous neuropathy can be defined in the Cockayne

syndrome (Moosa and Dubowitz, 1970), and some examples of the Leigh syndrome, which have been included here under the heading herein of progressive conditions presenting with ataxia. In *axonal neuropathies*, where the primary disturbance of function is in the axon, the nerve conduction velocity is either normal or only slightly reduced. These have included not only such disorders of the anterior horn cells as have been already outlined, but also *vincristine* toxicity, and at one time that of *thalidomide*, as well as genetic factors (e.g. in the hereditary sensory neuropathies), or even thiamine deficiencies in appropriate rice-dependent areas of the world.

Marked slowing of nerve conduction also characterizes other sources of segmented demyelination confined to peripheral nerves. The Guillain-Barre syndrome may involve the relevant age period, but both the hereditary hypertrophic polyneuropathy of Dejerine-Sottas, or peroneal muscular atrophy, do not present fully until late childhood or adolescence. In its manifestation in earlier childhood, the concomitant *wasting* of peroneal muscles is usually difficult to identify, but slow nerve conduction in both child *and one or other parent* will confirm the diagnosis in such dominantly inherited polyneuropathy.

# Central Positive Myelinolysis (CPM)

This rare disorder primarily affects alcoholics but may also occur as a reversible condition in children and adults suffering

severe electrolyte disorders, liver disease, malnutrition anorexia, burns, Addison's disease, cancer, sepsis and Wilson's disease.

Typically, it evolves within days or weeks of a severe illness, especially following, by one to three days, a period of profound hyponatraemia, in turn followed by rapid osmolar correction of more than 20 mEq/L. After a phase of lowered consciousness, with functional corticospinal interruption at the level of the pons, *hypotonic* or *hypertonic tetraparesis* may ensue.

This is associated with bulbar disturbance of speech and swallowing.

Abnormality exposed by CT or MRI, revealing an area of decreased signal in the pons, may achieve diagnosis in life. Limited recovery may follow electrolytic correction, especially of sodium balance, raising the serum sodium by less than 12 mmol/L, but some remain tetraplegic.

## Formimino Glutamic Aciduria (FIGLU: McKusick 22910)

In the metabolism of histidine, the first step involves elimination of ammonia to form urocanic acid which is then catabolized to produce FIGLU. The formyl group is then transferred to tetrahydrofolate with the production in turn of 5-formimino tetrahydrofolate and 5,10-methenyl tetrahydrofolate. Two groups of FIGLU tranferase deficiency are thus believed to be implicated (Rowe, 1983).

1. The first group of methionine-dependent (or Co-factor deficiency) was first introduced by Russell et al., manifesting hypotonia and an autistic-like variant of psychomotor retardation in a relatively mild clinical presentation. Underlying the basic defect or deficiency of glutamate formiminotransferase, there is a deficiency of co-factor methionine as one of its three main co-factors, vitamin B12, folate and methionine. This co-factor lack is illustrated in the immediate elimination of the excessive urinary excretion of Figlu, reaching over thirty times its normal levels by oral supplementation with methionine. of its excessive urinary excretion of FIGLU.

2. A more severe mental and physical retardation associated with cortical atrophy attends the so-called second group. Although there is only partial deficiency of glutamate formimino-transferase with less marked excretion of FIGLU, it is suspected to be coupled with severe deficiency of formimino tetrahydrofolate cyclo-deaminase.

### Impaired Remethylation of Homocysteine by 5-methyl-tetrahydrofolate

The conversion of Methionine to homocysteine is an important sequence in the provision of methyl groups for a range of important metabolic reactions. It is important to recall that the brain and CNS are deeply involved insofar as these reactions include inactivation of calecholamine neurotransmitters and creatinine synthesis. The *demand* for such *methylation* usually exceeds the Methionine *supply*, so that a remethylation cycle involving two remethylation reactions are called into play to convert homocysteine back to Methionine. One is Betaine as the methyl donor, the other 5-methyltetrahydrofolate.

# Methylmalonic Acidaemias and
# Combined Homocysteinuria and Methylmalonic Aciduria
## (McKusick 27740 and 27741)

Recurrent episodes of ketosis and acidosis expressed in vomiting and dehydration leading on to failure to thrive are associated primarily with peaks of methylmalonic acidaemia in concentrations of 2.6 to 34 mg/dl, and secondary hyperglycinaemia, due to a block or defective activity at L-methylmalonyl CoA mutase. The defect is within the mutase itself or in any of several transport and catalytic proteins involved in the biosynthesis of adenosylcobalamin - the mutase co-enzyme derived from vitamin B12. The classification therefore divides the disorder into *vitamin B12 responsive or unresponsive*, the latter more likely to manifest symptoms in the neonate. The appearance of large amounts of methylmalonic acid in the urine either alone or with 3-hydroxypropionic and methylcitric acids that stem from propionyl-CoA is a sensitive diagnostic marker. It is accompanied by simultaneous losses of potassium and of sodium which are to be met by sodium bicarbonate supplementation at 2-3 mmols/kg. Potassium supplements may be indicated during recovery. A critical episode is often ushered in by infection to which these infants are unusually prone. Intolerance to the usual level of dietary protein, or more specifically to the amino acids: isoleucine, valine, threonine and methionine, may precipitate such an attack. Hypoglycaemic reactions have been ascribed to inhibition of pyruvate carboxylase by methylmalonic acid, or to inhibition of mitochondrial transport of malate, 2-ketoglutarate and isocitrate.

Striking *growth-failure* and *osteoporosis* are also regularly found. *Anorexia* is usually severe enough to justify tube feeding. Developmental retardation in infancy is characteristic, but it is difficult to separate the influences of illness and *extreme hypotonia* in their interference with motor development. A frog-like position again illustrates the depth of the hypotonia in this infantile metabolic disorder.

The multiple amino acid toxicity reflects the fundamental defect in the activity of methylmalonyl CoA which catalyses conversion to succinyl CoA, an enzyme which lies on the direct degradative pathway for these same amino acids: isoleucine, valine, threonine and methionin and all major sources of methylmalonate in these children. In each of this family of distinct entities, there is defective activity of methylmalonyl CoA mutase. A defect is the apoenzyme itself may be the source, or a defect in the synthesis of its co-factor, 51-deoxyadenosylcobalamin, when responsiveness to high dosage of Vitamin B12 would be expected. Deficiency thereof interferes with the vital step of metabolization of methylmalonyl CoA to succinyl CoA. In a third category of the disorder, the defect in adenosylcobalamin biosynthesis also leads to deficiency of methyl B12, necessary for conversion of homocysteine to methionine. It is therefore also accompanied by elevated concentrations of homocystine and cystathionine in both blood and urine, linked to hypomethioninaemia. In the combined form of methylmalonic aciduria and homocysteinuria, the presentation is often later, and accompanied by severe central nervous system dysfunction, i.e. with *hypotonia, conspicuous developmental delay, epileptiform reactions* and *microcephaly*. Children with methylmalonic acidaemia should first be tested for responsiveness to Vitamin B12. If confirmed, weekly injections of the infant, likely to be vomiting and feeding poorly, of B12 (1-2 mg/day for five days). On the basis of a low protein diet, this programme can achieve active and healthy development. Even prenatal therapy with Vitamin B12 (Ampola et al., 1975) could successfully avert neuropathic changes before birth. If unresponsive to B12, therapy would be directed, as in propionic acidaemia, to treating shock expressed in profound hypotonia, as well as acidosis, hypoglycaemia and hyperammon-aemia. In addition, dietary restriction should be imposed of propiogenic amino acids to the amounts essential for normal growth and development. Alanine and possibly carnitine supplements are also indicated.

All forms are inherited genetically as autosomal recessive, probably diagnosable in utero. But its gene locus has already been successfully located on chromosome 6, with the implication in the long-term that gene therapy holds out promise for the future.

# HYPOTONIA: INITIAL AND TRANSITORY

## Syndromes of Chromosomal or Cytogenetic Anomaly

A growing number of disorders stemming from gross chromosomal aberration rather than a basic genetic component are being defined, of which a prominent initial clinical expression is a greater or lesser degree of *generalized hypotonia*. The greater the enploiding from XXY to XXXXY, the more severe the hypotonia, growth and mental deficiency, as well as the hypogenitalism and other components.

### XXXXY Syndrome

*Typical hypotonia* and joint laxity is associated with shortness of stature, marked by retarded osseous maturation, and severe mental deficiency, $\propto$ levels revealing a mean of 34.

Of craniofacial features, the sutures are sclerotic, the hypoteloric eyes show an upward slant with epicanthic folds. Strabismus is common, and the nasal bridge is low with wide or upturned nasal tip. There is prognathism of the mandible and the ears are large, low set and malformed. A small penis and testes, with hypoplastic and deficient Leydig cells, mark the characteristic hypogenitalism.

## Down's syndrome

Down's syndrome due to underlying regular Trisomy 21, 14:21 and 21 balanced translocation 21/13, initial floppiness and hypotonia is perhaps the best known example. As in so-called benign congenital hypotonia, there is a gradual lessening of the degree of hypotonia especially beyond infancy and during the 3rd and 4th years of life.

## Prader-Willi Syndrome

In the Prader-Willi syndrome of ultimate obesity, growth failure, mental retardation, hypogonadism and kyphoscoliosis, there is an initial severe degree of *generalized hypotonia*. *This* is associated with feeding difficulties linked to impaired sucking and swallowing from birth and an early stage of "failure to thrive". But despite persistent although lessening hypotonia, the appetite typically becomes voracious at a year or so of age. More recently, many but not all of these subjects (about 50% is the present assessment) have revealed a very small deletion (bands q11 q13), very close to the centromere in the long arm of Chromosome 15.

## Tetrasomy 12p or Pallister-Killian Syndrome

This more recently defined chromosomal anomaly associated with *hypotonia from birth* in an infant typically with disproportionate shortness of upper and lower extremities. Severe or profound motor and mental retardation become manifest from early infancy. The relative dysmorphism is distinctive with the coarseness of facies becoming more pronounced with age. The frontal bossing and high frontal hairline is in fact accompanied by temporo-frontal

alopecia and sparseness or absence of lateral or medial eyebrows and eyelashes. Later in infancy, patchy depigmentation of skin becomes apparent, but occasionally hyperpigmentation instead (detectable on Woods light examination). Hypertelorism is linked to features suggesting Down's syndrome: upward and outward slanting palpebral fissures, and epicanthic folds. Ears are low set and dysplastic. Exophthalmos has been reported, as has occasional cataract. The nasal bridge is flat and the nose itself small with upturned nares, and the philtrum long. The tongue enlarges during infancy, and protrudes, again as in Down's syndrome. The mouth is large with downturned corners, the lips becoming thicker as infancy advances. The neck is short and, like the Turner or Noonans syndrome in the male, is often webbed and with excess nuchal skin. Associated diaphragmatic defects are frequent, and detection during pregnancy has led to prenatal diagnosis of the syndrome.

## 5p or Cri du Chat syndrome (Lejeune et al., 1963)

The underlying chromosomal aberration is a partial deletion of the short arm of Chromosome 5. This hypotonic syndrome of a low birth-weight with microcephaly and mental deficiency is strikingly distinguished in the neonate or early infant by a mewing high-pitched cry reminiscent of the choked mewing of a cat, and stems from a small narrow and hypoplastic larynx. This effect becomes less pronounced with the increasing age of the child (Breg et al., 1970). As in the previous cytogenetic abnormalities, *hypotonia* is learly identifiable in early childhood but tends to disappear.

Deep tendon reflexes are exaggerated, and there may be ankle clonus. Later in this instance, it may be occasionally replaced by hypertonicity (Platt and Holmes, 1967).

Low in birth-weight for their gestational age, *failure to thrive* then ensues accompanying continuing *retardation of growth* as well as of cognitive and motor development. The cranio-facial dysmorphis is also characteristic. A round or moon-shaped face soon becomes long and narrow - as if flattened from side to side - and it is usually asymmetrical with ears poorly formed and low set. The hypertelorism is linked to epicanthal folds, anti-mongoloid orbital slant, and divergent strabismus may persist. A broad nasal bridge and a short philtrum surmount an often exceptionally large mouth and high-arched palate, with micrognathia and upheaping of the metopic suture frequent. Speech seldom develops, and the hair shows premature greying. The extremities are often marked by short metacarpals as well as clinodactyly and simian creases.

**4p syndrome: Partial deletion of short arm of 4 or Wolf-Hirschhorn syndrome** (Wolf et al., 1965; Hirschhorn et al., 1965)

The basic defect is a short arm deletion of the B-group, Chromosome No. 4 (Guthrie et al., 1971). Careful differentiation is required from the 5p syndrome since both share the *distinctive initial hypotonia* which is probably prenatal in onset, with no head control, and later appreciation of mental and growth retardation, retarded bone age, and anti-mongoloid ocular slant. The 4p pattern, however, includes colobomata of the iris and midline facial defects. To which in the

male can be added the hypospadias and cryptorchidism. Although the cry is also noticeably weak and plaintive in 4p, the cat-like cry of the 5p syndrome is still distinctive. Indeed weakness of foetal movement may already be recognized prenatally.

In 4p, the defect in mental motor and social development is profound, and they seldom if ever smile or respond socially. Generalized seizures are common. Cranio-facial dysmorphism is again characteristic with a high sloped forehead - although microcephaly is usual - and the nose unduly prominent although typically symmetrically flattened and misshapen. The glabella is prominent, with midline facial defects the rule with clefts of lips palate or both, often linked to a posterior mildline cleft of the skull. The philtrum is unusually short often accompanied by eversion of pulled-up centre of the upper lip. Together with the angles of the mouth being downturned, the micrognathia and short philtrum, the fish-like mouth is conspicuous. Hypertelorism is especially prominent as are ocular epicanthic folds, anti-mongoloid slant, strabismus and iris deformity, and low-set large ears.

**9p Monosomy syndrome**

The chromosomal anomaly consists of deletion of the distal portion of the short arm of Chromosome 9. The prominent craniostenosis involves the metopic suture, its upheaving producing a trigonocephalic defect, along with upslanting palpebral fissures, hypoplastic supraorbital ridges and midfacial hypoplasia with depressed nasal bridge, short nose and anteverted nares.

Micrognathia is also present and the ears are posteriorly rotated and defectively formed with hypoplastic adherent ear lobes.

## 18p Syndrome (Schinzel et al., 1974)

Deletion of the short arm of Chromosome 18 is involved. A broad variability in the phenotype includes in addition to the relatively mild hypotonia, moderate growth deficiency and mental deficiency linked to minor microcephaly. The craniofacial pattern embodies ptosis, epicanthal folds, low nasal bridge, hypertelorism, micrognathia downturning angles of mouth and large protruding ears.

Alopecia is an occasional burden. There is also pectus excavatum, and acromicria, or relatively small hands and feet. An immunological defect, IgA absence or deficiency, is usually asymptomatic and occasionally a more severe cranial defect, holoprosencephaly or arhinencephaly, emerges. Behavioural problems typically comprise undue restlessness, emotional lability, fear of strangers and lack of concentration capacity.

## Trisomy 13 Syndrome (Warkany, Passarge and Smith, 1966)

In this chromosomal trisomy syndrome, serious CNS defects include the holoprosencephaly type defect with degrees of incomplete development of forebrain, olfactory and optic nerves. An analysis in seven examples clarifying correlationships between these cerebral and facial correlationships was undertaken by Russell, Butler, France and Snodgrass in 1967.

Craniofacially, there is typically in more than 50% of such children, moderate microcephaly with sloping forehead accompanied by wide sagittal suture and fontanelles. Micropthhalmia bilaterally is associated with colobomata of the iris and retinal dysplasia. The ears show abnormal helices, and lax skin marks the back of the neck. The hands demonstrate the characteristic, the typical fisting, with flexion of fingers with or without overlapping and camptodactyly, polydactyly existing in the hands and sometimes in the feet. Characteristic rocker-bottom or heel prominence is another feature.

Occurring in less than 30%, there is congenital hypoplasia associated with either hypotonia or hypertonia. Agenesis of the corpus callosum may be present, and other major underlying defects of the brain including fusion of the basal ganglia and cerebellar hypoplasia. There is hypertelorism and the supraorbital ridges are shallow, palpebral fissures are slanting, and the eyebrows are absent. Anophthalmos is occasional. The philtrum may also be absent, and the tongue cleft together with micrognathia. In the hands and feet, there may be a retroflexible thumb, ulnar deviation at the wrist and even radial aplasia amongst numerous other defects. Associated cardiac anomalies may be particularly serious, from anomalous venous return, overriding aorta and/or hypoplastic aorta, pulmonary stenosis, and atretic mitral and/or aortic valves.

## Trisomy 20 Syndrome (Schinzel, 1980)

Hypotonia, ataxia and tremor are characteristic of this syndrome attributed to familial rearrangements. The craniofacial anomalies again include brachycephaly associated with blepharophimosis, upslanting palpebral fissures, a flat nasal bridge and anteverted nares. The ears are large and poorly formed. Of skeletal anomalies, cubitus valgus is prominent, and the fingers are small and tapering, with clinodactyly of the fifth digit. The nipples are small and widely spaced, herniae are present, umbilical and/or inguinae, and there is genital hypoplasia with cryptorchidism.

# Miscellaneous Disorders of Unknown Aetiology

## Hypermobility of Joints

A separate section on the significance of this phenomenon has been added (Chapter 4). Excessive joint mobility may be present independently but association with hypotonia is not uncommon and the relationship of these two components should be carefully appraised. Apart from the lack of resistance to passive movement the paucity of spontaneous activity in hypotonic states is conspicuous.

A key point is whether the hypotonia is allied to a parallel decrease in muscle strength. When raising the infant in the air, note his ability to maintain the extremities in an anti-gravity position, or the ability to resist slipping down when held in the axillae.

## Camptomelic Dysplasia

The term "Camptomelic" was derived by Maroteaux and colleagues (1971) from a Greek term indicating "bending" or curvature of bones, especially of tibia, fibula and femur. Pretibial skin dimples are regularly associated. Even the scapulae are hypoplastic and early scoliosis may exist in the presence of vertebral osteoporosis. The underlying primary defect appears to reside in a severe *prenatal* impairment of cartilage and bone. The thorax is also abnormally narrow. Polyhydramnios has also been frequently associated. Severe dwarfing results especially from shortening of the lower extremities. But in addition, these neonates are already *severely hypotonic*, with cyanosis and poor respiratory function even evident at bith. Such respiratory distress persists to ensure the infant's early death.

A diagnostic pattern links the general osseous anomalies with a characteristic craniofacial dysmorphism, a prominent occiput being associated with upheaping of the frontal metopic suture, flat facies, hypertelorism, low-set ears, a small mouth and micrognathia. Cartilaginous proliferation of metaphyses is grossly reduced. The respiratory distress itself may stem from hypoplasia of the cartilaginous rings of the tracheobronchial tree (Lee et al., 1972).

# INITIAL HYPOTONIA FOLLOWED BY SPASTICITY OR ACCOMPANIED BY INTERMITTENT HYPERTONIC REACTIONS AND/OR ATAXIA

This neuropathic constellation characterizes a long list of *progressive "Degenerative"* or *Metabolic disorders including*:

Urea cycle defects and congenital hyperammonaemia

Non-ketotic hyperglycinaemia

Lysosomal enzyme disorders

Early infantile Gaucher

Tay-Sachs disease

Sandhoffs disease

Congenital amaurotic idiocy

Early infantile $GM_1$ gangliosidosis

Early infantile Niemann-Pick

Infantile neuronic ceroid lipofuscidosis

Lowe's (oculo-cerebro-renal) syndrome

3-hydroxy-3 methyl glutaric aciduria

Glutaric aciduria Type II

3-methyl glutaconic aciduria

3-ketothiolase deficiency

Dihydrolipoyl dehydrogenase deficiency

Peroxisomal disorders

1. Glycogenosis Type II (Pompe's disease)

2. Zellweger's disease

3. Mevalonic aciduria

Other inborn metabolic disorders may also manifest acutely or intermittently, that is even periodically or cyclically like the Krebs urea cycle defects, sometimes intensifying often temporarily, or regressing within a multifocal syndrome of other clinical and biochemical features.

The role of the major forms of congenital hyperammonaemia and maple syrup urine disease in this context will be outlined first of all. Other metabolic disorders with which we are becoming increasingly familiar, even in the neonate, include hyperglycinaemia, both of the ketotic (propionic acidaemia) and the non-ketotic type, isovaleric acidaemia, methylmalonic aciduria, congenital lactic acidosis, the severe form of sulphite oxidase deficiency, congenital fructose intolerance, galactosaemia and pyridoxine dependency.

Other disorders, not regarded as genetically-determined, embrace the hyperkinetic hypotonic syndromes of hypocalcaemia and hypomagnesaemia, also expressed in tetany, or hypoglycaemia (which may occur in at least eight disorders of infancy) typically expressed in convulsions, but also in the interlude in apathetic states, later in flaccidity in infancy. Severe forms of congenital adrenal hyperplasia may also be expressed in profound sodium deficit, or rather hyperpotassaemia, as well as hypoglycaemia...

Difficulties in swallowing or feeding have in my experience often been the first hint of trouble, and may be sufficient to encourage tube feeding. Vomiting may be the next consequence of feeding, with diarrhoea a later expression of food intolerance. Fretfulness and dissatisfaction with food lead onto failure to thrive. More specific disturbance of CNS function is expressed in unpatterned twitches, tonic contractions, twitching of face and hands, sudden arrest of respiration and emergence of convulsions. These may be punctuated by several moments of unresponsiveness and stillness of limbs. Respiratory difficulties may appear early as in the neonatal phase of our case of maple syrup disease necessitating exchange transfusion

(Russell and Statter, 1982). These were preceded by feeding difficulties during the infant's first five days, as well as periodic apnoea. Whilst there *may be frequent opisthotonic (decerebrate) movements of neck and even trunk, hypotonia* may be a more constant feature. Concomitant lethargy extending through stupor to coma is a common characteristic. Cerebral damage can be a consequence of hypoglycaemia if prolonged and severe, especially if in combination with hypoxia and metabolic acidosis.

## Hyperammonaemia/Urea Cycle Defects and Intermittent Extensor Hypertonicity and Transitory Ataxia

The underlying state of congenital hyerammonaemia was observed for the first time by Russell et al. (1962) initially as the clinical expression of ornithine transcarbamylase (OTC) deficiency, in an infant of 20 months. But throughout infancy, it had already produced cyclical episodes of vomiting and alleged "collapse" really made up of a sequence of lethargy to stupor to coma. These are also marked by intermittent opisthotonus of neck and trunk, alternating flaccidity and tonic spasms of the limbs masking extensor hypertonus,

hyperreflexia, Babinski responses, spontaneous ankle clonus, and even repetitive hand-waving movements recalling the "hand-flaps" typical of the hyperammonaemia associated with adult liver failure. Another clinical expression of hyperammonaemia is ataxia, and several days of ataxia may indeed characterize the conclusion of the episodes. This aspect is dealt with more fully in the subsequent section on predominantly ataxic manifestations (Chapter 19).

## HHH Syndrome

Operation of the urea cycle within the hepatocyte involves the mitochondrial ornithine transporter, being responsible for transport of ornithine into the mitochondrium. This is believed to be defective leading to discharge therefrom of citrulline in the HHH syndrome, comprising

hyperammonaemia, hyperornithinaemia (which is relatively modest at 0.4-0.9 mol/l, and homocitrullinaemia.

The hyperammonaemia appears to be the result of deficiency in the mitochondrial ornithine impeding the urea cycle and leading to some orotic aciduria. To what extent the mitochondrial ornithine oxoacid amino transferase is responsible for ornithine synthesis and degradation is involved remains to be more precisely defined but ornithine catabolism continues within the mitochondria to increase the extramitochondrial ornithine, whilst homocitrulline is synthesized directly from lysine, its output increasing with the plasma lysone concentration and the load on the urea cycle. A mild urea cycle disorder is the outcome, with the typical sequence of intermittent hyperammonaemia. In addition, spasticity becomes conspicuous in some of the older children.

A demonstration of this reduced rate of incorporation of [$^{14}$C] ornithine into cell protein can be effected by phytohaemagglutin-stimulatedlymphocytes on cultured fibroblasts.

## Lysinuric Protein Intolerance

Functional deficiency of ornithine in the hepatic mitochondria is postulated as the source of lysinuric protein intolerance. The plasma concentration of ornithine, argenine and lysin are low, but citrulline concentration is increased. Hyperammon-aemia is intermittent. Protein restriction and arginine supplementation, rather than citrulline, is effective therapy.

Hyperextensible joints are also found in lysinuric protein intolerance associated with hyperelastic skin, lens opacities and sparse scalp hair. Ornithine aminotransferace, a pyridoxal phosphate-requiring enzyme, and a small proportion of patients respond to large doses of pyridoxal.

## Non-Ketotic Hyperglycinaemia

*Metabolic hypotonia* is one consequence of non-ketotic hyperglycinaemia. In most cases, this defect derives from failure in enzymatic conversion of glycine to serine with primary accumulation of glycine in the brain and to a lesser extent in the bloodstream.

*Extreme hypotonia at birth* marks such neonates suffering "glycine encephalopathy". Even diminished movement of the foetus has been noted by some mothers. Their *hypotonia of intercostal and presumably* *diaphragmatic musculature* may impede respiration. Survivors of this precarious introduction live on despite profound hypotonia and brain damage, also expressed in epilepsy of myoclonic type, as well as in the pathognomonically great elevation of CSF glycine.

The remarkable response of muscular tone, and the even more dramatic tolerance of such babies to *strychnine* are especially significant. That strychnine specifically antagonises glycine's neurotransmitter effects, supports the hypothesis that *the profoundly lowered muscle tone derives from excessive glycine concentration in the cord.*

*Hypotonia progressing to spasticity*, also characterizes this inborn error. The hyperglycinaemia and hyperglycinuria are linked to an abnormally raised CSF:plasma glycine ratio, and a defective glycine cleavage enzyme system. The absence of organic acid accumulation distinguishes this disorder from the ketotic hyperglycinaemia syndrome that arises with propionic acidaemia. The associated overwhelming illness early in life has been repeatedly detailed (Trauner et al., 1981).

A lack of spontaneous involvement except for myoclonic jerks may be already noted in the neonatal period with failure to thrive, and of mental development to follow. Undue lethargy may be noticeable from the first days of life and the hypotonia persists so that by the third year the child is diffusely hypotonic, unresponsive to social stimuli and incessantly turning the head from side to side. Generalized seizures are recurrent, the myoclonic type being especially characteristic, and there is no head control. Persistence of hiccuping which may reflect a seizure equivalent.

Most of these infants thus remain hypotonic from an early stage. Should survival extend beyond 8 to 12 months, hypertonicity takes over, opisthotonic posturing recurs, and hyperreflexia prevails.

The EEG in myoclonic infants displays periodic bursts of large amplitude sharp elements on a low voltage background in a so-called "burst suppression" pattern akin to that of hypsarrhythmia.

Neuropathologically, on exploration of the diffuse postnatal alterations in myelination *vacuolation in myelin* is found to be followed by loss thereof and gliosis. Analogous changes have been identified in other amino acidopathies including propionic acidaemia, PKU and Maple Syrup Urine syndrome.

A very different presentation, with a neurodegenerative evolution like Tay Sachs or Krabbe disease, could provide a difficult diagnostic differential from CP in the second half of the first year of life when progressive cerebral deterioration sets in.

Raised concentrations of glycine in the blood ranging from 6 to 12 mg/dl, or with a mean of 7.5 mg/dl, are diagnostic, and the level of glycine in the CSF is particularly high in non-ketotic hyperglycinaemia. Its ratio of glycine concentration to that of the plasma is greater in non-ketotic hyperglycinaemia than in hyperglycinaemic patients with organic acidaemia. The activity of the glycine cleavage system, as measured by the exchange of $14CO2$ with glycine is active in the brain but virtually absent in the brain of subjects with non-ketotic hyperglycinaemia.

The remarkable tolerance of infants to strychnine (Gizelmann and Steinmann, 1978) permitted a convincing demonstration of the dramatic influence of strychnine which is a specific antagonist of glycines, in restoring muscle tone. This supports the view that the fall in muscle tone is a consequence of excessive glycine levels in the spinal cord.

## Lysosomal Enzyme Disorders

Clinical components simulating those of cerebral palsy or of progressive disturbances of movement, balance and tone are expressed in each member of this group of such disorders already manifesting in infancy and early childhood.

## Tay-Sachs (Early Infantile GM$_2$-Gangliosidosis) Disease

*Axial hypotonia* becomes a cardinal feature in the second half of the first year of life after neuropathic signs emerge during the first month or two. It is an autosomal recessive hereditary disorder occurring primarily in Jewish children derived from a deficiency of Hexosaminadase. This leads to an intraneural accumulation of GM$_2$-ganglioside, which is increased throughout the grey matter, with myelin loss and gliosis in cerebral white matter. The *hypersensitive acousticomotor reaction* to sounds - and sometimes to light flashes and tactile stimuli - is the first sign of functional derangement of neurones in the very first weeks of life.

Psychomotor deterioration becomes manifest after 4 to 6 months, with inability to sit up soon obvious. Loss of both projected and purposeful movements follows, and *after several months*, the axial hypotonia is marked, but combined with pyramidal signs and *spasticity* of the limbs, and even opisthotonic reactions. Visual failure is first expressed in pendular nystagmus as early as the fourth month, at which point the macular cherry-red spot may already be identifiable, with blindness inescapable by the end of the first year.

## Sandhoff's Disease (GM$_2$-Gangliosidosis, type 2)

Closely related to Tay-Sachs, it is also characterized by an increased concentration of GM$_2$-ganglioside in the nervous system. It differs in that there is a deficiency of both Hexosaminodase A and B in all cells, but is otherwise identical in its age of onset, and in both neurologic and ophthalmologic manifestations.

## Congenital Amaurotic Idiocy (Hagberg et al., 1965)

A severe neurological syndrome present at birth and in the neonatal period, is associated from the outset with *hypotonia*. Its microcephaly is associated with hydrocephalus, and the optic atrophy is attended by almost complete absence of retinal vessels.

The existence of prenatal pathology has been a feature of several lipidoses such as Tay-Sachs, Niemann Pick Disease, GM$_1$-gangliosidosis and Krabbe's leukodystrophy.

386

# Early Infantile GM₁-Gangliosidosis (type 1)

*Hypotonia* and *hypoactivity* are also expressed in feeding difficulties and poor sucking in the first weeks of life. Underlying this is an already prenatal accumulation of both a neuro-visceral GM1-ganglioside and keratin sulphate-like mucopolysaccharide, due to deficiency or defect of lysosomal GM₁-ganglioside

β-galactosidase. The facial dysmorphism and oedema is very characteristic, alongside psychomotor deterioration, macular cherry-red spots and hepatomegaly. As the months pass, head control is achieved but the child fails to sit up without support, or to crawl. *The hypotonia gives way to spasticity* with hyperreflexia and tonic spasms.

# Infantile Niemann-Pick Disease

Neurovisceral accumulation of sphingomyelin attributable to *deficit of sphingomyelinase* lead to feeding difficulties and failure to thrive from the first weeks of life. Hepatomegaly may already be identifiable in the neonate, if not during the first three months, when hepatospleno-megaly will be clearly established. Progressive cerebral deterioration may already manifest by 6 months. Neurodevelopmental regression may be

clear, even before head control is achieved, and neurogenic impairment of swallowing accentuates the feeding difficulties. A combination of *axial hypotonia and bilateral pyramidal signs* is prominent, but as the disorder progresses, there is increasing opisthotonus and rigidity.

Helpful in more specific diagnosis is the finding of sea-blue histiocytes and foam cells in the marrow.

# Infantile Neuronic Ceroid Lipofuscidosis or Polyunsaturated Fatty Acid Lipidosis

In this group of lysosomal storage diseases, the defective enzyme has not yet been identified. The earlier the onset the more destructive is the effect upon the brain, and the more conspicuous the visual failure and seizures with oncoming *hypotonia* and *ataxia*, etc., *leading to ultimare spasticity*. In these original cases, primarily of Finnish origin, ataxia of limbs and trunk, of a cerebellar character, is attended between 2 and 4 years by generalized hypotonia during the first half of the second year of

life. *Not unlike the hypotonia of the cerebral palsies, particularly* in the *ataxic* form, *hyperreflexia* is associated. Myoclonic jerks are also a constant feature. The cerebral cellular accumulation of complex molecules with characteristics of both ceroid and lipofuscin leads to widespread and rapidly developing destruction of neurones especially cortical astrocytes, as well as of glial cells and macrophages. The encephalopathy is reflected in cortical atrophy. Arrest of brain growth follows so that microcephaly becomes evident by the second year, with the head circumference never exceeding 45-47 cm. This is paralleled by mental and developmental deterioration, which may already be reflected in apathy and mental dullness by eight months, and later by retinal degeneration with hypopigmentation and visual failure reflecting optic atrophy. Whilst the Tau fraction in the CSF progressively falls, arachidonic acid is increased in both serum and cerebral tissue, where an abnormal pattern of phosphoglycerides prevails. Conjunctional biopsy and ultrastructural analyses of myenteric neurones can help identify the underlying ceroid lipofuscinosis by the third year. *Spasticity* and hyperreflexia with intermittent tonic spasms ultimately predominate.

Complete loss of contact with the surroundings simulates autism, and a gestural stereotype of knitting movements is characteristic.

Neuroxonal dystrophy is a related disorder to be considered later in childhood when symptoms begin with difficulty in walking.

## Lowe's Syndrome (Oculo cerebro renal syndrome)

This is an hereditary disorder of unknown aetiology affecting males. It comprises three principal areas of pathology. It is only after the age of 6 months that the sensori-motor retardation becomes obvious. *Generalized hypotonia* is marked, accompanied by exaggerated passive mobilisation of joints and absent or depressed deep tendon reflexes. The ocular expression is mainly of bilateral cataracts and glaucoma linked often to megalocornea and buphthalmus. Corneal opacities appear later, and amblyopia accounts for the random oscillatory movements of the eyes. Slow movements of the hyperextended fingers to rub and press on the eyes, is sometimes attended by a characteristically high-pitched cry. This feature is central to the unusual facial pattern which has already become conspicuous by the second half of the first year of life: frontal prominence, sunken eyes, buphthalmos because of increased tension, and possibly retrognathism. The striking skin pallor is accentuated by the anaemia, and the long bones exhibit diffuse demineralization and the deformity of typical rachitic metaphyseal swelling. The renal lesion becomes evident after a few months or years comprising renal tubular acidosis, with decreased ammonia production or defect in bicarbonate reabsorption, proteinuria and hyperaminoaciduria.

## 3-Hydroxy-3 Methylglutaric Aciduria

A disorder of leucine metabolism (Przyrembel et al., 1976) presenting with recurrent or persistent neonatal infantile hypoglycaemia and metabolic acidosis in a clinical pattern punctuated by *hypertonic extensor spasms* resembling that of Reye's syndrome. There is no ketonuria during the acute illness which may serve to distinguish it from other organic acidurias such as propionic acidaemia or methylmalonic acidaemia. Diarrhoea and vomiting may usher in an episode marked by dehydration, somnolence to pallor, cyanosis and apnoea, culminating in stupor to coma. *Initial hypotonia or floppiness* is striking, with *concomitant dyspnoea* and *hypothermia*, later interrupted by the hypertonic extensor spasms. As in Reye's syndrome, these may be related to an intense hyperammonaemia, again frequently associated with a specific disorder of organic acid metabolism. Plasma ammonia concentrations of 388 and 500 $\mu$M/L have been recorded (Leonard et al., 1979), and even a level as high as 1370 $\mu$M/L has been documented in a recent case. *An increased intake of leucine can precipitate the attack*. Glutaric and acipic acids have been identified in the urine, with increased lactic acid in serum. The defect of activity of 3-hydroxy-3-methylglutaryl CoA lyase was demonstrable (Gibson et al., 1982) in cultured fibroblasts, leucocytes and liver.

Exchange transfusion or peritoneal dialysis may serve to overcome the critical hyperammonaemia, with the exploitation of sodium benzoate as supplementary. Less severe episodes of hypoglycaemia and acidosis should respond to parenteral glucose, fluid and electrolytes. A high carbohydrate diet and supplementation with glucose polymers could help but avoidance of long fasts and frequent feedings cannot avert the hypoglycaemia. Restriction of protein intake and especially of leucine is indicated.

## Multiple AcylCoA Dehydrogenase Deficiency (MADD) or Glutaric Aciduria Type II

Presentation has been in the neonatal period, so far only in males, with life-threatening illness. Tachypnoea was already striking at two hours of age in one such infant, rapid development of persistent metabolic acidosis ensuing in spite of parenteral fluid therapy and bicarbonate. An acrid odour of "sweaty feet" was characteristic. Non-ketotic hypoglycaemic convulsions are usual and a considerable degree of hyperammonaemia consistent. Since the acidosis arises only during occasional incidents of encephalopathy with vomiting and ketosis, organic acids are infrequently examined and the diagnosis is missed.

There is underlying fatty infiltration of the liver, renal tubules and myocardium. There is also cystic disease of the kidneys (as also characterizes the Zellweger syndrome, the prototype of peroxisomal disorder). Dysmorphic features are relatively specific including low-set malrotated ears, semilunar folds beneath the eyes, disproportionately large head with widely spread cranial sutures and anterior fontanelle (head circumference 75 percentile), high forehead, depressed nasal bridge and short anteverted nose and long philtrum. A Potter-like facies, as well as anomalies of abdominal wall and genitalia have also been described. The hands are short and broad, with bilateral Simian creases.

*Hypotonia is generalized*, and in addition extremities are *hypermobile* because of joint laxity. Bilateral hip clicks and patellar dislocation were also noted in one case. Pallor may become conspicuous, and macrocytic anaemia with an haemoglobin concentration of 9.1 g/dl was identified in one of the infants studied by Nyhan and Sakath (1987).

Biochemically, it is marked by the accumulation and excretion of compounds derived from the substrates of flavoprotein dehydrogenase that transfer the electrons to ETF. The most prominent organic acid elevation in plasma and urine was of lactic acid, glutaric acid and 3-hydroxy glutaric and occasionally glutaconic acids. But many other decarboxylic and hydroxyacids can be found, including ethylmalonic, butyric, methylbutyric, isobutyric and isovaleric acids. Most of these are also elevated in the plasma. Of significant relationship to the coexisting hyperammon-aemia, the levels in plasma and urine of citrulline, lysine, ornithine and proline are also raised, and that of arginine is particularly high. Its neuropathology is marked by *loss of neurones in the putamen* and lateral aspect of the caudate nucleus (Leibel et al., 1980).

That the above disorder can be differentiated from the neurodegenerative condition defined as *glutaric aciduria Type I*, has been shown by Goodman et al. (1975) in infants showing both glutaric acidaemia and glutaric aciduria.

The basic defect is an inherited deficiency of glutaryl-CoA dehydrogenase which oxidises and decarboxylates glutaryl CoA to crotonyl-CoA. Diagnosis has already been established in utero by both the high level of amniotic glutaric acid enzyme assay on cultured amniotic cells.

With more recent refinement of technique it has been possible to define specific deficiency in ETF dehydrogenase in three infant examples of this disorder, also showing congenital anomalies. Two infants without such anomalies proved to be solely deficient in ETF. It appears that both clinical types are inherited as autosomal recessive traits.

The neonatal diagnosis is usually confirmed by the characteristic organic aciduria, alongside non-ketotic hypo-glycaemia, acidosis and the odour of sweaty feet. Many of the accompanying excreted compounds such as ethylmalonic acid, glutaric acid, isovalerylglycine and sarcosine are clearly related to the substrates of flavoprotein/dehydrogenases. The functional deficiency of fatty acyl-CoA dehydrogenase in MADD indicates that the B-oxidation process generally is extra-mitochondrial and possibly peroxisomal.

The rapid termination of life is attributed to the cardiomyopathy that may stem from an impaired supply of glucose and ketone bodies to a tissue which cannot oxidise long chain fatty acids, its normal substrates. Since there is urinary loss of large amounts of ocylcarnitine esters, secondary carnitine deficiency may also be a pathogenic factor which could be readily overcome by carnitine supplementation. If the accumulation of compounds like glutaric and 3-hydroxyvaleric acids is strongly pathogenic, the administration of an artificial electron acceptor like methylene blue has been suggested (Goodman, Lenick and Frerman, 1985), especially when the presentation is later in life.

# 3-Methyl Glutaconic Aciduria

This is caused by deficiency of 3-methylglutaconyl CoA hydratase (Narasawa et al., 1986). Presentation is in older children so that retardation of speech development was disproportionately conspicuous in the first two examples. This had however been preceded by delay in motor development, with walking first attained at the age of 2 years. Long fasting - for 18 hours - induced hypoglycaemia and mild metabolic acidosis. The urine showed high excretion of 3-methylglutaconic acid, 3-methylglutaric acid and 3-hydroxy isovaleric acid.

Once protein-containing foods have been introduced, lethargy develops, attended by anorexia and failure to feed or suck, followed by progression to stupor and coma. Vomiting is not prominent. The infant becomes *flaccid and hypotonic* as well as completely unresponsive to stimuli, with apnoea ultimately necessitating artifical ventilation.

Another group of children with 3-methylglutaconic aciduria followed a distinctively different course. After ostensibly normal development for some months, progressive neurological deterioration follows. *Hypotonia* with bizarre posturing of one arm was described in one case, apart from self-mutilative behaviour. Two such affected siblings developed *spastic paraparesis and choreo-athetosis* as well as optic atrophy and neurogenic impairment of hearing. Another two unrelated infants were soon victims of "failure to thrive". Indeed after three to four months of normal development, psychomotor regression followed, again alongside marked hypotonia, spastic paraparesis and optic atrophy (Hagberg et al., 1983). A specific defect or deficiency of 3-methylglutaconyl CoA hydratase was not identified in these infants.

# 3-Ketothiolase Deficiency

This is also reflected in recurrent acute episodes of vomiting and lethargy with underlying ketosis and acidosis due to deficiency of 2-methylaceto acetic acid 3-ketothiolase. Typifying the classic presentation of the organic acidaemias, these are recurrent episodes of acute illness embodying massive ketosis and acidosis, which are ushered in by vomiting, with lethargy and hyperventilation leading on to dehydration and coma. Neutropenia and thrombocytopenia may already present at three months, or possibly earlier. Early development is slow, but head control was sustained well by 7 months, and sitting unsupported by 13 months. Walking could be attained by 2½ years.

The specific organic aciduria is diagnostic, 2-methyl-3-hydroxykutyric and 2-methyl acetoacetic being the key metabolites. The molecular defect is in the mitochondrial short-chain length-specific thiolase, 2-methyl acetoacetyl CoA thiolase.

Restriction of the intake of isoleucine is considered prudent in the management of the child subject of this disorder.

Victims of propionic acidaemia are distinguishable by the excretion of hydroxypropionic acid and methylcitric acid. But it may be necessary to give a load of 100 mg/kg isoleucine in the absence of ketosis in order to clarify the organic aciduria. Tiglylglycine is another metabolite of isoleucine that may be found in urine; butanone and 2-methylglutaconic acid may also be present.

A method permitting the analysis of 2-methyl-3-hydroxybutyric acid in amniotic fluid should be helpful in rapid *prenatal diagnosis* and possible prevention.

## Dihydrolipoyl Dehydrogenase Deficiency

This defect was first suggested in three siblings of an American Indian family (Haworth et al., 1976) whose chronic metabolic acidosis was associated with mental retardation together with seizures and neurological manifestations. Another example exhibited *intervals of hypotonia* alternating with hyper-irritability and hypertonia from the age of 8 weeks. Subnormal blood glucose was noted on occasion. Plasma concentration of alanine and glutamate which may be produced by transamination of pyruvate or α-ketoglutarate were consistently raised.

Subsequent biochemical findings were highly suggestive of a lesion involving some aspect of oxidative decarboxylation common to several substrates.

Enzyme studies unequivocally established a deficiency of E3. E1 and E2 of the PDH complex are different proteins from those of the KGDH complex. That of E1 of the KGDH complex does not catalyse decarboxylation of pyruvate (Koike et al., 1974). The same E3 component is also shown by the branched-chain α ketoacid dehydrogenase(s). Deficient activity of this complex has been elucidated in several forms of Maple Syrup Urine Disease wherever the three branched-chain amino acids, leucine, valine and isoleucine, and their α-keto analogues accumulate. The above condition might therefore be regarded as a new variant of "Maple Syrup Urine" disease.

The studies of Blass et al. (1976) led to the thesis that decreased activity of E3 or *dihydrolipoxl* dehydrogenase constitutes the underlying mechanism in Friedreich's ataxia.

## ∝-Thalassaemia: X-linked Mental Retardation Syndrome

Four forms of ∝-thalassaemia occur corresponding to deletions of one, two, three or all four of the ∝-globin genes present in normal individuals. Deletion of all the ∝-globin genes accompanied by a total absence of ∝-chain synthesis produces the most severe form of ∝-thalassaemia. Severe hypoxia and hydrops, or massive generalized oedema, are already evident in the neonate.

Deletion of three of the four ∝-globin genes is associated with a thalassaemia intermediate-like syndrome, Hb H disease. The microcytic anaemia is accompanied by abnormal red cell morphology with prominent intracellular inclusions following supravital staining. Haemoglobin H is highly unstable and identifiable by electrophoresis. These and other ∝-thalassaemia syndromes are found in specific population groups. In African-Americans ∝-thalassaemia genes are prevalent with most individuals revealing a deletion arrangement (-,∝) that produces a single ∝-locus chromosome. Chromosomes with deletions of both the ∝-loci (-,-) prevail in both Mediterranean and Asian populations, so that Hb H disease occurs in both groups.

*Persisting hypotonia* is to be found in a relatively specific X-linked form associated with severe mental retardation and a characteristic flat mid-facies, depressed nasal bridge and open mouth, reminiscent of hypothyroidism, also linked to scoliosis and marked club foot. An X-linked gene interfering with the ∝-globin locus is presumed.

## Metachromatic Leukodystrophy

The late infantile form is the variant most likely to be encountered in the age period relevant to this context. In the new category introduced as an example of Torsion Dystonia by Russell and Yatziv (1985), it was on the basis of a differing permutation of arylsulphatase defects, principally of arylsulphatase A with approximately 50% deficiencies of iso enzymes B and C. As another *progressive* expression of dystonia, the differentiation from choreo-athetoid CP would depend solely upon its pathognomonic movement disorder, primarily an intention dystonia. In the infantile form presenting at about 18 to 24 months of age, neuromuscular development is profoundly delayed in the presence of generalized *hypotonia*. There is also progressive loss of the limited speech achieved, and ataxia emerges to ultimately end in spastic tetraparesis. Within about 5 years, a rapid downhill course begins. Optic atrophy and blindness also become conspicuous in the juvenile entity of later onset.

Because of the underlying deficient activity of arylsulphatase A readily measured with p-nitrocatechol sulphate as substrate, there is accumulation of metachromatically staining sulphatide material in neuronal tissue, illustrated diagnostically by positive involvement of the sural nerve. On biopsy, failure of arylsulphatase cleavage has led to the Schwann cell accumulation of cerebroside sulphates, a process associated with progressive segmental demyelination. The deficient activity of the arylsulphatase A in cultured fibrblasts can be enhanced to normal levels by addition of the heat-stable protein activator.

# Mucolipidosis: Type IV

This rare affliction, combining cardinal clinical features of both the lipidoses and the mucopolysaccharides, has as yet emerged solely in Ashkenazi Jews. It was first diagnosed by me in London in 1966, my first three patients being Israeli children who presented as tetraparetic and retarded in wheelchairs. Attention was drawn to the cornea in the first child by the recurrent episodes of ophthalmic pain linked to headache and peripalpebral and fronto-temporal erythema on the left side. Although already 7 years of age, a clear history of psychomotor retardation dated back to his first year. Cloudiness of the cornea was then identified bilaterally, although it has already been found during the first year in other examples, including my fourth patient.

Diminishing muscle tone was also recognizable early in infancy, but a progressive hypertonicity appears later along with heightened deep tendon reflexes and bilateral Babinski. No retinal degeneration was definable although documented in other cases. Underlying developmental regression is the end course.

The intelligent Kibbutz father not unnaturally took pride in recognizing the identical condition associated with corneal opacity in two siblings of another Israeli family a week later. Corneal biopsies (Dr Keith) revealed unequivocal mucopoly-saccharide deposit. Bone marrow histiocytes were also found to contain Sudanophilic PAS-positive bodies showing weak metachromasia in toluidine blue, and lipid-like inclusions and clear vacuoles were exposed in the whole cellular range. Similar grossly abnormal storage bodies also characterized cerebral cells as well as cells of liver, conjunctivae and fibroblasts. The skin fibroblasts, in particular, demonstrated typical lamellated and multivesicular membrane bodies. A partial deficiency of ganglioside sialidase activity has been suggested, but a primary role has not yet been confirmed.

These three children were first presented together at the Hadassah Medical Centre in Jerusalem, in the course of a symposium on "The Cornea as a Mirror of Metabolism". My fourth case next appeared in my ward as an *hypotonic* developmentally retarded infant with poor vision soon ascribed to the conspicuous bilateral corneal opacities. After confirmation of the clinic diagnosis, and subsequent corneal biopsy (Dr Marin), this infant was reported by Berman and Shapiro, and a prenatal diagnostic technique by electronmicroscopic identification in cultured amniotic cells was evolved with the help of teratological colleague, Asher Ornoy.

# PEROXISOMAL DISORDERS

*Plasmalogens* are particularly important in myelin membranes and if there is failure of their synthesis in peroxisomes, the sequel is *hypo-myelination.*

An *excess of pipecolic acid*, believed to be a principal product of lysine in the brain, is also typical of these important defects of peroxisomal biogenesis. *That it competes for the receptor of GABA* within such a lysine-pipecolic pathway has been indicated by the work of Takahama et al. (1982), suggesting furthermore that it is possibly one element of a major pathway competing with GABA.

A striking corollary of this, as shown in the experimental animal, is that injection of pipecolic acid itself can induce profound *hypotonia,* such as has also been a consistent presenting feature of these peroxisomal disorders.

## Glycogenesis Type II (Pompe's Disease)

This form of glycogen storage disease is due to a deficiency of 1,4-glucosidase (acid maltase) first clinically manifest in the early months of life. It is the only one in which there is considerable anatomic "storage" of glycogen within the central nervous system. This brings about *profound hypotonia with depressed deep tendon reflexes* presenting in the first months of life. Glycogen accumulation also permeates skeletal muscle and heart so that there is also progressive muscular weakness with an EMG myopathic pattern, and an expressionless face from which the enlarged and glycogen-engorged tongue protrudes. The resultant cardiomegaly is also progressive so that cardiac failure brings life to a close by the end of the first or in the second year of life. Vacuolated lymphocytes in blood and oligosaccharides in urine associated with the specific enzyme in lucocytes or more reliably in cultured skin fibroblasts will complete the diagnosis. Prenatal diagnosis also offers the preventive possibility of elective termination of an affected foetus.

## Zellweger's Disease
### (Cerebro-hepato-renal transport defect)

Although typically lethal within a few months, the *profound hypotonia*, with sucking and swallowing difficulties necessitates tube feeding from the outset. The absence of motor progress and of deep tendon reflexes, still initially challenge a differential diagnosis from atonic cerebral palsy. The total lack of progress in mental and motor development during earliest infancy sharpens the distinction.

This widespread disorder appears to stem from a defect in a peroxisomal biosynthetic pathway, marked primarily by an absence of morphologically distinct peroxisomes in the liver and elsewhere. It includes both *malformations* and *"degenerative processes" in different organ systems*, making up an unique combination of facial dysmorphism, profound muscle hypotonia and weakness, associated with widespread anomalies in tissue organization. Categorized broadly, these can include renal cortical cysts and heterotopic grey matter in the brain as well as regressive changes such as liver fibrosis, cerebral white matter degeneration and chorio retinopathy. It also involves *the eyes*, in terms of visual fixation, cataracts, corneal opacities, glaucoma and rudimentary optic nerves with absent pupillary light responses and poor following. Later, say at 2.5 years, optic atrophy can be clearly identified, with clumping of pigment throughout the retina. The electroretinogram is extinguished. The *liver* is predominantly affected with fibrosis/cirrhosis and dysfunction reflected in significant hepatomegaly. *Cranio-facial growth* shows dysmorphic development attending the microcephaly: a high forehead, upraised metopic suture, shallow supraorbital ridges, hypertelorism, epicanthal folds, abnormal helices of low-set posterior angulated ears with hypoplastic lobule, a highly arched palate and hypoplastic mid-face. Patellar calcification is a peculiarly characteristic stigma.

*Of laboratory findings*, the raised blood levels of bile acid intermediate e.g. 185$\mu$mol/l (n< 17 $\mu$mol/l) and elevated concentration in serum, urine and CSF of pipecolic acid, a metabolite of lysine, have been the most consistent, current evidence pointing to an important role of peroxisomes in the metabolism of pipecolic acid, of bile acids and synthesis of plasmalogens. A defect in mitochondrial metabolism, and especially in the first phase of the oxidative respiratory pathway, has been identified in muscle, liver and also in cerebral mitochondria. *In fibroblasts* were found an accumulation of very long chain fatty acids and decreased activity of acyl CoA, dihydroxyacetone phosphate acyl transferase. The resultant neuropathology reveals abnormalities in cerebral *cortex, cerebellum and inferior olives secondary to interruptions of neuronal migration.* The white matter lesions also demonstrate astrocytic hyperplasia. Whatever the primary genetic metabolic defect may prove to be, it profoundly interferes with prenatal cerebral development.

But the combination of liver fibrosis, chorio retinopathy or optic nerve dysplasia and diffuse encephalopathy is shared by at least three other disorders outlined in this context *because of their association* with hypotonia: Hyperpipecolic acidaemia, neonatal adrenoleukodystrophy and infantile Refsum. New evidence has even suggested that these three disorders represent milder variants of the Zellweger syndrome.

## Mevalonic Aciduria

*Failure to thrive* is apparently secondary to poor feeding and is accompanied by developmental delay and retardation of growth. So that by 19 months of age in one child, height, weight and head circumference were all 4 to 8 standard deviations below the mean for age. There was virtually no subcutaneous fat. Despite the microcephaly, closure of both fontanelle and sutures was delayed. Central cataracts were already recognizable at 2 months of age.

*Hypotonia* and muscle weakness are persistent but in association with *increased deep tendon reflexes.* Extension was also found to be incomplete at both elbows and knees. Underlying the hypotonia and developmental delay, there is evidence of *cerebral atrophy* and diffuse slowing of the EEG.

Dysmorphic features included dolichocephaly, a high prominent forehead, low-set receding ears, a small mouth and jaw and long philtrum with thin lips and mild hypognathia. The conspicuous anaemia was sufficiently severe to necessitate several blood transfusions. There was also significant hepatosplenomegaly.

On organic analysis of the urine, an abnormally high peak of mevalonic acid was identified, and the trimethylsilyl (TMS) derivative yielded a huge peak on gas chromatography. Mevalonic acid is regarded as occupying a central place in intermediary metabolism with sources in leucine, a precursor of HMG CoA (3-hydroxy-3-methylglutaryl CoA) which plays a key role in ketogenesis, i.e. in the formation of aceto acetic acid as a direct product of fatty acid oxidation.

It has an important function in many vital metabolic processes. It is, for instance, a precursor in the biosynthesis of cholesterol and yet serum cholesterol levels remained low (1.8 mmol/L). It is also a precursor of other sterols, as well as of nonsterol isoprenes participating *in membrane formation*, the glyosylaton of proteins, the respiratory chain and the replication of DNA.

The molecular defect is in the enzyme *mevalonate kinase*, the activity of which was 1 to 2 $\mu$mol/min/mg protein, levels intermediate between patient and control being assayed in lymphocytes from both father and mother.

*During gestation, at 17 weeks, the mother's* urine already showed an *abnormal peak of 8.7 $\mu$mol/mol creatinine of mevalonic acid.* High levels in amniotic fluid in a subsequent pregnancy reached 408 uM/L which could afford reliable prenatal diagnosis.

*CT scanning* defined a moderately *widened ventricular system* especially of the *fourth ventricle,* underlying cerebral atrophy.

# INITIAL HYPOTONIA FOLLOWED BY
# CHOREO-ATHETOSIS

## Purine Disorders

Neurological disturbances are cardinal to two X-linked purine disorders transmitted as autosomal dominants to male children as outlined below. Firstly, the Lesch-Nyhan Syndrome, where complete HEPRT deficiency is associated with compulsive self-mutilation and *choreo-athetosis*, and secondly, PRPS superactivity. Where the defect is severe, *hypotonia* and *developmental retardation* are already evident in the first months of life. In addition to the subsequent inability to walk is the convergent strabismus and nerve deafness. In both disorders, there is uric acid overproduction, with raised plasma and urine uric acid levels.

Neuropathy akin to that in severe Lesch-Nyhan, *including spastic paresis*, also mark purine nucleoside phosphorylase (PNPI) deficiency, where paradoxically enough HGPRT - the enzyme in deficit in Lesch-Nyhan - cannot function without its PNP substrate.

It is of relevance that muscle weakness, rather than disorders of tone or movement, can have a specific metabolic basis. It characterizes deficiency of myo adenylate deaminase (M-AMPDA) an enzyme concerned with re-utilization of ATP degradation products of muscular work. These disorders are transmitted to males as a sex-linked autosomal dominant, or are inherited in an autosomal recessive manner.

### Lesch-Nyhan or Congenital Hyperuricaemia

In this X-linked disorder of purine metabolism, a defect of hypoxanthine guanine phosphoribosyl transferase (HRPTase) leads to *overproduction of uric acid*, and thence to an unique neurological syndrome: *athetosis* alongside developmental motor and mental retardation accompanied by the pathognomonically *compulsive oral self-mutilation*.

There may be *initial hypotonia* together with recurrent vomiting and the already *delayed motor development* of the first six months. The *involuntary movements appear after 12 months*, although *predominantly choreiform*, with facial grimacing, and *sometimes superadded athetosis*. Especially in severe examples, axial hypotonia is prominent by the end of the first year of life, although pyramidal signs with *spastic paresis and tonic spasms* supervene. Painful oral automutilation, produced biting of the lips, tongue and cheeks, appears between the ages of 2 and 4 years. Finger biting is another facet, their self-mutilatory preoccupation, which is also a co-feature of the Gilles de la Tourette syndrome with its compulsive tics, abusive foul language and myoclonic reactions.

The coexisting mental retardation is of variable degree, whilst speech remains limited with dysarthria usually severe.

*Classical spasticity* together with hyperreflexia, clonus and positive Babinski have emerged by the second or third year of life. Some of the children learn to walk by 3 to 5 years of age, others remain wheelchair-bound.

The hyperuricuria is often sufficient to give an orange colouration to the diapers. The hyperuricaemia is constant, the serum urate concentrations reaching 7 to 10 mg/100 ml. Assay of low HGPRTase in erythrocytes or cultured fibroblasts confirms the diagnosis.

Where deficiency of HGPRTase is partial, the neurological manifestations may be less striking and the automutilative behaviour even absent. Nevertheless, mild *athetosis, choreiform movements* or *spasticity* may remain prominent. In milder cases, medical recognition may finally depend upon renal failure, perhaps preceded by obstructive nephropathy, or even gouty arthritis.

A diminished increment of norepinephrine in plasma *on assuming a sitting position* attributed to the relative disuse from infancy in the Lesch-Nyhan subject of the sympathetic nervous system because of diminished or lack of demand for noradrenergic responsiveness to a standing posture. There was consequently a lessened need for synthesis of norepinephrine and its synthetic enzymes.

The deficit in passive avoidance learning characterizing Lesch-Nyhan children (Anderson et al., 1977) is in part overcome by intranasal administration of a long-lasting vasopressin analogue, a finding successfully extrapolated from experimental studies in the rat. Whilst a combination of 5HT and carbydopa was not convincingly effective in modifying behavioural disturbance in Lesch-Nyhan, it greatly reduced the self-mutilation and tics in the "Gilles de la Tourette" syndrome (Van Woct et al., 1977).

## Other Disorders of Purine Metabolism

### Phosphoribosylpyrophosphate (PRPS) Synthetase

Elevated intracellular concentrations of PRPP synthetase (even three times that of the normal enzyme) are characteristic and are associated with hyperuricaemia and urieosuria. Indeed the urine in infancy may be noted to be persistently pink. Intermittent crystalluria and haematuria from 8-16 months was conspicuous. Gouty arthritis and nephropathy may emerge later. Sensorineural deafness is paralleled by strabismus and general neurodevelopmental retardation expressed in delayed motor progress with head lag and retarded speech maturation. EEG reveals generalized slowing, with spindle activity reported over the right hemisphere. Early infantile hypertonicity was definable, but later at 2-3 years of age generalized hypotonia was present. Allopurinol is the treatment of choice in such overproduction of hyperuricaemia. PRPP synthetase has already been coded by a gene on the long arm of the X chromosome. In some families, the defect may be fully expressed in the heterozygous female, whilst in others it may appear fully recessive, possibly expressing different degrees of lyonization.

## Combined Xanthine oxidase/Sulphite oxidase (XOD/SO) Deficiency

Wherein uric acid is replaced in plasma and urine by xanthine and hypoxanthine. Neonatal seizures are an early manifestation. More serious expressions of SO deficiency include *ataxia* and *spastic paresis* as well as ocular lens subluxation such as also characterizes homocysteinuria, and a form of molybdenum co-factor deficiency in which *cystic degeneration of the cerebral cortices* is also represented.

**Defects of enzymes involved in re-utilization of ATP degradation** produces (a) AMPSL deficiency, associated with severe autistic features (produced during muscle work), and (b) myo-adenylate deaminase deficiency associated with muscle weakness.

# Mitochondrial Myopathy

Two main groups of such disorder are implicated.

## 1. Defects of Mitochondrial Oxidation

Where there have been recurrent subacute attacks of muscular 'weakness', especially if following physical stress, or if associated with nausea and vomiting, mitochondrial myopathy or primary and secondary forms of carnitine deficiency should be suspected. Repeated episodes of temporary paralysis would especially point to mitochondrial myopathy, provided that hypokalaemic, hyperkalaemic and normokalaemic forms of periodic paralysis have been excluded. Hypokalaemia of whatever cause such as chronic diarrhoea and vomiting, renal tubular acidosis, congenital alkalosis of gastro-intestinal source and galactosaemia may produce similar *episodes of hypotonia linked to areflexia* and muscular weakness.

Defects in the enzymatic steps of the complex process of complete mitochondrial oxidation of pyruvate or of fatty acids to $CO_2$ and $H_2O$, may be involved along with the parallel synthesis of ATP. Confirmation of a specific defect of a stage in mitochondrial oxidation requires accurate measurement of the activity of nine enzymes of mitochondrial fatty acid ß-oxidation in addition to the carnitine palmitoyl transferase and carnitine acyltranslocase steps needed for the oxidation of saturated fatty acid.

When fatty acids have been converted to acyl-CoA esters in the matrix of the mitochondria this may be either by:
(a) carnitine-dependent transfer through its inner membrane of the mitochondria (long-chain fatty acids); *or*
(b) by the acyl-CoA synthases of the matrix (short-chain fatty acids), which are normally ß-oxidized to acetyl-CoA by the ß-oxidation enzymes present in the matrix.

### Acyl-CoA Dehydrogenase Deficiency

Of the inborn errors at several steps in the pathway of fatty acid oxidation, the most common is medium chain acyl CoA dehydrogenase deficiency. This reflects a deficiency of one of the three different acyl-CoA dehydrogenases which have been identified with different and overlapping chain length specificities. It is in general a relatively common entity, occurring in 1:6500 of the population, thus equalling the prevalence of PKU. It has already been incriminated in sudden infant deaths, or in early infantile hypoglycaemic episodes. It is vital to inhibit mobilisation of fatty acids especially in the long chain disorders. Additional therapy with the sometimes rapid metabolic carnitine is also employed here to help in reversing decompensation in such disorders of medium chain fatty acids, and the otherwise inevitable encephalopathy. In one female example at 4 years of age manifesting persistent anorexia, *generalized hypotonia* was associated with progressive skeletal myopathy and marked muscle weakness. *Arreflexia* was also striking and the combination of mild equinovarus with contractures can wrongly suggest an underlying cerebral palsy.

### Enoyl CoA-hydratases (Erotonases)

A deficiency of one of two known erotonases has been associated with a female infant of 5 months who presented with marked *floppiness due to profound muscle weakness* rather than hypotonia. Muscle biopsy revealed massive lipid droplets. This short chain erotonase also reacts with branched-chain enoyl-CoA esters, indicating that the enzyme is active in the breakdown of branched-chain amino acids and other compounds.

### 2. Defects of Mitochondrial Respiratory Chain Complexes

The cytochromes of these have iron-porphyrin prosthetic groups which undergo oxidation and reduction by release and uptake of electrons. These will be included subsequently in this chapter amongst disorders presenting clinically with *ataxia*. Weakness and exercise intolerance are also frequent symptoms as well as ophthalmoplegia and myoclonic epilepsy.

Abnormal muscle biopsies may expose "ragged red" fibres on light microscopy, and bizarre mitochondria on electron microscopy. Either increased in size or number, proliferation of the inter-mitochondrial membrane with tightly packed or whorled crystal, paracrystalline arrays and osmophilic, lipid or glycogen inclusions.

## Infantile Refsum (Phytanic acid storage disease)

Although it does not fully manifest in cerebellar ataxia superimposed upon sensory ataxia and weakness until well into the first and second decade of life, the symptoms of this autosomal recessive polyneuropathy, especially of *weakness and hypotonia, may exist from birth, and emerge* *before 10 years in one third*. Its constituent pigmentary tapeto-retinal degeneration may also be identifiable from infancy, and consequent *night blindness* is often its first sign. One witnesses a slowly evolving sensorimotor distal atrophic *areflexic* syndrome with frequent remissions.

Associated disorders include cataract, sensorineural deafness, and ichthyosis or rough scaly thickening over extremities, especially palms and soles, and sometimes on the trunk.

The tissue accumulation, and urinary excess of *phytanic acid* is derived from ingested exogenous plant sources containing the chlorophyl molecule, this disorder being attributed to a defect in the first step of catabolism, i.e. the alpha-oxidation of the terminal carboxyl group *due to deficiency of phytanic acid* α-*hydroxylase*. Diagnosis may be based on fatty acid quantitation in serum by gas chromatography: only trace amounts of phytanic acid are found normally whereas it may reach 30% in Refsum.

Schwann cells show characteristic onion-bulb formations and other inclusions. Hepatocytes show lipid inclusions in cultured fibroblasts. The failure of phytanic oxidation can be demonstrated. Bile acid intermediates are found in increased concentration. The CSF protein is increased, which is also an almost constant feature of metachromatic leukodystrophy, Austin's mucosulfatidosis and globoid body leuko-encephalopathy.

*Extreme slowing of motor conduction* reflects the *basic peripheral neuropathy*. But after reduction of the serum phytanic acid level achieved by an appropriate diet lacking phytenate and calorically high, there is a lowering of serum and tissue level followed by a *significant improvement*. In the experience of Eldjarn et al. (1966), this is from the pre-treatment level of 7 m/s to 19 m/s one year later. The earlier this treatment begun, especially before significant demyelination, the more likely is "reversal" of the neuropathy.

# OTHER MISCELLANEOUS RARE METABOLIC ABNORMALITIES WITH CLINICAL EXPRESSION IN INITIAL HYPOTONIA AND OTHER DISORDERS OF MOVEMENT, POSTURE AND BALANCE

1. Increased levels of lysine and histidine in urine associated with an *hypotonic "floppy baby syndrome"* with presumptive myopathy and weak proximal muscles, together with weak suck, expressionless face, and congenital ophthalmoplegia.

2. *Lysinuric protein intolerance* where marked muscular *hypotonia* is associated with difficulties in feeding, episodic vomiting and chronic diarrhoea, linked to retardation of growth and mental development.

3. *Hyper ß-alaninaemia* in association with excessive urinary excretion of ß-alanine, ß-amino butyric acid and taurine. *Hypotonia together with hyporeflexia*, lethargic failure to thrive, and intermittent seizures.

## Aspartyl Glucosaminuria

Characterized by an accumulation of 2-acetamide-1(B-L-aspartamide)-1,2-dideoxy-B-Dglucose(AADG), it probably reflects a defect in the catabolism of glycoproteins due to deficiency of N-aspartyl-β-glucosaminase. There is insidiously gradual regression of mental function from early childhood. Speech development in particular remains poor or is never achieved. There is delay or initially severe behavioural upset with *alternating hyperactivity and apathy*. Deterioration of motor function remains mild, with *movements clumsy* and minor evidence of disorder in corticospinal tracts. Differentiation from non-progressive cerebral palsy states may therefore prove difficult except for subtle non-neurological signs. Their coarse facies would be comparable with that of Hurler, whilst even the hepatomegaly, abdominal herniation, and Hurler-like deformation of the thoraco-lumbar vertebrae, heighten the resemblance.

Levels of AADG are elevated in urine and CSF, whereas there is significantly decreased activity of N-aspartyl-β-glucosamindase in plasma and cultured fibroblasts (as well as in brain, liver and spleen).

## Menkes' Kinky Hair Syndrome

This is a progressive degenerative X-linked recessive disorder of the central nervous system leading to early death. A disturbance of copper homeostasis is involved. Severe deficiency in copper has been identified mainly because of inability to absorb copper from the gastro-intestinal tract, and a presumptive inability to use the available copper effectively as an enzyme co-factor. It exclusively affects males, and premature birth is common. Clinical onset is within the first three months of life, and is marked by neurodevelopmental arrest. Significant neonatal jaundice is typical, associated with slow feeding, poor weight gain and instability of body temperature. Drowsiness and lethargy insidiously worsen at 4 to 6 weeks. Early seizure activity is markedly myoclonic, and there is a gradual increase in *hypotonia* or *hypertonia*. Such *variability in tone*, and a *lack of spontaneous movements* become more conspicuous, whilst hypothermia persists. The failure of acquisition of smiling or its rapid loss marks an expressionless face. The characteristic facial appearance (Danks et al., 1974) also includes pallid "pudgy" or dry thickened skin, puffed out cheeks, and a cupids' bow upper lip.

The clinical hallmark is the appearance of the tangled horizontal eyebrows and sparseness of scalp hair, the hair shafts being relatively depigmented and wiry. Secondary growth of hair is lacking in lustre and is relatively depigmented. Hair strands break off easily leaving short stubbles, imparting a feel of "steely" hair. The characteristic twisting, or pili torti, is well illustrated microscopically. Spasticity in association with bilateral pyramidal signs eventually prevails.

There is conspicuous abnormality of the vascular system, with elongation and tortuosity of arteries. Wormian bone formation mark both posterior sagittal and lambdoidal sutures. Neurological deterioration is rapidly progressive culminating in death between 6 months and 3 years. Extensive neuronal degeneration, gliosis and optic degeneration underlie this pattern. Striking vascular pathology co-exists, marked by fragmentation and splitting of the internal elastic lamina, with intimal proliferation followed by narrowing and occlusion of the lumen.

Underlying the defect in the gastro-intestinal absorption of copper, a considerable increase in the copper content of the intestinal mucosa is evidently the result of a defect in its intracellular transport including that through the serosal antiluminal aspect of the cell membrane. Analogous impairment of placental transport or cortex has been suggested.

Diagnosis is supported by the following findings which may not appear until five weeks:

1. *Hair* - Washed out colour, with strands that fracture easily producing short or miniature follicles, pili torti, and monilethrix in a skull biopsy specimen. Looks and feels like kinky or steel hair in apt comparison with a pad of well-used steel wool.

2. *Serum* - Low copper (e.g. 19ug/100ml at 21 days) and reduced ceruloplasmin levels. Both rise rapidly in *normal* infants to reach near adult levels by age 1 month. Serial measurement would expose its failure to rise, a copper deficiency which can be alleviated by parenteral administration of copper.

3. Low *liver* copper content, e.g. 14 ug/g dry weight, requiring liver biopsy and assays of the low copper contrasting sharply with what is normally an eightfold increase in infantile over adult values.

## Spongy Degeneration of Nervous System White Matter: (Canavan-Van Bogaert-Bertrand Disease)

In this recessive autosomal hereditary disorder, a progressive degenerative disease mostly affecting infants of Jewish extraction and fair complexion, *early hypotonia* is the cardinal clinical feature already apparent between 2 and 6 months of age, and attended by lack of motility. Tonic spasms and seizures recur in the midst of rapid neurodevelopmental regression or absence of any advance, marked by early mental deterioration. There is gradual failure of head control, or it is lost during those first 2 to 6 months when lassitude and lethargy are early characteristics. Even earlier, difficulty in sucking soon accounts for failure to thrive. Seizures and decerebrate stiffness supervene. *The head undergoes rapid enlargement* (macrocephaly), usually reaching between two to four standard deviations above the norm, and blindness supervenes on the basis of optic atrophy somewhere between 8 and 18 months, and sometimes preceded by squint and pendular nystagmus.

The *early floppiness and flaccidity* gives way *to tonic extensor spasms with full pyramidal signs of hypertonicity*, exaggerated deep tendon reflexes and positive Babinski. This pattern is interrupted repeatedly by opisthotonus with legs extended and arms flexed. Both hands and feet often adopt postures and motion akin to choreoathetosis.

The neuropathology is unique with the brain showing considerable increase in weight, although myelin is absent especially in the convoluted white matter. A peculiar spongy vacuolization of this white matter replaces lower parts of the cerebral cortex and subcortical regions as well as the cerebellar cortex. Vesicular astrocytic nuclei are conspicuously enlarged to constitute Alzheimer Type II cells.

# Neurobiological Disorder:
# Peroxisomal Defect of Neuronal Migration

**Sudanophilic Leukodystrophy with Deficient Hepatocellular and Renal Tubular Peroxisomes (Zellweger's cerebro-hepato-renal syndrome)**

Cerebellar heterotopia and olivary dysplasia may also be associated with polymacrogyria and pachygyria. Defective synthesis of the plasmalogens in myelin membranes leads to hypomyelination. Defective genesis of peroxisomes is also the basis of neonatal adreno leukodystrophy, also leading to profound demyelination and ultimately to profound hypotonia and seizures. Renal peroxisomal deficiency in hepatocytes in Refsum's disease is expressed in cerebellar ataxia.

# Neurobiological Disorders of Uncertain or Unknown Aetiology

Three profound disorders of this source have to be considered in relation to *marked hypotonia*:

**Meckel-Gruber Syndrome** (Jones, 1988)

The microcephaly is grossly modified by the sloping forehead and dorsal encephalocele, the dysmorphic feature below including micropththalmus, slanting eyes, hypo- or hypertelorism as well as micrognathia and a high arched palate. The neck is short and both cardiac and renal defects may co-exist. Cerebral and cerebellar hypoplasia are the underlying defects.

**Cerebro-oculo-facio-skeletal (COFS) Syndrome** (also described by Jones, 1988)

Sometimes known as "neurogenic arthrogryposis", reduction in cerebral white matter being the underlying factor. Again *hypotonia is marked* and accompanied by hypo- or arreflexia, in part the result of severe flexural contractures. the microcephaly is linked to bilateral microphthalmia and cataracts, the ocular depression being accentuated by prominence of the root of the nose.

### Neu-Laxova Syndrome

Granulation is the site of defect. The result is marked hypotonia; like COFS, it is also associated with flexural contractions. Microcephaly and hypertelorism linked to microphthalmus (but with the eyes protruding without lids), a flattened nose, cleft lip, micrognathia, and both a short neck and short limbs.

This early neurobiological defect has been found in association with atrophy of cerebellum and pons, as well as absence of corpus callosum and olfactory bulbs.

# DISORDERS WITH CONSPICUOUS CARDINAL CLINICAL FEATURES OTHER THAN HYPOTONIA

Although hypotonicity is a frequent feature in the following syndromes and disorders, the associated history and clinical and morphological components are sufficiently conspicuous and pathognomic to almost immediately differentiate the condition from cerebral palsy.

*Achondroplasia* and its characteristic short-linked dwarfism is too dramatically distinctive to warrant differential diagnostic detail in respect of the associated initial hypotonia. Likewise the *Blepharophimosis* syndrome, with its specific ocular features, mainly short papebral fissure with lateral displacement of the inner canthi, and ptosis of eyelids and strabismus (Kohn and Romano, 1972).

## Coffin-Siris Syndrome (Coffin and Siris, 1970)

The significant or severe hypotonia is associated with mild microcephaly, with coarse facies, mental retardation, mild to moderate growth deficiency of prenatal onset, general hirsutism but often sparse scalp hairs, and hypoplastic to absent fifth finger, and toenails.

## Generalized Gangliosidosis Type I (Kaback et al., 1973)

Already touched upon in the text, it includes several features of the Hurler syndrome, including the coarse facies but of prenatal onset. There is severe early developmental failure, associated with hypotonia and incoordination, later producing spasticity.

# Miller-Dieker Syndrome (Lissencephaly Syndrome)

The incomplete brain development with smooth surface and heterotopias linked to severe mental deficiency with initial hypotonia and subsequent opisthotonus and tetraplegia has already been referred to in the text.

The distinctive craniofacial facies include the microcephaly, yet variably high forehead, with vertical soft tissue ridging and furrowing including that of the central forehead, and of the upper lip particularly conspicuous during crying. The nose is small and nares anteverted. Low-set ears show posterior angulation of the auricles.

The coarse facies include the broad nose with low nasal bridge and flaring alae nasi, frontal bossing, long philtrum and hypertrophied alveolar ridges linked to the prominent maxilla and slight macroglossia. In early infancy, these features may be obscured by facial and peripheral oedema. There is also a mild limitation of joint movement with especially thick wrists, "claw hand" and contractures of elbows and knees.

# X-Linked Hypophosphataemic or Vitamin D Resistant Rickets

This severe nutritional form of rickets is associated with significant hypotonia. Mild to moderate growth deficiency with diminished rate of new bone formation and associated bowing of lower limbs, waddling of gait and coxa vara. The radiological evidence of rickets is unresponsive to physiological amounts of vitamin D, but will respond to adequate dosage. There is underlying hypophosphataemia with reduced renal tubular reabsorption of phosphorus and calcium from the gastro-intestinal tract.

# Rieger Syndrome

The Rieger eye malformation embodying dysplasia of the iris, filling-in of the angle of the anterior chamber, occasionally in association with glaucoma, microcornea, corneal opacity, ectopia lentis and even optic atrophy. The mental deficiency and hypotonia may be linked with hypodontia and partial anodontia or coexist in other syndromes. Whilst the characteristic facies includes a broad nasal bridge with maxillary hypoplasia, a thin upper lip but everted lower lip.

## Stickler Syndrome or
## Hereditary Arthero Ophthalmopathy (Herrman et al., 1975)

*In these hypotonic children, the flat facies is distinctive.* It includes a depressed nasal bridge together with midfacial and mandibular hypoplasia. There are also clefts of hard and/or soft palate. Occasionally the uvula is also cleft, and the micrognathia simulates the Robin complex. Associated ocular anomalies comprise myopia, together with retinal detachment and/or cataracts.

This is another syndrome embodying hyperextensible joints adding to the cardinal muscular hypotonia. The prominent large joints may be conspicuous from birth, and the underlying arthropathy already recognizable in childhood. The hip subluxation so common in cerebral palsy is associated with spondyloepiphyseal dysplasia not seen in CP. In addition, the long bones have disproportionately narrow shafts.

## Thanatophoric Dysplasia Syndrome (Maroteux, 1967)

In describing this hypotonic condition often confused with achondroplasia, the Greek term thanatophoric (death-bringing) was used by Maroteux (1967) because of their inevitably tragic death shortly after birth.

Growth failure is associated with a large cranium and fontanelle which shows a short base of skull and small foramen magnum.

The nasal bridge is correspondingly low and the facies small. The extremities are conspicuously short and bowed with fingers also small and "sausage-like", and their metaphyses are cuffed, demonstrating spur-like irregular flaring. The vertebral bodies are short and flattened although the intervertebral disc spaces are relatively wide.

## William's Syndrome (Bennet, La Veck and Sells, 1979)

Mild growth deficiency is already prenatal, and average IQ rarely exceeds 56%. The unusually friendly, outgoing, loquacious personality with prominent protruding lips and hoarse voice is characteristic. In addition, the dysmorphology is distinctive, with flaring of medial eyebrows, short palpebral fissure and epicanthal folds. The nasal bridge is depressed and nares anteverted. There is

periorbital fullness of subcutaneous tissue. The iris shows stromal patterning, and bladder urography reveals diverticulae.

In the main, these features are associated with supravalvular aortic stenosis, and vascular stenoses elsewhere are classically combined in this syndrome: peripheral pulmonary artery, pulmonic valvular stenosis, etc. Ventricular and atrial septal defects also coexist. Hypercalcaemia has been infrequent, but the underlying aberration of calcium metabolism still requires determined study and explanation.

## Foetal Aminopterin Syndrome (Shaw and Steinbach, 1968)

Hypotonia is an occasional component of this multifocal malformation syndrome that can follow the abortifacient use of the folic acid antagonist, Aminopterin. This has been given between 4 and 10 weeks of gestation at a dosage level of 12-30 mg. Similar toxic effects may stem from the analogous use of methotrexate - the methyl derivative of Aminopterin.

Profound growth deficiency and microcephaly begins prenatally. All limbs are short, especially the forearms (mesomelia). The severe craniofacial malformation is made up of hypoplasia of frontal, parietal, temporal and occipital bones, and the fontanelles are wide. Synostosis of coronal or lambdoidal sutures coexists. The supraorbital ridges are shallow, the nasal bridge broad, the ears low set, maxillar hypoplastic as well as micrognathia. There is also talipes equinovaries and hypodactyly.

## Hyperthermia-induced Spectrum of Defects

Experimental studies in the guinea pig have in the past (Edwards, 1969) confirmed that elevation of maternal temperature of 1.5°C above normal tends to arrest growth of neuronal mitotic cells in the ependymal layer of the developing brain, whereas elevation of 3.0°C or more kills those cells. In the human, most of the relevant cases of maternal hyperthermia in studies which were entirely retrospective, have been tentatively related to febrile illness, with the patient's temperature reaching 38.9°C or higher. Its duration was several days.

Even sauna bathing of 30-45 minutes was involved in two cases. A tentative correlation has been found with 170 cases of neural tube defects (Smith and Jones, 1982).

Apart from significant facial defects including microphthalmia, interference with frontal lobe growth produced a small midface and deficit of movement leading to micrognathia. The major neuromuscular abberation was hypotonia, although about half the cases showed hyperactive reflexes (so-called "hypotonic diplegia").

## Fabry Syndrome (Wallace, 1973)

The CNS consequences of this X-linked syndrome of ceramide trihexosidase deficiency which normally degrades ceramide trihexoside may include spastic diplegia with typically initial hypotonia. Headache, hypotonia, vertigo and hemiplegia are more consistent manifestations. Mental deficiency and even optic atrophy are occasionally associated.

But the basic clinical features firstly include the attacks of burning pain in hands and feet which may begin in childhood which are precipitated by heat, cold, exercise or fever. The cutaneous expressions which are not often visible after 10 years of age are clusters of minute dark nodular angiectases around umbilicus, genitalia, knees and hips. Mucous membranes are also involved. Superficial corneal opacities are usual, mild opacities being also evident in the heterozygous female with ceramide trihexosidase levels intermediate between that of the affected normal male. There is also progressive renal insufficiency leading to proteinuria and variable red and white cells, and evolving to a fixed specific gravity of the urine.

## Shprintzen Syndrome (Velo-Cardio-Facial) (Shprintzen et al., 1981)

These children with short stature (usually below the 10th centile), share multi-focal features from conductive hearing loss secondary to cleft palate, with the cleft of the secondary palate either overt or submucous. Although the nose is prominent, the alar base is narrow as are the downslanting palpebral fissures, the malar areas hypoplastic, the mandible and chin retruded, with vertical maxillary excess and long Madiglioni face. There is a generalized muscular hypotonia with slender and hyperextensible limbs and fingers.

## Osteogenesis Imperfecta Syndrome Type I (McKusick, 1956)

This generalized disorder of connective tissue is encountered in four to six types. The commoner version includes the classically blue sclerae due to their thinness and translucency as well as of the skin. The thin fragile bones are subject to frequent fracturing partly as a result of which the limbs may appear unduly short in these children of already short stature.

Occasionally the calvarium is soft and thin and the fontanelles are wide and display wormian bones. There is also bulging of temporal and frontal regions, linked to platybasia.

In addition to the associated *overall muscular hypotonia*, this also constitutes another example of the type of hyperextensibility referred to in Chapter 4.

# Pena-Shokeir II Syndrome:
# COFS Syndrome: Centro-Oculo-Facial Skeletal
(Pena- Shokier, 1974)

In the majority, the phenotype is already recognizable at birth. The *generalized hypotonia* and hypo- or a-reflexia is associated with reduced cerebral white matter and grey mottling apparently derived from a degenerative disorder.

Microcephaly is associated, with ocular anomalies, blepharophimosis, microphthalmia, cataracts and nystagmus. The root of the nose is especially prominent, the pinnae of ears enlarged and the upper lip overlapping the lower lip.

## Langer-Giedion Syndrome (Hall, 1974)

There is multiple exostosis of the long bones and less often of ribs, scapulae and pelvis. *Hypotonia* is associated with *winged scapulae*. There is mild to moderate mental retardation but disproportionate delay in speech, and the microcephaly is linked to distinctive facies, with bulbous nose and thickened alae nasi and septum, large laterally protruding ears, prominent and elongated philtrum and thin upper lip with receding mandible. There is also redundancy and looseness of the skin in infancy which regresses with age. Cone-shaped epiphyses of the fingers become evident at about 3-4 years of age.

## Marfan Syndrome (McKusick, 1956)

The tendency towards a tall stature is associated with long lean limbs and fingers, joint laxity with kypho-scoliosis and pectus excavatum. Other pathognomic features especially include ocular anomalies: subluxation of the lens, usually upward, and occasionally retinal detachment, colobomata of the iris and secondary glaucoma. Apart from occasional thrombo-embolic vascular complications, cardiovascular anomalies include dilatation with or without dissecting aneurysms of the aorta, especially ascending, but also occasionally of thoracic and abdominal segments. Homocysteinuria may be associated.

# References

Ampola MG, Mahoney MJ, Nakamura E, Tanaka K. (1975) Prenatal therapy of a patient with Vitamin B12-responsive methylmalonic acidemia. New Engl J Med 293: 313-317

Anderson LT, Dancis J, Alpert M, Herrmann L. (1977) Punishment learning and self-mutilation in Lesch-Nyhan. Nature (London) 265: 461-463

AndreThomas AJ, Chesni Y, Dargassies SA. (1960) The neurological examination in the infant. Little Club Clin Dev Med 1. No. 1 (London) Medical Adviser Committee of National Spastics Committee

Bennett FC, La Veck B, Sells CJ. (1979) The Williams' elfin facies syndrome. Pediatrics 61: 303

Blass JP, Kark RAP, Menon NK. (1976) Low activities of the pyruvate and oxoglutarate dehydrogenase complexes in 5 patients with Freidreich's ataxia. New Engl J Med 295: 62-67

Breg WR et al. (1970) The cri-du-chat syndrome in adolescents and adults. J Pediatr 27: 782

Coffin GS, Siris E. (1970) Mental retardation with absent fifth fingernail and terminal phalanx. Am J Dis Child 119: 433

Danks DM, Cartwright E, Stevens BJ, Townley RRW (1972) Menkes' kinky hair disease: a further definition of the defect in copper transport. Science 179: 1140-1141

Donner M, Rapola J, Somer H. (1975) Congenital muscular dystrophy: a clinico-pathological and follow-up study of 15 patients. Neuropädiatrie 6: 239

Dubowitz V. (1985) Muscle Biopsy. A practical approach. 2nd Ed. Balliere Tindall, London

Dubowitz V, Davies K. (1991) Pontocerebellar hypoplasia. Neuromuscular Dis 1: 81

Edwards MJ. (1969) Congenital defects in guinea pigs. Prenatal retardation of brain growth of guinea pigs following hyperthermia during gestation. Teratology 2: 239

Eldjarn L et al. (1966) Dietary effects upon serum phytanic acid levels and clinical manifestations. Lancet 1: 691-693

Fenichel GM. (1983) Myasthenia gravis. In: Emery AEH, Rimoin DI (Eds) Principles and Practice of Medical Genetics. Churchill Livingstone, Edinburgh. Ch. 34

Gibson KM, Sweetman L, Nyhan WL, Page TM, Green C, Cann HM. (1982) 3-hydroxy-3 methyl glutaric aciduria. A new assay of 3-hydroxy-3 methylglutarye CoA lyase. Clin Chim Acta 126: 171

Gizelmann R, Steinmann B. (1978) Non-ketotic hyperglycinaemia treated with strychnine: a glycine receptor antagonist. Helv Paediat Acta 32: 517-525

Goodman SI et al. (1975) Glutaric aciduria. A "new" disorder of amino acid metabolism. Biochem Med 12: 12

Guthrie RD et al. (1971) The 4p-syndrome. Am J Dis Child 122: 421

Hagberg B, Hjalmarson O, Lindstedt S, Ransnas L, Steen G. (1983) 3-methylglutaconic aciduria in two infants. Clin Chim Acta 134: 59

Hagberg B, Hultquist G, Ohman R, Jvennerholm L. (1965) Congenital amaurotic idiocy. Acta Paediat Scand 54: 116-130

Hall BD et al. (1974) Langer-Giedion syndrome. Birth Defects 10: 147

Haworth JC, Perry TL, Blass JP, Hansen S, Urquhart N. (1976) Lactic acidosis in three siblings due to defects in both pyruvate dehydrogenase and α-ketoglutarate dehydrogenase complex. Pediatrics 58: 564-574

Herrman J, Opitz JM. (1974) Naming and nomenclature. Birth Defects 10(7): 69 (Hermann in text - page 18)

Herrman J et al. (1975) The Stickler syndrome of hereditary arthro ophthalmopathy. Birth Defects 11: 76

Hirschhorn K, Cooper HL, Firschein IL. (1965) Deletion of short arms of chromosomes 4-5 in a child with defects of midline fusion. Humangenetik 1: 479

Jones KL. (1988) Smith's recognizable patterns of human malformation. 4th Edn. Saunders, Philadelphia

Kaback MM et al. (1973) GM$_1$ gangliosidosis type I: In utero detection and fetal manifestations. J Pediat 82: 1037

Koike K, Hamada M, Tanaka N, Otsuka K, Ogashara K, Koike M. (1974) Properties and sabunit composition of the pig heart 2-oxoglutarate dehydrogenase. J Biol Chem 249: 3836-3842

Kondo K, Tsubaki T, Sakamoto F. (1970) The Ryukyuan muscular atrophy. J Neurol Sci 11: 359

Lecky BRF et al. (1986) Congenital myasthenia: Further evidence of disease heterogeneity. Muscle Nerve 9: 233-242

Lee FA. Isaacs H Jr, Strauss J. (1972) The "camptomelic" syndrome. Am J Dis Child 124: 485

Lejeune J et al. (1963) Trois cas de deletion partielle du bras court d'un chromosome 5. CR Acad Sci(D) Paris 257: 3098

Leonard JV, Seakins JWT, Griffin NK. (1979) ß-hydroxy-ß-methylglutaric aciduria presenting as Reye's syndrome. Lancet 1: 680

McKusick V. (1956) Hereditable Disorders of Connective Tissue. Mosby, St. Louis

Maroteux P, Lang M, Robert JM. (1967) Le nanisme thantophere. Presse Med 75: 2519

Maroteaux P et al. (1971) Le syndrome campomelique. Presse Med 79: 1157

Moosa A, Dubowitz V. (1970) Peripheral neuropathy in Cockayne syndrome. Arch Dis Child 45: 674

Narasawa K, Gibson KM, Sweetman L, Nyhan WL, Wadman SK. (1986) Deficiency of 3-methylglutaconyl-CoA hydrolase in two siblings. J Clin Invest 77: 1148

Nyhan WL, Sakath NO. (1987) Diagnosis and Recognition of Genetic Disease. Lea and Febiger, Philadelphia. p. 223

Pena SDJ, Shokier MHK. (1974) Autosomal recessive cerebro-oculo-facio-skeletal (COFS) syndrome. Clin Genet 5: 285

Platt M, Holmes LB. (1967) Hypertonia in older patients with the 5p-syndrome. Lancet 2: 1429

Poswillo D. (1966) Observations of fetal posture and causal mechanisms of congenital deformity of palate, mandible and limbs. J Dent Res 45: 584

Pruzanski W. (1966) Variants of myotonic dystrophy in pre-adolescent life (syndrome of myotonic dysembryoplasia). Brain 89: 563

Przyrembel H et al. (1976) Glutaric aciduria Type II. Clin Chim Acta 66: 227

Reynolds SE, Blass JP. (1970) A possible mechanism for selective cerebellar damage in partial pyruvate dehydrogenase deficiency. Neurology 26: 625-628

Robinson BH. (1983) Inborn errors of pyruvate metabolism. Biochem Soc Trans 11: 623-626

Rowe PB. (1983) Inherited disorders of folate metabolism. In: The Metabolic Basis of Inherited Disease, 5th Edition. JB Stanbury, JB Wyngaarden et al. (Eds). McGraw-Hill, New York. pp 498-521

Rowland LP. (1983) Molecular genetics, pseudogenetics and clinical neurology. Neurology 33: 1179-1195

Russell A, Levin B, Oberholzer VG. (1963) A form of infantile hypoaldosteronism. A reversible salt wasting syndrome of the newborn and infant. Arch Dis Child 38: 313-325

Russell A, Butler R, France N, Snodgrass (1967) The D(13-15) Trisomy syndrome: analysis of cerebral and facial correlationships in seven examples. Arch Dis Child 41: 250-261

Russell A, Levin B, Oberholzer VG. (1963) A form of infantile hypoaldosteronism. A reversible salt wasting syndrome of the newborn and infant. Arch Dis Child 38: 313-325

Russell A, Perlman M. (1992) Neonatal diagnosis of Riley-Day syndrome. Unpublished communication

Russell A, Shapiro Y. (1994) Fixed "open mouth" syndrome due to prenatal impact upon mandibular growth of congenital myasthenia gravis. Arch Dis Child: in press

Russell A, Statter M. (1982) Maple syrup disease: presentation in the neonate. Unpublished observation

Russell A, Yatziv S. (1985) A metabolic basis for idiopathic torsion dystonia: a new variant of metachromatic leukodystrophy. World Pediat Child Care 1: 25-29

Schinzel A et al. (1974) The 18p-syndrome. Arch Genetik 47: 1

Schinzel A. (1980) Trisomy 20pter-q11 in a malformed boy from a t(13:20) p11,q11 translocation carrier mother. Human Genet 53: 169

Shaw E, Steinbach HL. (1968) Aminopterin-induced fetal malformation. Am J Dis Child 115: 477

Shprintzen RJ et al. (1981) The velo-cardio-facial syndrome: a clinical and genetic analysis. Pediatr 67: 167

Smith DW, Jones KL. (1982) Recognizable Patterns of Human Malformation. Genetic, Embryologic and Clinical Aspects. W B Saunders & Co., Philadelphia and London. pp 430-431

Spiro AJ, Fogelson MH, Goldberg AC. (1967) Microcephaly and mental subnormality in chronic progressive spinal muscular atrophy of childhood. Dev Med Child Neurol 9: 594

Takahama K et al. (1982) A new type of $\alpha$-amino acid possessing bicuculline-sensitive action in the mammalian brain. Brain Res 239: 294-298

Trauner D, Page T, Greco C, Sweetman L, Kuloritch S, Nyhan WI. (1981) Progressive neurodegenerative disorder in a patient with non-ketotic hyperglycinemia. J Pediat 81: 272

Van Woct MH, Yip LC, Balis ME. (1977) Purine phosphoribosyl-transferase in Gilles de la Tourette syndrome. New Engl J Med 296: 210-212

Vincent A et al. (1981) Congenital myasthenia: End-plate acetylcholine receptors and electrophysiology. Muscle Nerve 4: 306-318

Wallace HG. (1973) Anderson-Fabry disease. Br J Dermatol 88: 1

Walton JN. (1956) Amyotonia congenita: a follow-up study. Lancet 1: 1023-1028

Walton JN. (1957) The limp child. J Neurol Neurosurg Psychiat 20: 144

Warkany J, Passarge E, Smith LB. (1966) Congenital malformations in autosomal trisomy syndromes. Am J Dis Child 112: 502

Wolf U et al. (1965) Defizienz an der kuzen armen eines Chromosoms Nr 4. Humangenetik 1: 397

# 19

# SYNDROMES PRESENTING WITH ATAXIA,

# PRECEDED OR ACCOMPANIED BY HYPOTONIA,

# OR WITH CHOREO-ATHETOSIS INTERPOSED

**Ataxia: Clinical and Patho-Physiology**

**Sensory Ataxia Sometimes with Initial Hypotonia and Arreflexia**

    Dejerine-Sottas Disease
    Hypertrophic Polyneuropathy
    Roussy-Levine Syndrome
    A beta Lipoproteinaemia
    Friedreich's Ataxia

## Nutritional and Toxicological Disorders with Peripheral Neuropathy and also Presenting with Cerebellar Ataxia and Arreflexia

Vitamin E Malnutrition: Primary and Secondary
>    *Preterm and Term Malnutrition*
>    *Secondary Forms of Vitamin E Deficiency*
>    *Syndromes of Progressive Neuronal Degeneration due to Vitamin E Deficiency*
Lead Encephalopathy
Phenytoin Overdosage

## Metabolic Disorder with Ataxia, Choreiform Movements and Intermittent Pyramidal and Spastic Syndrome (Extensor Thrusts), Hyperreflexia and Clonus

Krebs Urea Cycle Defects and Congenital Hyperammonaemia

## Transient Initial and Intermittent Hypertonicity with Pyramidal Signs linked to later Ataxia

Ornithine Transcarbamylase (OTCO Deficiency (Russell Type II Congenital
>    Hyperammonaemia)
Argininosuccinic Acidaemia
Citrullinaemia
Hyperornithinaemia with hyperammonaemia

## Sudanophilic Leukodystrophies expressed in the Cerebellar type of Ataxia, with later association of Choreo-athetosis and Hypertonicity with Pyramidal Involvement

Early Infantile Sudanophilic Leukodystrophy
Late Infantile or Juvenile Sudanophilic Leukodystrophy
Familial forms including Orthochromatic Leukodystrophy with Diffuse
>    leptomeningeal angiomatosis
Pelizaeus-Merzbacher Disease

416

## Sensory and Cerebellar Ataxia, and Proximal Muscle Weakness

Generalized Glucose Phosphate Isomerase (GPI) Deficiency, and Mixed Sensory
and Cerebellar Ataxia

## Ataxia Preceded by Initial Hypotonia and often Later Hypertonicity

Lactic Acidaemias and Deficiency of the Pyruvate Dehydrogenase Complex
(PDHC), etc
Pyruvate Dehydrogenase Deficiency
Decreased Activity of Pyruvate Oxidation especially in relation to Ataxic
Disorders
Leigh's Disease

## Ataxia Preceded by Initial or Persistent Hypotonia

α-Hydroxybutyric Aciduria
Multiple Carboxylase Deficiency: Holocarboxylase Synthetase and Biotinase
Deficiency
Isovaleric Acidaemia
Valine Metabolic Defect with Deficiency in 3 Hydroxy CoA Diacyclase
Maple Syrup Disease: Late Onset Episodic Variant
Tryptophanuria
Carbohydrate-Deficient Glycoprotein Syndrome associated with Hypoplasia
of Segments of Cerebellum
Mitochondrial Cytopathy
*Defects of Mitochondrial Respiratory Chain Enzymes*
*Kearns-Sayre Syndrome*
*Infantile/Juvenile Refsum's Ataxia*

## Initial Ataxia Ending in Spasticity

Late Infantile $GM_2$ Gangliosidosis
Juvenile $GM_2$ Gangliosidosis
Peroxisomal Disorder
Adrenoleukodystrophy
De Sanch's-Cacchione Syndrome (Xeroderma Pigmentosa Idiocy)

## Ataxia Occasionally Associated with Choreo-Athetosis

Ataxia Telangiectasia (Louis-Bar syndrome)

## Miscellaneous Conditions of Unknown of Uncertain Genesis associated with Ataxia

Rett Syndrome
Congenital and Genetically-determined Ataxia
Other Genetically-determined Cerebellar-type Ataxia
*Fraser Sanger-Brown and Marie*
*Lafora: Familial Progressive Myoclonic Epilepsy and Ataxia*
*Strumpel-Lorain Familial Paraplegia*
*Sjogren-Larsen Disease*
*Familial Ataxic Diplegia*
Periodic Ataxia (of dominant inheritance)
Ataxia associated with Hydrocephalus
Oculo-Dento-Digital Dysplastic Syndrome
Cockayne Dwarf Syndrome
Alper's Syndrome or Progressive Degeneration of Cerebral Grey Matter
Hartnup Disease
Batten-Bielchowsky-Jansky Disease (BBJD): Late Infantile Amaurotic
Idiocy or Myoclonic Variant of Cerebral Lipidosis,
Ceroid Lipofuscinosis
*Spielmeyer-Vogt-Sjogren*
Marinesco-Sjögrens Ataxic Syndrome
Biemonds Syndrome
Congenital Hypothyroidism

## References

# ATAXIA:
# CLINICAL AND PATHO-PHYSIOLOGY

The first recognizable elements of ataxia may not emerge until late in the first year of life, usually as part of a generalized disorder of coordination evident in reaching for objects and other hand movements, as well as in sitting. Later the unsteadiness will be conspicuous in standing or attempts at walking. In any case the onset is often insidious and usually found in conjunction with other signs or symptoms which may provide clues as to the basis of the ataxia, whether of the early prenatal cerebral or cerebellar damage in cerebral palsy·(CP) or a metabolic or related source in a disorder of progressive nature. It may thus be associated with a motor defect as in ataxic CP, or the syndrome of ataxia, spastic diplegia and dysequilibrium, or linked to anatomical abnormality such as the Arnold-Chiari malformation or posterior fossa cysts. On the other hand, chronic cerebellar-type ataxia later to be attended by a conspicuous dysequilibrium, associated with dyssynergia and "scanning" speech may be the clinical expression of a host of metabolic disorders such as will be outlined subsequently, including infantile Refsum's disease, retinitis pigmentosa, peripheral neuropathy, anosmia, ichthyosis, Maple Syrup disease or Hartnup's syndrome. Other examples of progressive disorders associated with ataxia whether of metabolic, chromosomal or neoplastic basis, may also be listed for the time being. These encompass ataxia-telangiectasia and the late infantile lipidoses, wherein ataxia is generally the first sign, as well as other hereditary disorders, such as Bielchowsky's disease wherein myoclonus and seizures are earlier and major features, and those like A-ß-lipoproteinaemia, metachromatic leukodystrophy and hydrocephalus, to craniopharyngioma and occult neuroblastoma in which ataxia also eventually becomes prominent.

Further diagnostic criteria, and neurophysiological data are covered in Chapter 4.

# SENSORY ATAXIA SOMETIMES WITH INITIAL
# HYPOTONIA AND ARREFLEXIA

## Dejerine - Sottas Disease (Type III HMSN)

This is an autosomal recessive trait most often apparent as soon as the child starts walking which is always delayed until approximately 18 to 36 months of age. It is often found that the child had been floppy in infancy and that the ability to sit up was also delayed. It is a severe *diffuse sensorimotor polyneuropathy* marked by an increase of CSF protein. Early in the disease, all tendon reflexes are abolished. Involvement of the upper limbs rapidly follows the weakening of the legs. Sensory deficits especially affects proprioceptive sensation so that a variable degree of *sensory ataxia* supervenes.

Cranial nerves may be affected, and miosis, impaired pupillary light reflexes and nystagmus may ensue. Peripheral nerves become significantly enlarged in diameter with segmental demyelination and onion-bulb changes of the Schwann cells which are typically not detectable until beyond 10 years of age. An earlier criterion may be the extremely low motor nerve conduction velocities.

## Hypertrophic Interstitial Polyneuropathy

*In other congenital causes of Hypertrophic Interstitial Polyneuropathy*, such as those described by Anderson (1973), the affected infants are *hypotonic and arreflexic* with markedly early delay in motor development.

*Arthrogryposis-like* defects of hands and feet may sometimes have been recognizable from birth. The CSF protein is raised, and on nerve biopsy there are characteristically concentric Schwann cell whorls.

## Roussy-Levine Syndrome

A "tabetic" form of sensory ataxia in childhood (Lapresie and Salisachs, 1973) may prove to be the presentation of this autosomal dominant trait. Arreflexia is found along with sensory loss, primarily in the legs, but weakness is minimal. On nerve biopsy, "onion bulb" changes within Schwann cells are again characteristic.

In metabolic disorders especially of the age period 1 to 4 years of age, ataxia attributable to vestibular disorder is uncommon in childhood. However, a

complaint of vertigo in the older child, either spontaneous or elicited, alerts one to this possibility.

Ataxia of station, or its marked exaggeration on closing of eyes whilst standing with the feet, together constitutes a positive Rhomberg sign, indicative of *sensory ataxia*. There may be accompanying abnormality of involuntary movements such as the athetosis, or choreiform movements, or complex combination of them, appearing in ataxia-telangiectasia.

## A Beta Lipoproteinaemia

This autosomal recessive disorder is marked by the unique absence of low

density lipoproteins (β-lipoproteins). It also lacks all apo-β-containing lipoproteins as well as chylomicrons, VLDL and LDL both in plasma and in intestinal mucosa - the source of synthesis of the chylomicrons. Levels of plasma cholesterol (0.6-3mmol/l), triglycerides (usually <0.4 mmol/l) and of total phospholipid concentration are invariably very low. The clinical pattern dependent upon the absorption defect of the intestinal mucosa presents with bulky stools, steatorrhoea, vomiting and abdominal distension. This already emerges in early infancy, even from birth, although tending to subside after a few years.

Depressed tendon reflexes may already expose the *peripheral neuropathy* during the child's second year of life but the *ataxia* may not appear until the fifth to the tenth year when it is attended by an array of incoordination, proprioceptive sensory loss, dysarthria and other cerebellar signs. A positive Babinski is usual, and weakness of legs occasional, followed ultimately by the gradual evolution of pes cavus and kyphoscoliosis. These findings are accounted for by a loss of myelinated fibres in the posterior columns, in the spino-cerebellar tract, and related to the Purkinje

and granular cells of the cerebellum and to a lesser extent of the corticospinal tract.

A superimposed pattern of oculomotor paralysis is sometimes found, presenting with ptosis, night blindness, pigmentary degeneration and constriction of visual fields. Facial weakness and tongue atrophy have also been reported. Large amounts of lipofuscin are identified in the cortical cells.

The spiky or thorny erythrocyte abnormalities of acanthocytosis are a constant and early diagnostic finding, best found in preparations of fresh blood suspended in Dacie's solution. Other haematological changes include low sedimentation rates and lack of Rouleaux formation. To the neurological analogy with Friedreich's ataxia is added several cardiological features: cardiomegaly, arrhythmia and ECG aberrations. In the intestinal tract, lipid droplets mainly consisting of triglyceride fill the mucosa, although the villi are revealed to be normal on jejunal biopsy, of course unlike the coeliac situation.

## Friedreich's Ataxia

Inherited as an autosomal recessive trait, it manifests before the age of 10 years in more than half of the patients of Mollard, even as early as 3 years. Ataxia of gait typically emerges first. Incoordination and clumsiness of the hands soon follow, with dysarthria either preceding or following The ataxia displays both a sensory or "tabetic" component, showing dependence on vision with a positive Romberg sign, and

a cerebellar component, which typically predominates. A so-called "static" element is evident insofar as it manifests most clearly whilst the child is sitting or standing, presenting as tottering and swaying of the body and nodding of the head. The child reels when walking, trying to overcome the imbalance by adopting a wide stance. When the eyes are closed, unsteadiness of posture and of the outstretched fingers is accentuated. There is dysdiadokokinesia, and finger-nose and heel-knee-shin tests evoke asynergia and dysmetria as well as intention tremor. The ataxia even extends to respiratory, facial and lingual movements which accounts for the slow, sometimes staccato, explosive speech. Tendon reflexes are gradually lost, but the plantar reflexes are extensor. Position and vibratory senses are diminished, whilst tactile sense is lost.

Cardiomyopathy may also be a feature together with a systolic murmur, typically the result of subaortic stenosis. Cardiomegaly is to be expected as well as hypertrophic obstruction.

Pathologically, the basic process appears to reflect cellular degeneration or regression, mainly leading to atrophy with death of dorsal root ganglia, and of medullated fibres of the posterior columns. Especially this involves the spino-cerebellar tracts and Clark's column, with the peripheral nerves affected concurrently. Anterior and lateral corticospinal tracts are also affected. The paradoxical abolition of deep tendon reflexes is mainly because of the loss of such proprioceptive neurones. Purkinje cells are also sparse, particularly in the anterior cerebellar lobes and superior vermis. Widespread necrosis of cardiac muscle fibres impose an additional threat.

# NUTRITIONAL AND TOXICOLOGICAL DISORDERS WITH PERIPHERAL NEUROPATHY AND ALSO PRESENTING WITH CEREBELLAR ATAXIA AND ARREFLEXIA

Whilst the proportion of hereditary ataxias which have a recognizable metabolic defect is considered small, and in the order of 5% or less, a careful elucidation of the progressive metabolic and related progressive disorders cited here may well come to raise this figure. In other words, we postulate that ataxia is a major neurological sign or presentation in a variety of inborn errors, including several lipid storage diseases, aminoacidaemias, urea cycle defects, disorders of pyruvate metabolism, and lactic acidosis, quite apart from nutritional deficiencies considered to be rare in the Western world.

## Vitamin E Malnutrition: Primary and Secondary

### Preterm and Term Malnutrition

Unless supplemented with Vitamin E, formula-fed infants show a persistently low serum vitamin E concentration during at least the first six months (Martin and Hurley, 1977), the level at one month being one-fourth of that originally in colostrum.

Deficiency of Vitamin E may also be expressed in haemolytic anaemia of prematurity. This may be attributable to several conditioning factors, including a high unsaturated fat diet together with low dietary *selenium* such as is believed to be endemic in mountainous regions of China. This may still obtain in the West despite the threefold level of selenium in human milk compared to that in infant formula milk. Alternatively, a *combination of Vitamin E and selenium* may protect the infant from the high maternal intake of polyunsaturated fat diet.

**Secondary Forms of Vitamin E Deficiency**

Malabsorption may be a factor as has been found in a-ß-lipoproteinaemia. It has also been reported in chronic cholestasis, and has been associated with progressive myopathy, when it is treatable with high dosage of the vitamin (Guggenheim et al., 1982). It has also been found in a child with autosomal recessive neuropathy and ataxia (Burck et al, 1981) and even in Werdnig-Hoffman disease.

**Syndromes of Progressive Neuronal Degeneration due to Vitamin E Deficiency**

In another case presented by Hardinge et al. (1985) *cerebellar-type ataxia* was a cardinal feature, and occurred in association with arreflexia which was one clinical expression of the peripheral neuropathy. Paradoxically there was no evidence of the fat malabsorption that could be expected in the absence of Vitamin E. On the contrary, hyperlipaemia may co-exist with the Vitamin E deficiency. Depressed Vitamin E levels were identified in several members of the patient's family. Conversely, in pregnancy, a strikingly high serum lipid concentration correlates with a serum level

of Vitamin E considered double that in non-pregnant women.

The reported incidence of isolated vitamin E deficiency in a progressive degenerative form of ataxia is one example. Progressive spino-cerebellar syndromes embodying progressive ataxia, arreflexia and diminution of proprioceptive and vibration sense secondary to vitamin E deficiency have been identified. Pronounced muscle weakness has also emerged in atypical cases. In the absence of fat malabsorption, isolated vitamin E deficiency can lead to a progressive neurological syndrome of ataxia resembling Freidreich's ataxia. Selective impairment of intestinal absorption of vitamin E has been exposed as one cause, a deficiency of an hepatic vitamin E binding protein being suggested.

The girl of 6 years described by Rayner et al. (1993) was characterized by intoeing gait and early pes cavus with bilateral tightness of the tendo Achilles. Arms and legs were incoordinated, deep tendon reflexes equivocal. Subsequently, her gait became increasingly ataxic, the Romberg test was positive and a bilateral intention tremor appeared. Proprioceptive and vibration sensation became impaired in her legs. Widespread discrete yellowish-white spots, apparently patches of atrophy, marked her peripheral retinae, presumably attributable to long-term vitamin E deficiency (Berger et al., 1991). Low circulating serum levels of vitamin E are confirmatory and its estimation should be included in the study of all children with unexplained progressive ataxia, or even in unexplained *non-progressive* ataxia. This finding is especially important since such neurological deterioration has proved to be treatable in several cases (Rayner et al., 1993).

*The treatment given* is generally *Tocophery*l acetate 500 mg daily, gradually increasing to 800 mg. The fasting serum vitamin concentrations reached within four months were within the normal range (26 umol/l) which could be sustained by 500 mg daily.

## Lead Encephalopathy

Manifestations of lead encephalopathy have been recognized from the first year of life with *elements of ataxia* evidenced in early efforts at sitting or walking. Hyper-irritability not infrequently culminates in convulsions alternating with drowsiness, when papilloedema may already be identified, leading ultimately to coma.

Signs of increased intracranial pressure may already be associated in infancy with megalocephaly accompanied by sutural separation and elevation of the anterior fontanelle. Eventual cerebral oedema may necessitate the use of mannitol or dexamethasone, apart from the addition of lead-chelating agents such as calcium edentate (EDTA) and 2,3-dinercapto succinic acid (effective orally), if not penicillamine in less severe examples.

In childhood, *incoordination of hand movements and reaching out* may be apparent before the ataxia is first evident when sitting is attempted. The imbalance of ataxia may also become more obvious when walking is attempted, and when foot-drop in expression of peripheral neuropathy associated with weakness of the tibialis anterior muscles, may be superadded. If the peroneal nerve is also affected, the foot is inverted when the child walks. Attempts to compensate for foot-drop may lead instead to dragging the foot in a *steppage gait* with exaggerated lifting of the lower extremity. The toe is then slapped down before the heel strikes the floor. The footfall sounds split *as in sensory ataxia*. A similar gait also distinguishes the neuropathy of the common peroneal which may be of traumatic or other origin, being seen in later childhood or adolescence in the early stage of progressive peroneal muscle atrophy or the Charcot-Marie-Tooth syndrome.

*Plumbism* has also been implicated in a pattern of early infantile autism. An appropriate history of chronic exposure to lead may be ascertained in relation to *ingestion* whether of lead-laden paint surfaces of toys, furniture and walls, etc., or of water from lead pipes, even from the one-time use of lead nipple shields, or *inhalation* through atmospheric petrol pollution, or burning of batteries. The routine *application* to the eyes, including direct conjunctival involvement of cosmetics containing "surma" or lead salts still constitutes a danger to children of Asian families.

Metaphyseal "lead lines" may be revealed radiologically even in association with rachitic changes. Blood lead levels or measurement of blood level of haem precursors, or erythrocyte "stippling" may be the basis of screening for early lead poisoning.

## Phenytoin Overdosage

A constellation of new clinical features *including ataxia* in a child who has been exposed long-term to anti-convulsant therapy, should raise suspicion of drug intoxication. This would especially apply to new neurological and personality aberrations, and in the kindergarten or older child, deterioration in performance, behavioural changes, unsteadiness and alterations in gait. The abnormal gait closely resembles that in cerebellar ataxia. Other parallel features may point to such specific drug intoxication, including the gum hypertrophy, or co-existence of nystagmus, hiccoughs, slurred speech and rashes. Specific diagnosis can be confirmed by monitoring blood levels assayed by gas-liquid chromatography with peak levels ranging from 62.2 to 66.6 ug/ml whereas reported peak levels in phenytoin intoxication range between 42.6 and 46.6 ug/ml (Abe et al., 1980). Its toxicity may be due to arene oxide metabolites generated by a murine hepatic microsomal system and not the parent drug, as was demonstrated in human lymphocytes by Spielberg et al. (1981).

# METABOLIC DISORDER WITH ATAXIA, CHOREIFORM MOVEMENTS AND INTERMITTENT PYRAMIDAL AND SPASTIC SYNDROME (EXTENSOR THRUSTS), HYPERREFLEXIA AND CLONUS

## Krebs Urea Cycle Defects and Congenital Hyperammonaemia

Enzymes of the urea cycle convert waste nitrogen into relatively innocuous urea. The sequence of these inborn errors have been characterized since identification of the first in 1962 (Russell et al., 1962). Excesses of both blood ammonia and glutamine which are neurotoxic are the cardinal attributes of all derangements of the Krebs-Henseleit urea cycle. Hyper-ammonaemia is therefore the crucial orienting clue, but additional biochemical assays (including orotic and uridinuria) and specific individual enzyme assays of liver or duodenum, even rectal mucosal material, may be justifiable to provide the specific diagnosis.

# TRANSIENT INITIAL AND INTERMITTENT HYPERTONICITY WITH PYRAMIDAL SIGNS LINKED TO LATER ATAXIA

## Ornithine Transcarbamylase (OTC) Deficiency
## (Russell Type II Congenital Hyperammonaemia)

This congenital hyperammonaemic disorder, first defined by Russell et al. (1962) as the clinical expression of OTC deficiency, and indeed of all the Krebs urea cycle defects yet to be identified, is inherited as a sex-linked dominant trait. It presents in the homozygous male in a rapidly lethal neonatal form due to complete deficiency of OTC. Heterozygous females present less severe partial deficiencies, possibly of different mutations of the OTC molecule, which may begin to manifest in early infancy, late infancy or in the juvenile period.

Apart from blood ammonia levels in the range of 200 to 1200 $\mu$g/100 ml, accentuated by the introduction or increased intake of protein or amino acid hydrolysates, and extreme elevation of serum transaminases, enzymatic diagnosis can be confirmed on assay material from liver or jejunal mucosa (Russell et al., 1962). Discrete recurrent episodes of intense headache, vomiting, and even haematemeses, irritability, lethargy, stupor to coma, may initially mimic severe migraine or so-called cyclical vomiting. The manifestations may be strictly confined to the three major components of migraine: ocular, vomiting and headache, in the partial deficiency of OTC in the female, as they were exhibited to an intense degree in both mothers who were sisters during their gestation of patients I and II (Russell, 1973).

*Spastic* diplegia may be simulated in the infantile form or in discrete intensive episodes recurring in later infancy or childhood. The transitory hypertonic manifestation linked to opisthotonic episodes, hypertonic extensor spasms of the legs, and ankle clonus may persist in the homozygous examples with intermittent intensification. Uniquely transitory impact upon the pyramidal system, may include spontaneous clonus, hyperreflexia, as well as bilateral Babinski response comparable to the acute infantile expression of Reye's encephalopathy also often linked to hyperammonaemia and extreme elevation of serum transaminase. Temporary focus of the ammonium concentration upon hypersensitive areas of the upper brain stem has been suggested as a source of the episthotonic spasms and the temporary signs of decerebrate rigidity. Transient ataxia with a different although closely adjoining localization or zone of impact upon colliculo-vestibular-cerebellar pathways may emerge solely in the recovery phase.

Apart from the routine use of a low protein intake and aspartate in acute situations (Russell and Levin, 1967) sodium benzoate is most widely used (at 250 mg/kg/day) conjugated with glycine to form hippurate, approximately one mole of nitrogen being eliminated for each mole of sodium benzoate. Phenylbutyrate (also at 250 mg/kg/day) metabolised in vivo to phenylacetate is more effective, two moles of nitrogen being excreted after conjugation with glutamine (to form phenylacetyl glutamine) for each mole of phenylbutyrate. Becoming an essential amino acid, arginine supplementation at the level of 100 mg/kg/day in frequent small doses, is also necessary except in arginase deficiency, raising this to 500-700 mg/kg/day during acute illness of subjects of Citrullinaemia and Argininosuccinic aciduria.

*Reye's syndrome* may reproduce an analogous clinical picture of acute metabolic encephalopathy with conspicuous intermittent hypertonic extensor spasms, transitory hyperreflexia and clonus, apart from the associated hyperammonaemia. Hepatic transaminases also show extreme elevation.

## Argininosuccinic Aciduria:
## with intermittent episodes of ataxia or
## choreiform movements in late-onset type

The more frequent late-onset type pursues a much more benign course than the malignant early-onset, even neonatal form. The extremely slow psychomotor development has been conspicuous, although already preceded by a history of difficult feeding in infancy. Superimposed upon the basic lethargy and recurrent seizures in almost half the cases, there are intermittent episodes of ataxia or choreiform movement lasting from several days to one or two weeks. The degree of ataxia may be particularly disabling after a series of generalized seizures.

In remittent attacks first evident between 2 and 6 years of age, impairment of alertness or more severe disturbance of consciousness also attended by ataxia of limb movements and gait, with less abnormality of coordination persisting between attacks, may be punctuated by seizures coupled with impairment of alertness or more severe disturbances of consciousness corresponding to the underlying theme of lethargy-to-stupor characteristic of all the Krebs urea cycle defects. Associated mental retardation is usually severe, and there are classical features such as the rough dry skin and irregular growth of the dry and fragile scalp hair giving a ruffled appearance. Microscopically, the hair is identical with trichorrhexis nodosa, attributable to deficiency of arginine. Hepatomegaly occasionally co-exists.

Identification can be simply by systematic amino acid screening, but can be firmly confirmed by enzyme assay of liver or duodenal mucosal biopsy material.

## Citrullinaemia

In this disorder, due to deficiency of argininosuccinic synthetase activity, high blood urine and CSF levels of citrulline are associated with hyperammonaemia which is accentuated post-prandially. Only rare examples of its more benign form with signs of chronic neurological dysfunction in episodic exacerbation, may be implicated in the differential diagnosis of CP. Recurrent episodes of vomiting beginning after the first few months of life are accompanied by psychomotor regression, with *tremor* and *pyramidal signs* associated, as in argininosuccinic aciduria, with dysequilibrium.

## Hyperornithinaemia with Hyperammonaemia

Intermittent ataxia was also a clinical expression of hyperammonaemia and hyperornithinaemia in a young boy documented by Shih et al. (1969) in association with mental retardation and seizures.

# SUDANOPHILIC LEUKODYSTROPHIES EXPRESSED IN THE CEREBELLAR TYPE OF ATAXIA, WITH LATER ASSOCIATION OF CHOREO-ATHETOSIS AND HYPERTONICITY WITH PYRAMIDAL INVOLVEMENT

Their common underlying neuropathological theme is demyelination of the CNS. The "liberated" sudanophilic lipids accumulate in astrocytic and other cells of the white matter so affected. Particular types of myelinopathy can be roughly subdivided as outlined below.

Head control and sitting up with support is finally achieved by some children. Significantly enough, mental deterioration only emerges in terminal stages, seldom after 5 to 7 years, the speech having become dysarthric before this.

*Gross cerebral and cerebellar atrophy* marks the cerebrum, internal capsule, brain stem and cerebellar peduncles. Small islets of preserved myelin are interspersed in larger areas of patchy demyelination and accumulation of sudanophilic degradation products in nerve cells and axons.

Electronystagmographic studies and CSF ultrasediment examination may provide specific findings.

**Several significant variants exist:**

### Early Infantile Sudanophilic Leukodystrophy

Onset is before 3 months and is usually terminal within 2 years. Neurological dysfunctions include hypertonic paralysis, optic atrophy and blindness, and occasional seizures. True microcephaly with the head circumference even 3 SD below the mean for age is to be expected.

### Late Infantile or Juvenile Sudanophilic Leukodystrophy

This form usually emerges between 3 and 7 years of age. A diffusely progressive cerebral disease manifests. Mental deterioration is soon apparent, and meanwhile, a triad of incoordination, spasticity and occasional involuntary movement slowly become manifest. The process is often so slow that differentiation from non-progressive congenital encephalopathy or cerebral palsy is difficult.

### Familial type Leukodystrophy

Another familial type first reported by Norman and Tingey (1963) was marked by spastic diplegia together with nystagmus and microcephaly associated with mental retardation and large ears. Pachygyria coexisted with the leukodystrophy.

### Familial type "Orthochromatic" Leukodystrophy

Familial type "orthochromatic" leukodystrophies with diffuse leptomeningeal angiomatosis, of infantile and juvenile types first defined by van Bogaert (1970). Additional neuropathology includes intracortical necrosis and diffuse demyelination. Pyramidal hemiplegia is also accompanied by *tremor*, *dysarthria* and *pseudobulbar symptoms*.

## Pelizaeus-Merzbacher Disease

The only sharply defined entity in this group of demyelinating encephalopathies, this is a sex-linked recessive genetic disorder, predominantly affecting males. *Disorder of movement* is striking from the outset in the neonate or first month of life. *Tremulous movements of the eyes* mainly constitute rapid irregular *pendular* nystagmus. Intermittent pendular or shaking movements of the head take the form of *spasmus nutans*. The arms later demonstrate different types of choreiform or athetotic movement, but *voluntary movements are usually ataxic*. Regression of whatever initial psychomotor development had been attained dates from 3 months onwards. Pyramidal involvement is invariable, with hypertonicity and hyperreflexia.

Spasmus Nutans is defined as a triad of head-nodding, nystagmus and head tilt. The nodding is rhythmic and involuntary, disappearing during sleep. There may be spread to the shoulders and trunk. It is to be differentiated from the "bobble-head doll" syndrome commonly associated with a third ventricular cyst, and thus may precede hydrocephalus and other evidence of intracranial hypertension. The to and fro or side to side head bobbing is more dysrhythmia and less constant than in spasmus nutans with onset tending to be later in life.

The onset of Pelizaeus-Merzbacher manifestation may also be somewhat later in certain families but with the identical

pendular nystagmus and head nodding. Ataxia of cerebellar type and choreo-athetosis also emerge later, as does the spasticity and pyramidal signs. Progression of pes cavus and kyphoscoliosis follows.

# SENSORY AND CEREBELLAR ATAXIA, AND PROXIMAL MUSCLE WEAKNESS

## Generalized glucose phosphate isomerase (GPI) Deficiency, and Mixed Sensory and Cerebellar Ataxia

In this rare complex syndrome ultimately associated with ataxia, there is a general lowering of the specific activity of *glucose phosphate isomerase* (GPI). This principally involves the *erythrocytes* to produce an *haemolytic anaemia* apparent clinically in pallor and a mild jaundice, granulocytes with lowering of bactericidal activity, and the *central nervous* and *neuromuscular systems*. The latter leads to psychomotor retardation manifested mainly in a disturbance of logical thinking, immature or inappropriate behaviour and impaired school performance. *Feeding difficulties* had however been troublesome from birth and repeated attacks of impaired consciousness was attributed to epileptiform

reactions. Myopathy affected the proximal extremities, so that standing on one leg was possible for only a short period of time and the extended arms fell quickly. The weak facial expression was associated with mild ptosis and down-turned corners of the mouth.

The late onset ataxia was both sensory and cerebellar, with ataxia during standing and grasping. Myoclonic jerks were superimposed upon *athetoid* movements. Statural states was at the 10th percentile. The degradation of the GPI-deficient musculature is demonstrable histo-chemically.

# ATAXIA PRECEDED BY INITIAL HYPOTONIA AND OFTEN LATER HYPERTONICITY

## Lactic Acidaemias, etc: Deficiency of the Pyruvate Dehydrogenase Complex (PDHC), etc.

Ataxia is a prominent clinical feature of these disorders even if preceded by hypotonia. But the cardinal clinico-pathological pattern associated with the progressive spino-cerebellar ataxia is no less conspicuous. Firstly, the consistent hypotonia, then the recurrent hyperventilation linked to acidosis, underlying pulmonary hypertension, developmental retardation and failure to thrive. The elevated concentrations in blood and urine of lactate, pyruvate and alanine will be discussed subsequently. In the related myopathies, the clinical pattern differs especially in the insidious onset or episodic muscle weakness, neural deafness together with proximal or muscular dystrophy linked to facial muscle weakness and extraocular muscle impairment which may include ptosis. The early symptomatology may also include poor exercise tolerance which may lead to muscle cramps and even myoglobulinuria.

The lactic acidaemias make up a family of metabolic disorders embodying a considerable variety of known enzymatic deficiencies including those involved in pyruvate metabolism and the organic acidaemias as well as in the mitochondrial myopathies. Most of these disorders manifest initially, and in more advanced stages, with progressive or episodic disorders of tone, movement and balance simulating entities of cerebral palsy.

The normal arterial lactate is 1.0-1.5 mmol/L whilst the venous level is 1.0-2.0 with a pH of less than 7.37 in the absence of other causes of acidosis. A lactate concentration in blood of over 2 mM (18 mg/dl) is considered abnormal and constitutes lactic acidaemia. Although most children with its congenital form reveal concentrations exceeding 5 mM, underlying lactic acidosis would also be reflected in an increased anion gap and lowered plasma bicarbonate $(NA^+ + K^+)-(HCO_3^- + Cl^-)$. The anion gap is normally between 12-15 mEg/L, but values above 25 mEq/L are clearly abnormal and usually indicative of organic acidaemia. But lactic acidosis is identified definitively by measure of blood lactic acid, preferably from an arterial source to obviate blood stasis and the erythrocytic production of lactate. When lactic acidaemia is authenticated, therefore, disorders of pyruvate metabolism and levels of pyruvate should first be explored, although considerable concentrations of pyruvate are seldom seen because of their rapid conversion to lactate, or transamination to alanine, levels of which should also be assayed.

Pyruvate is a key intermediate in major metabolic pathways involving anaerobic glycolysis, gluconeogenesis and alanine formation so fundamental to muscle metabolism. In the acquired metabolic disorders, an increased anion gap plus an

431

increased lactate/pyruvate ratio in the absence of obvious pulmonary or cardiovascular disorder, would be important diagnostically. Several primary inborn errors of pyruvate metabolism which are responsible for chronic neurological impairment relevant in this context will be subsequently outlined. Clearly they must be considered in the differential diagnosis of cerebral palsy, with at least their progressivity as a distinguishing feature.

*Before embarking on a full work-up of pyruvate enzymology,* however, it must be appreciated that hyperlactic acidaemia in the infant may also be the product of hypoxia, hypoventilation, shock and hypoperfusion, or of other clinical situations without primarily metabolic associations that need be excluded such as sepsis, cardiac, pulmonary, hepatic disease, and severe anaemia, although pancytopenia may be one facet of a metabolic acidosis. In addition, apart from mitochondrial encephalo-myopathy, there are other groups of syndromes such as Fakahara disease, the Kearns-Sayre syndrome, as well as the organic acidaemias which will be outlined later, such as propionic and isovaleric acidaemias, or 3-hydroxy-3 glutaric, pyroglutaric and decarboxylic acidurias, all of which may present with a triad of *lactic acidaemia* alongside *muscle weakness* and *significant hypotonia.*

Three basic groups of acquired and inherited disorders of pyruvate metabolism can lead to such lactic acidaemia. These include:
1. Those interfering with operation of the pyruvate dehydrogenase complex.

2. Those interfering with pathways of gluconeogenesis.

3. Those interfering with the tricarboxylic cycle.

A mutual pattern of the clinical manifestation of specific causation embodies *initial hypotonia* associated with the muscle weakness. The earliest expression may even be prenatal with decreased or delayed foetal movement. It is followed usually by hypertonia and initially heightened deep tendon reflexes, but later depressed. *Ataxia,* intermittent or recurrent episodes, then take over alongside recurrent episodes of acidosis with hyperventilation. It may last for days or weeks, often precipitated by stress such as intercurrent infection, with clumsiness perpetuated between attacks. An unusual odour is recognizable. Episodes of unexplained vomiting may actually herald the onset of symptoms. In some categories, acute symptomatic hypoglycaemia may arise, and be responsible for convulsions. Hyperammonaemia may also be found at this point. Any such patient with chronic lactic acidaemia may produce progressive pulmonary hypertension.

Presentation in infancy will often include overall *failure to thrive. Retardation of growth* is eventually evident, incidentally often out of proportion to the degree of depression of the serum concentration of bicarbonate. Frequently but by no means invariably, psychomotor retardation becomes apparent. Microcephaly and even optic atrophy may be associated. Other ocular signs may include ophthalmoplegia and cataracts.

Recognizable dysmorphism has been described in association with a small subgroup of these deficiencies of PDH complexes (Nyhan and Sakath, 1987). The forehead is high and bossed, the nose anteverted and ears large. Hip dislocation was associated with limbs in extreme external rotation with feet in typical ballerina position.

Some of these children suffer more specific behavioural disorders, as in Leigh's syndrome, or subacute necrotizing encephalomyelitis. The significance of a close histopathological resemblance to Wernicke's encephalomyelitis with involvement of brain stem, basal ganglia and cerebellum, has not yet been evaluated. One distinguishing feature is that the mamilliary bodies are spared in Leigh's syndrome. But CT or MRI scanning has clarified striking hypodensity of both caudate nucleus and putamen (Schwarz, Hutchinson and Berg, 1981). The striatal and cerebellar involvement is important in terms of the pathogenesis of a movement disorder, and including choreo-athetoid manifestations and even dystonic posture whereas the superadded cerebellar involvement would appear to account for the characteristic ataxia.

The principal group of disorders of pyruvate metabolism are listed below and those relevant in this context are outlined in turn:

**Defects of PDH complex**
Pyruvate decarboxylase E1
Lipoamide dehydrogenase
Pyruvate dehydrogenase phosphate phosphatase

**Defects of Gluconeogenesis**
Deficiencies of:
Glucose-6-phosphatase
Fructose 1,6, diphosphatase
Phosphoenolpyruvate carboxykinase
Pyruvate carboxylase
Multiple carboxylase

**Defects of Pyruvate Oxidation**
of Respiratory chain
Redux lactic acidaemias
Kreb's cycle turnover defects

What is important to realise even in the context of the foetus, perinatal or early neonatal situations is that the most clinically significant causes of lactic acidosis, particularly involving asphyxia and shock are acquired disorders associated with impaired tissue oxygenation as in hypoxia and/or ischaemia. The shift to anaerobic metabolism induces lactate production. *"Mitochondrial toxins"* also exist that inhibit oxidative phosphorylation apart from many other mitochondrial findings. The two most common inhibitors of mitochondrial function show a challenging clinical association, Reye's syndrome and salicylism.

## Pyruvate Dehydrogenase Deficiency

The major pathway in oxidative metabolism of pyruvate is its conversion to acetyl-CoA by the pyruvate dehydrogenase complex (PDHC) consisting of three primary enzymes and two regulatory enzymes. The essential cofactors are thiamine CoA and

433

lipoic acid. Pyruvate dehydrogenase of E1 (which is also termed pyruvate decarboxylase (PDC), decarboxylates pyruvate, transferring the acetyl moiety to dipoamide. The regulatory function of PDHC is crucial, since any disorder leading to inhibition of pyruvate oxidation results in accumulation of pyruvate and thus lactate. Furthermore the PDHC provides substrate for the tricarboxylic acid cycle, as well as for lipid and acetylcholine synthesis.

Clinical manifestations of such decarboxylase (E1) deficiency (Blass et al., 1970; Robinson and Sherwood, 1984) with E1 activity in cell-free preparations of fibroblasts found in only 20% of controls, range from intermittent neurological dysfunction including *ataxia* and *choreo-athetosis* to an acute fatal lactic acidosis. The first of the *remittent episodes of ataxia* may begin early in the second year of life, typically after a febrile illness or other stress. The *ataxia is of cerebellar type*. The *associated choreo-athetosis is relatively mild* and occasionally complicated by dystonic posturing. Intellectual status was considered "high average". Irregular "wandering" eye movements have also been noted.

The enzymatic defect within this complex is also expressed clinico-metabolically in systemic acidosis (the so-called "cerebral lactic acidosis"). But there is a fundamental and extensive cerebro-pathological association: *agenesis of the corpus callosum, absent pyramids* and *ectopic olivary nuclei*. The significance of this remains a challenging problem. Most commonly, cystic changes and demyelination of cortex and brain stem were also found, and in some examples severe hydrocephalus as well as hydrancephaly. *Demyelination and cavitation is also prominent in discrete areas of the basal ganglia, thalami and brain stem* in combined defects of the α-keto acid dehydrogenase complexes.

Diagnostic support can stem from a recognizable manifestation of metabolic myopathy in this subgroup, some with neural deafness or cortical blindness, if not the emergence of early cataracts and/or impairment of extraocular movement, in addition to a dysmorphic syndrome comprising craniofacial features: *narrowed microcephalic head, high-bossed forehead, anteverted nose, with flared nares and large ears. Hip dislocation* is frequent, with the gross bilateral external rotation at the hips producing a striking ballerina positioning of the feet. In this context, the presence of muscle weakness or proximal muscle "dystrophy" has been emphasized, whereas in other examples the weakness is episodic, and there is a picture of ataxic CP apart from neurodevelopmental delay.

Clinically, delayed motor and neurological development is associated with the acidosis, including examples with distinct microcephaly and ataxic episodes, or with symptoms analogous to those of Leigh's syndrome. Pyruvate dehydrogenase is close to rate-limiting in provision of oxidative energy for the brain. Depression or lack of activity incurs a drop in cellular high energy phosphate stores (i.e. in creatine phosphate and ATP), and thence to stimulation of excessive glycolysis and rapid accumulation of lactic acid. Other possible consequences appear to be an inability of neurones to generate enough acetylcholine wherein the PDHC plays a significant role as a substrate source to fulfil demands for acetylcholine production. The most vulnerable areas of brain to such influences are those most dependent upon oxidative energy, e.g. basal ganglia, so crucial to evoking choreo-athetoid manifestations, as well as the thalamus and brain stem where indeed the demyelination was especially focussed in the combined defect of the α keto acid dehydrogenase complex.

An important therapeutic note was sounded by Matalon et al. (1982) in deficiency of lipoamide dehydrogenase, when lipoic acid administration produced a convincingly favourable response. A finding that would also be worthy of therapeutic exploration is the activation to a normal range of pyruvate dehydrogenase phosphate deficiency in the presence of Ca++ and Mg++.

Neurological manifestations which could also be consistent with the diagnosis of Leigh's necrotizing encephalomyelopathy are already conspicuous during the first year in the infantile form of pyruvate carboxylase deficiency (PC), emerging during the first two years of life. The correlationship between PC deficiency and Leigh's disease remains controversial.

After vomiting and diarrhoea in early infancy undue irritability, lethargy and mental retardation are noticeable. *Axial hypotonia* can be identified although interrupted occasionally by tonic spasms, whilst the *deep tendon reflexes are depressed*. Relatively slight hypoglycaemia is associated with generalized aminoaciduria and consistently minor increase of blood pyruvate (0.3 mM) and lactate (34 mM), normal basal levels of pyruvate and lactate being 0.2 mM and 2.0 mM respectively. These raised levels in the presence of elevated values for pyruvate and lactate indicate impairment of gluconeogenesis. This concept is supported by the finding of only 1% of activity of pyruvate carboxylase in liver.

## Decreased Activity of Pyruvate Oxidation especially in relation to Ataxic Disorders

*Ataxia* is the main neurological sign in many other inborn errors of metabolism including several lipid storage diseases, and amino acidurias apart from disorders of pyruvate metabolism. Carbohydrates are the major source of energy in brain, yet its PDH activity is only twice that needed to catabolize a normal pyruvate load. So that even a moderate reduction in PDH activity can lead to CNS dysfunction.

The studies of pyruvate oxidation in muscle slices by Kark and colleagues (1974) revealed significant reduction in 7 of 19 patients with *spino-cerebellar degeneration* including 4 patients with Friedreich's ataxia and in 8 of 19 patients with motor neuropathy. Levels were reduced to 19-21% of controls.

With onset in the second and third years in a juvenile form, difficulties in walking first present complicated by severe neuropathic manifestations, including cerebellar incoordination and significant *slowly progressive ataxia*. Intellectual regression slowly becomes apparent, as does dysarthria. Oculomotor disturbances of lateral and vertical gaze are also noticeable, together with intermittent abnormality in respiratory rhythm and hyperventilation.

## Leigh's Disease

In *Leigh's disease*, the infantile encephalomyelopathy is marked by *necrosis of striatum and cerebral white matter* together with multiple bilateral symmetrical foci of incomplete necrosis, spongy degeneration and concomitant increased stromal cellularity with gliosis in brain stem and basal ganglia. The *striatal necrosis* in infantile examples has been observed by Adams and Lyon (1982). Brain stem dysfunctions may nonetheless be relapsing, the prolonged remissions sometimes lasting up to two years. This is strikingly similar to that in Wernicke's encephalopathy attributed to thiamine deficiency, and even more closely resembles thiamine deficiency in the macaque monkey. And indeed, an inhibitor of thiamine pyrophosphate has been identified in the urine in some cases, ATP phosphoryl transferase, which catalyses the formation of thiamine triphosphate. Symptoms are mainly of *ataxia* and muscle weakness, *hypo-* or *hypertonic difficulties in sitting, feeding and walking*, and absent papillary reaction to light. Additional clinical features such as ophthalmoplegia, other cranial nerve signs, respiratory irregularities or central hypoventilation - or central apnoea - can complete a more specific diagnosis. Ultimately spasticity prevails, often with a positive Babinski, although there is depression or even loss of deep tendon reflexes later in the course.

This clinical pattern has been associated most commonly with impaired gluconeogenesis especially related to deficiency of pyruvate carboxylase, although also described in the syndrome of pyruvate dehydrogenase complex (PDHC) deficiency. The associated lactic acidosis, implying a blood lactate concentration of more than 2mEq/L characterizes several other conditions we have outlined: Mitochondrial myopathy, Pyruvate decarboxylase deficiency, Cytochrome oxidase deficiency, and a congenital lactic acidosis of an idiopathic or unknown nature. Administration of Glutamine (150 mg 3 hourly) plus pyridoxine (25 mg q.i.d.) has produced significant clinical improvement together with reduction in urinary lactate. At the same time as becoming more alert and active, there has been a significant *lessening of the later phase of hypertonicity.*

436

# ATAXIA PRECEDED BY INITIAL OR PERSISTENT HYPOTONIA

## δ-Hydroxybutyric Aciduria

In this autosomal recessive disorder, the central neuropathic feature was again *ataxia of trunk and limbs*, which was responsible for instability in sitting or even crawling. Muscular *hypotonia* was also marked, with *intention tremor* and general retardation of motor development from infancy also being cardinal manifestations of the first case reported by Jacobs and colleagues (1984) and in all subsequent cases. Inability to stand, walk or speak marked the second half of the second year of life in these children.

In addition to undue ocular mobility described as *ocular apraxia*, and a diffusely abnormal EEG, brief convulsions recur between 6 and 12 months. The CT scan confirms cerebral atrophic changes. *Both the hypotonia and the ataxic gait* persisted certainly until 5 years of age. Without any progressive intensification to this point, the deep tendon reflexes were difficult to elicit. Of the original early cases, two displayed striking conjunctival telangiectasia, calling to mind the classical syndrome of ataxia telangiectasia. Improvement in cerebellar symptoms may come about over a period of years.

Excessive urinary excretion of δ-*hydroxybutyric acid* - documented by gas chromatographic-mass spectrometry - was consistent in all child subjects. Likewise it was high in the CSF, indeed at 600 $\mu$m/L equalling 60% of that in the plasma. δ-*aminobutyric* acid or GABA was also increased in the CSF.

The molecular defect is in the enzyme *succinic semialdehyde hydrogenase*, a key enzyme in δ-aminobutyric acid (GABA) metabolism. Direct assay of this enzyme with 14C-labelled succinic semi-aldehyde yields about 4% of the control level. Increased excretion of succinic semi-aldehyde is also identified in the urine of these children, and is the product of the transamination of GABA. Normally it is converted to succinic acid, but is further metabolized in this disorder through the citric acid cycle.

## Multiple Carboxylase Deficiency: Holocarboxylase Synthetase and Biotinase Deficiency

There are two distinct disorders wherein multiple carboxylase deficiencies coexist. In the first form with holocarboxylase deficiency, *initial hypotonia* is followed by athetosis and hypertonus, whilst in the second, lacking biotinase, *ataxia* predominates, but may be intermittent yet sometimes so profound as to seriously interfere with ultimate walking.

*The first* is a neonatal or early infantile disorder. *Delay in motor development* can be averted if diagnosed early and treated promptly. Recurrent episodes of vomiting date from birth, and an erythematous scaly rash emerges at 6 weeks. Later unresponsiveness may suddenly attend massive ketosis and metabolic acidosis with an anion gap. In the infants with subnormal holocarboxylase synthetase (Burri et al., 1981) it may present from day 1 to 15 months.

*Immunological dysfunction* with diminution of T-lymphocytes, and in their *in vivo* response to candida. Neurological abnormality includes that of the EEG in a "burst suppression" pattern, and that of the *CT scan* of cerebral white matter *indicative of leukodystrophy*. The *hypotonia* may be massive *with absent reflexes* and loss of head control, although transient hypertonia may even precede the lethargy and coma characterizing the neonate. *Athetoid movements* have also been noted along with hypertonia, clenched fists, hyperreflexia with extensor plantar responses and opisthotonos (Leonard et al., 1981). Early spastic contractures of arms and legs may also be found.

*A more "indolent" late-onset, late infantile disorder* with onset also in infancy, although generally after 3 months of age, is ascribed to a *deficiency of biotinidase* (Wolf et al., 1981; 1983). Persistent vomiting and failure to thrive may progress to dehydration and deep coma. *The characteristic bright red scaly rash* usually involves the entire body, and resembles that of acrodermatitis enteropathica. Perioral *stomatitis* is regularly seen and there may be glossitis. Varying degrees of *alopecia* to alopecia totalis may prevail, with absence of eyelashes, eyebrows, lanugo and scalp hair. *Ataxia* may be intermittent, but may also be so profound as to seriously interfere with walking. *Myoclonus and intention tremor* may be superadded.

*The cerebellum* has been reported as showing gross atrophy in the region of the *superior vermis* (curiously enough similar to that in chronic alcoholism) and a virtually complete disappearance of the Purkinje cell layer. Neurosensory disturbance involving both optic and auditory nerves has also been observed. The associated optic atrophy or neurosensory hearing loss do not respond to biotin therapy, although most of the neurological manifestations do disappear in response to therapy with biotin. An immunological deficiency with decreased numbers of B and T lymphocytes resembles that seen in the Di George syndrome.

The associated lactic acidosis may be extremely high, and a full assay for other organic acids being indicated whenever chronic lactic acidosis is confirmed. Hyperammonaemia may also be present in young infants, and will subside just as rapidly as the acidosis and ketosis on a dosage of 40 mg or more of biotin daily. Skin lesions disappear and hair begins to grow. The high lactic acid and pyruvate levels are normalized. The levels of other organic acid metabolites usually decrease, although still remaining somewhat elevated in children with holocarboxylase deficiency.

At the same time the lethargy and convulsions are eliminated, *and both the hypotonia and ataxia disappear*. Even prenatal therapy can be effective (Packman et al., 982) as illustrated in a mother in whom the diagnosis of an affected foetus was confirmed prenatally (Burri et al., 1981).

## Isovaleric Acidaemia

Episodic illness is heralded by intense vomiting often strongly suggestive of pyloric stenosis. Its underlying ketosis and acidosis is the classical presentation of this autosomal recessive disorder. There is also the characteristic "sweaty tennis shoe" odour, the smell of a typical volatile short-chain organic acid, as well as urinary excretion of isovalerylglycine and 3-hydroxy isovaleric acid, stemming from *deficiency of isovaleryl CoA dehydrogenase*, the third step ion the pathway of leucine degradation. *Ataxia* may be a presenting sign, with mental retardation and microcephaly eventually ensuing.

*In early infancy, there may be prominent hyperammonaemia* (one such reading was 152 µg/dl), a special indication for exchange transfusion. Occasional hyperglycaemia may suggest diabetes mellitus. During the initial attack, leucopenia, thrombopenia and anaemia may be detected.

To enhance the otherwise major accumulation of isovaleric acid, its urinary excretion can be enhanced by an oral or intravenous combination of L-carnitine (100 mg/kg/day) and glycine (250 mg/kg/day), which are conjugated to produce isovalerylcarnitine and isovalerylglycine respectively. L-carnitine is also exploited to augment removal of aryl groups in other organic acidaemias: 3-methylcrotonyl glycinuria and glutaric aciduria Type I.

*Tone is very poor*, and *hypotonia* appears to be the only residual neurological abnormality after the acute ketotic episode. The sucking reflex is diminished as are the minimal deep tendon reflexes.

An accurate method for gas chromatographic-massspectrometryanalysis of 3-hydroxybutyric acid (Jacobs et al., 1984) should lead to *rapid* prenatal diagnosis with preventive implications. In treatment, a low protein regimen includes supplemental glycine and alanine, as well as carnitine.

## Valine Metabolic Defect with Deficiency in
## 3 hydroxy isobutyryl CoA diacyclase (Brown et al., 1982)

Underlying the accumulation therein of Methacrylyl CoA and conjugates, are profound structural anomalies of the brain, including *agenesis of corpus callosum and cingulate gyrus*. In one such *hypotonic* infant (McKusick 27708), the multiple malformations included dysmorphic facial features, vertebral anomalies and failure to thrive with poor feeding. It is of challenging pathogenetic significance that *exposure of pregnant rats to methacrylate* has reproduced the same anatomical anomalies in the progeny.

# Maple Syrup Disorder: Late onset episodic variant

Although the deficiency of the branched-chain ketoacid decarboxylase appears to be relatively less, the affected infants manifest intermittent attacks lasting several days of acute or subacute neurological disorder. Essentially this is expressed in mental confusion, lethargy to coma, and attended by repetitive vomiting followed by *intense ataxia* during recovery, a sequence comparable to acute attacks of hyperammonaemia precipitated by protein or amino acid. There is concurrent elevation of branched-chain amino acids and keto acids, valine, leucine, isoleucine and their keto acids in blood and urine. Accompanying this is an accentuation of the characteristic maple syrup odour of skin, sweat and urine during these episodes.

A large protein intake, or a surgical operation may induce such an attack apart from intercurrent febrile illness.

Underlying this disorder, a deficiency can be defined in leucocytes and cultured fibroblasts of the branched-chain keto acid decarboxylase. Other inherited disorders of branched-chain amino acid catabolism may be responsible for intermittent episodes of metabolic acidosis attended by severe neurological upset, although tending to occur later in life. This may include coma, but again *ataxia* is prominent and associated with involuntary choreo-athetoid movements. Such disorders include methylmalonic aciduria, isovaleric aciduria, β-methyl crotonylglycinuria and propionic acidaemia. The pathognomonic odour of the urine (like sweaty feet) distinguishes attacks of isovaleric aciduria and β-methyl crotonglycinuria.

# Tryptophanuria

*Cerebellar ataxia* has also been associated with dwarfism and mental retardation in tryptophanuria (Tada et al., 1963). A photosensitive dermatitis is also characteristic, rather like that in the Cockayne dwarf syndrome, or in porphyria and Sjögren's syndrome.

# Carbohydrate-Deficient Glycoprotein Syndrome associated with Hypoplasia of Segments of Cerebellar

Hypotonia in infancy and cerebellar ataxia in childhood characterized a brother and sister of 7 and 5 years respectively reported by Heckmatt et al. (1993). Independent walking had not been attained and there was also severe convergent squints bilaterally, although without intellectual maldevelopment. Neuroimaging had identified cerebellar hypoplasia established by more recent higher resolution

MRI to be *hypoplasia of the vermis* and *peduncles*, together with some *hypoplasia of the cerebellar hemispheres*, a small pons and mesencephalon.

It is of challenging significance that in addition there was an underlying familial metabolic disorder, "a carbohydrate-deficient glycoprotein syndrome". This was diagnosed on the basis of abnormal transferring electrophoresis. Although a severe neonatal onset variant of this disorder has already been recorded in Britain, examples of a less severe variant,

akin to the disorder in these children, have previously emerged in Belgium and Scandinavia.

To what extent this metabolic disorder contributes to and accentuates the ataxia is by no means clear. Such congenital defects of cerebellar vermis, peduncles and hemispheres should suffice to explain the disorder of balance, as it has done in two cases personally studied in the Hornsey (London) Centre for Cerebral Palsied Children (Russell and Lingam, 1993).

## Mitochondrial Cytopathy of Respiratory Chain Enzymes

Some examples of this mitochondrial myopathic category have revealed defects in one or more of the respiratory chain enzymes. Such underlying defects of Complexes I, II, III and IV are gradually being identified, especially by the Turnbull team from Newcastle. His most recent data includes 50 patients with respiratory chain disorders. Recently, deficiency of Complex III of the respiratory chain was diagnosed on the basis of muscle biopsy material in three children presenting within 36 hours of birth (Morris, Taylor, Birch-Machin and Turnbull, 1993) with already evident growth retardation and birth-weight below the 3rd centile (1.83-2.02 kg), hypoglycaemia, lactic acidosis with lactate levels reaching 3.1, 13.8 and 25 mM, and the Fanconi syndrome and proximal renal tubular acidosis. One infant in whom Complex III activity proved to be 37% of control values died after developing dystonic posturing and seizures. Treatment with menadione and ascorbic acid was ineffectual in all three infants. Usually these are demonstrable in electron microscopy of

muscle biopsy material (Clark et al., 1983), their cytochromes embodying iron-porphyrin prosthetic groups that undergo oxidation and reduction by release and uptake of electrons.

Defects thereof interfere with the transport of protons across mitochondrial membranes. The resultant very high lactic acidaemia is linked to severe lactic acidosis. Clinical consequences again include *ataxia*, which is transitory or progressive, movement disorder, developmental delay interrupted frequently by myoclonic spasms, seizures, and sudden infant death. Deafness is also chronically progressive. A maternal pattern of inheritance has been recognized, and is considered an index for suspicion of a mitochondrial enzyme defect.

Another kindred group of lactic acidaemic infants are typically overwhelmed in the floppy hypotonic neonatal phase by acidosis associated with severe muscle *Cytochrome oxidase* deficiency.

## Kearns-Sayre Syndrome

A syndrome of chronic progressive external ophthalmoplegia, retinitis pigmentosa, defects including those of intracardiac conduction associated with multiple defects of the cerebral or peripheral nervous system also encompassing *cerebellar ataxia, pareses of pyramidal tract source*, and meagre musculature. EMG findings of a general myopathy appear, and characteristic *ragged-red* and special mitochondrial clumps with paracristalline inclusions, are also demonstrable in other organs.

*Growth deficiency* is often considerable. The earliest manifestation in the first year of life may be *ptosis, progressive paralysis of external eye muscles* and, in some, progressive facial paresis and decreased hearing for high tones. However, the simulation of CP may be strong with ataxia and spasticity being pre-eminent, apart from oncoming signs of congestive cardiomyopathy.

## Infantile/Juvenile Refsum's Ataxia

Some of this account is repetitive in this context, because of the association with Ataxia supervening upon the initial Hypotonia (Chapter 18).

In this autosomal recessive disorder characterized by accumulation of phytanic acid in the central nervous system and other tissues, there is an underlying deficiency or defect of phytanic acid hydroxylase. A progressive polyneuropathy is the major consequence, with failure of vision associated with tapetoretinal degeneration and later with cataract, also accompanied by sensorineural deafness. A high concentration of phytanic acid is found in both serum and urine, and the CSF protein is high.

In more than one third of over 50 such cases recorded, the onset is apparent before the age of 10 years. But infants with Refsum's disease have more recently been recorded, and have survived to the second decade although with profound cognitive deficit. They are able to walk, although there is early hypotonia, but the gait may be characteristically ataxic and broad-based.

Dysmorphic features may include epicanthal folds, flat nasal bridge and low-set ears. Hepatomegaly is found with underlying micronodular cirrhosis, so its impaired function is to be expected. Small hypoplastic adrenals found on autopsy have been documented. Of laboratory features, there is moderate reduction of plasma cholesterol as well as of high and low density lipoprotein.

No malformations have been defined in the brain to account for the ataxia, except for the severe hypoplasia of the cerebellar granular layer, and ectopic displacement of Purkinje cells in the molecular layer.

In four such infantile subjects of this disorder, hyperpipecolic acidaemia was

442

identified in association with defects of peroxisomal biogenesis, the peroxisomes being diminished or absent. This feature recalled both the Zellweger syndrome and neonatal adrenoleukodystrophy.

# INITIAL ATAXIA ENDING IN SPASTICITY

## Late Infantile GM$_2$ Gangliosidosis

This differs from the classic infantile forms in terms of its later onset, between 12 and 18 months, slower course, and incompleteness of the clinical neurological syndromes. The cerebral accumulation is of GM$_2$ ganglioside due to a partial deficiency of hexosaminadase A. The cardinal manifestations are an *unsteadiness of gait and frequent falling* which have been found to be due to a mild slowly progressive cerebellar *ataxia, ultimately ending in spasticity*. This is also associated with arrest of speech and regression of other higher cerebral functions, with frequent disconcerting laughing spells in some cases as well as the pathognomonic macular degeneration with macular cherry-red spots and a perifocal area of pallor. Minor motor or generalized epileptiform episodes and myoclonic jerking emerge quite early. Hexosaminadase assays in leucocytes or serum should confirm the diagnosis.

## Juvenile GM$_2$ Gangliosidosis

Clinically this disorder resembles the Batten-Spielmayer-Vogt syndrome, although more likely to have early visual disturbances and retinitis pigmentosa. Assay of Hexosaminadase A best resolves the issue. A certain amount of genetic heterogeneity has been established amongst GM2 gangliosidoses. The first to be appreciated was Sandoff's disease wherein deficiencies of both Hexosaminadase A and B is associated with a phenotype indistinguishable from that of Tay Sachs. A more indolent phenotype that has been referred to as juvenile GM2 gangliosidosis tends to have its onset at about 2 years of age with *ataxia and incoordination*. Speech is lost and the extremities also lose strength. Thereafter, mental and motor deterioration are progressive, moving through hypertonicity to eventually end in decerebrate rigidity. Seizures also develop and death ensues within 5-16 years. Although they usually do not emerge, cherry-red macular spots may develop as well as optic atrophy and retinitis pigmentosa. Amounts of GM2 ganglioside is increased in the brain but not to the degree found in Tay Sachs. Likewise activity of Hexosaminadase A is deficient, but not to the same degree seen in Tay Sachs.

Another type of patchy demyelination is accompanied by striocerebellar calcification in the Cockayne-Neill syndrome outlined later.

443

# PEROXISOMAL DISORDER

(Schutgens et al., 1986)

As subcellular organelles, peroxisomes are responsible for diverse functions including:

- *peroxidation*;
- *synthesis of plasmalogens* involving Acyl CoA dihydroxy acetone phosphate acyltransferase (DHA PAT);
- *Degradation of bile acids*; and

- *Breakdown of very long-chain fatty acids* by β-oxidation (Wanders et al., 1987).

In adrenoleukodystrophy, there is believed to be a defect of a single peroxisomal enzyme, whereas the peroxisomes are absent in some forms of the Zellweger group of disorders.

## Adrenoleukodystrophy (ALD)

This tragic X-linked cerebral demyelinating disorder is confined to males between 4 and 8 years of age. It is associated occasionally with hyper-pigmentation of skin and other evidence of adrenocortical degenerative disease which may culminate in adrenal crisis. In the precipitation such crisis, an extragenic or immune factor may be superimposed. This Addisonian picture may present first and only later develop full ALD signs. An alternative presenting form is as adrenomyeloneuropathy, a gradually progressive spastic paraparesis linked to adrenocortical dysfunction. *Its neonatal type* is clinically a very different disorder which presents with *profound hypotonia*, accompanied by several recurrent seizures (Jaffe et al., 1982). Extensive demyelination, hepatic fibrosis and adrenocortical atrophy are its principal pathological features.

This is a peroxisomal disorder wherein biochemical features are indistinguishable from Zellweger syndrome and pipecolic aciduria. Most of the *juvenile* patients

undergo full progression of the cerebral manifestations without the clinical symptomatology of adrenal insufficiency, although signs thereof may sometimes antedate the neurological manifestation... especially with intermittent vomiting and sometimes identifiable hypotension. Inadequacy of response to ACTH of the plasma cortisol or of urinary 17-hydroxy steroid levels would be useful criteria.

*Presenting features* in the older child, mainly if not entirely in males in the full-blown form, are typically behavioural. Inattentiveness, poor concentration and failing memory insidiously become evident in his school work. Loss of acquired skills in speech and other *difficulties in communication*, aggression or belligerence may manifest in outbursts. Homonymous hemianopia has also been noted. There may be transient horizontal nystagmus in the early phase of progressive visual loss ultil ultimately hearing impairment follows. Later, unsteadiness and incoordination become conspicuous and he begins to fall.

*A classically ataxic gait* may be manifest from an early stage or the child is merely stiff-legged as well as unsteady. Increased deep tendon reflexes and positive Babinski may be found, possibly alongside *hemiparesis* as an earlier finding. Dysarthria and dysphagia may soon be associated, and *seizures* have become more frequent later in its relentless course. Eventually it culminates in *spastic tetraplegia*. Repeated CT scans over time may identify a caudal-rostral progression of the demyelination. The neuropathy is progressive over months or years, ranging from 9 months to 9 years, to a terminal decorticate state.

Recognized recently as one of the peroxisomal disorders, the single peroxisomal enzymatic defect is believed to be lignoceryl CoA synthetase. Location of the gene is in the Xq28 position close to that for red/green colour blindness.

Histologically, the nature of the disorder is clarified by the characteristic cytoplasmic inclusions in large glial cells or macrophages of the central nervous system as well as in adrenocortical cells. Such inclusions may also be seen in Schwann cells, so that sural nerve or even conjunctival biopsies may prove to be diagnostic. In the adrenals, there are inclusions of one crystalline trilaminar form made up of long-chain fatty

acids. Although the cortex of the brain is apparently unaffected, large areas of grey to brown translucent tissue replaces the centrum semi-ovale, and bilateral symmetrical demyelination involves the parieto-occipital region. The peripheral neuropathy is basically myelinoclastic. Visually evoked responses from the occipital cortex are reduced. There is also a characteristic accumulation in cultured fibroblasts and muscle cells of very long-chain unbranched fatty acids which are saturated or monounsaturated, particularly C26:0, C24:0, but without any elevation of bile salt intermediates. A ratio of C26 to C22 fatty acids of 0.76 appeared to be especially useful in diagnosis. The basic defect appears to be in the oxidation of the very long-chain saturated fatty acids, with impaired production of $CO_2$ (Singh et al., 1981). Oxidation of hexacosanoic (C26) was 14% of that of the controls. A characteristic leukodystrophy is identifiable on both CT scanning and MRI, especially marked in occipital areas. The ACTH test is concurrently raised and the teraco sactrin test positive.

Until the dream of gene therapy becomes realisable, a diet low in both crucic acid and oleic acid which can restore the C26:22 fatty acid ratio to normal levels, is being put to the test.

## De Sanch's-Cacchione Syndrome
## (Xeroderma Pigmentosa Idiocy) (Shimasaki et al., 1978)

This microcephalic mental deficient child showing slow developmental and growth progress from infancy as well as

neurological dysfunction including seizures, is characterized by sun hypersensitivity together with flat wart-like lesions and telangiectases to epithliomas and atrophy. The male shows small testes and there is variable hypogonadism in both sexes, attributed to primary hypothalamic insufficiency.

Incoordination, ataxia and variable spasticity ultimately reflect the underlying cerebral neuropathy.

# ATAXIA OCCASIONALLY ASSOCIATED WITH CHOREO-ATHETOSIS

## Ataxia Telangiectasia (Louis-Bar syndrome)

In this autosomal recessive syndrome, growth deficiency may be prenatal in onset although more commonly presenting in later infancy. Likewise, *the progressive ataxia* becomes evident in later infancy, usually also attended by *an element of choreo-athetoid movement* as well as by dysrhythmic speech. Other abnormalities include the drooling, the aberrant ocular movements such as fixation nystagmus. The posture is stooped and the facies dull and depressed, although the child may remain genial and pleasant. The instability or dysequilibrium may seriously disturb ambulation.

The pathognomonic telangiectasia first becomes conspicuous on the bulbar conjunctiva, whilst later involving the nasal bridge, auricles and elsewhere. Their frequent respiratory tract and other infections are apparently related to the associated defect in cellular immunity. Thymic hypoplasia is accompanied by hypoplasia of tonsillar and adenoidal lymphoid tissue. Lymphopenia is therefore characteristic, with low to absent serum gamma 1-A globulins. Their general features are ascribed to the severe pleiotropic effect of these pair of mutant genes. There are significant analogues with Blooms and Fanconi syndromes wherein there is also generalized growth deficiency, skin disorder, and a predisposition to lymphoreticular malignancy associated with a heightened frequency of chromosomal breakage in cultured leucocytes.

# MISCELLANEOUS CONDITIONS OF UNKNOWN OR UNCERTAIN GENESIS ASSOCIATED WITH ATAXIA

Amongst these miscellaneous disorders of unknown aetiology, I have given fuller treatment to the Rett syndrome because it is relatively frequent in incidence, and is commonly confused at different stages in its course with one or other category of cerebral palsy. This will be followed by an outline of so-called congenital or genetically-determined ataxias.

# Rett Syndrome

This syndrome of progressive cerebral deterioration exclusively afflicts girls and simulates both the initial hypotonia and the subsequent spasticity of cerebral palsy during at least two of the four developmental phases described by Hagberg et al. (1983). When first presented by Rett in 1966, he had previously associated it with hyperammonaemia ascribed to ornithine transcarbamylase (OTC) deficiency in a detailed letter to me in 1964 after my introduction of this disorder in 1962. I questioned the association and some of the plasma assays of ammonium, and a score of years later the occasional association with OTC deficiency was confirmed (Hyman and Batshaw, 1986). However, findings compatible with a carrier state for OTC deficiency have also been reported (Thomas et al., 1987).

A four stage clinical model illustrating clusters of characteristics make up a pattern and staging profile over the years. Normal skull growth and development proceeds for the first 7 to 18 months, after which there is regression with a progressive loss of cerebral functions. At that stage the behaviour is usually misinterpreted as autistic. Loss of previously acquired language, and of previously acquired purposeful hand skills have preceded stereotypies of hand-washing with the hands held in front of the chest or mouth, tightly fisted when not engaged in these stereotypies. These and *finger-mouthing* or *tapping of their teeth with the fingers* are immediately recognizable behavioural phenotypes. Self-mutilative behaviour may be added, with biting of forearm or arm. At the same time there is no sustained interest in persons or objects, the facial expression is flat, whilst an empty gaze with a sometimes whimsical twist of smile has sometimes earned them a Mona Lisa epithet.

Any unfamiliar situation is met with disproportionate apprehensiveness, hyperpnoea or hyperventilation and profuse sweating. Breath-holding or repeated brief apnoeic phases are also characteristic, but only during wakefulness. Oxygen hypo-saturation may be the result.

Spasmodic plantar flexion is an early sign. Jerky *ataxic-like* movements follow, and are sometimes myoclonic. About one-third learn to walk independently, although half later lose this skill, the gait on a wide base being described as apraxic or without "central" organization. *Initial hypotonia* is variable, and typically with progress through all stages of tone from hypotonia to rigidity. Signs of pyramidal tract involvement are gradually elicitable, moreover including increasing tone, hyperreflexia, often bilateral Babinski and ankle clonus *progressing to spastic tetraparesis. From about 3 to 4 years onwards* major epileptic seizures emerge and these may take the form of tonic posturing with some clonic movements. It is not surprising that the label of cerebral palsy is sometimes diagnostically applied, although the pattern of developmental unfolding and the specific stereotypies should be unmistakeably distinctive.

Ultimately, contractures may result, whilst the earlier plantar flexion merges into

447

equinovarus deformation. Scoliosis is another ultimate deformity. Another undeniably distinctive feature of this syndrome was the gradual unexplained wasting or atrophy of the lower limbs below the knees. This becomes increasingly conspicuous with an underlying peroneal muscular atrophy and *late onset denervation* reflected in a mild primarily distal axonopathy of peripheral nerves. A lesser degree of this lower motor neuropathy eventually touches the median nerve and involves the thenar, hypothenar, and interosseus muscles of both hands.

Speculation as to aetiology has centred upon insufficient stimulation by target-derived neurotropic factors ("nerve growth factors") (Levi-Montalcini, 1987), or of transmitters allowing synapses and receptors to form and continue development during the period of brain plasticity (Barde et al., 1987).

Familial cases were rare in the excellent comprehensive study of 109 examples in Sweden by Engerstrom (1990). Two half sisters were cited by her and one with an affected maternal aunt. Two other sisters have been personally studied (Russell and Green, 1991). One had a particularly intensive, even stormy, presentation and died at the age of 2½, whereas her sister of 5½ years still survives in the third stage of Rett's natural history.

Although diagnosis is considered only tentative until 3-5 years, Engerstrom has constructed a very helpful clinical staging system to facilitate the characterization of the clinical pattern applicable to different phases of this unfolding disease from infancy to adolescence.

**Stage I.** Early onset "stagnation" stage

The onset from ½ to 1½ years is marked by developmental arrest, personality deviation and diminished play interest. Hand-waving is as yet non-specific and episodic. Skull growth shows deceleration. *There is initial hypotonia.*

**Stage II.** Rapid destructive stage of 1-3 years duration

Developmental deterioration with Rett stereotypies becoming conspicuous, and preliminary or concurrent loss of hand skills. Clumsiness and apraxia culminates in *ataxia.* Respiratory aberrations include hyperventilation, breath-holding and apnoeic episodes.

**Stage III.** *Pseudo-stationary* stage lasting from pre-school to early school years

Some stabilization but unequivocal mental retardation. Gross motor dysfunction with pyramidal involvement and *spastic paraparesis and hyperreflexia. Gait apraxia* is then especially prominent, as is jerky truncal ataxia. Epileptiform symptomatology may become conspicuous.

**Stage IV.** *Late motor deterioration stage*, with duration from 5 years to 25 or more

Some decreasing mobility with a severe multihandicap syndrome - wheelchair bound. Para to tetraparetic signs take over. *Increasing lower motor neurone signs* appear, and both scoliosis and trophic foot signs intensify. Growth failure is clear, but ultimately there is normal puberty. There is some perceptible emotional contact, but with a characteristic staring unfathomable gaze. Cachexia often develops.

CT scans may show cerebral atrophy and PET (positron emission tomography) after 2-oxyglucose injection (Wagner, 1986) has exposed strikingly *reduced activity in the parieto-temporal cortex*, whilst injection with 11C-N-methylpiperal which binds to D3-dopamine receptors in the basal ganglia produced a result at the lower limit of normal. More recent studies of mitochondrial respiratory chain enzymes (Coker and Melnyk, 1991) revealed low levels of cytochrome-C-oxidase and of succinate cytochrome-C-reductase.

An inconstant feature can be the Raye ambient of organic concomitants of propionic acidaemia in the urine, which can be reduced by treatment with biotin. Neuropathologically, there is a diffuse and progressive depigmentation of the *substantia nigra* which is recognized on electron microscopy with reactive and degenerative changes in the axons. Together with the PET finding, this may indicate abnormality in *nigrostriatal dopaminergic function*. The

cerebellum shows atrophy with focal loss of Purkinje cells and astrocytic gliosis of the molecular and granular cell layer, and gliosis and loss of myelin in the white matter.

Chromosomal studies suggest an X-linked dominant gene that produces the syndrome in females, but leads to a failure of implantation or early abortion of the hemizygous male foetus. It is also suggested that the occurrence exclusively in females is due to a mitochondrial mutation, the greater defect in the male zygote ending in embryonic death.

The mitochondria in muscles of four subjects of Rett syndrome indeed showed structural aberrations including swollen dumb bell shaping (Eeg-Olofsson distension, vacuolation and membraneous bodies) (Rush et al., 1989). On the other hand, Coker and Melnyk (1991) recently identified deficiencies of the mitochondrial respiratory chain enzymes in the shape of reduced cytochrome and oxidase-succinate cytochrome with reductase.

## Congenital and Genetically-Determined Ataxias

These were believed to be a relatively rare form of CP although recent estimates have reached 25-30%. They are characterized by incoordination of voluntary movement and impaired balance, with hypotonia already manifest in the infant. Some infantile examples may appear well ahead intellectually from those in whom hypotonia is accompanied by global developmental delay. Deep tendon reflexes

may be normal or slightly reduced, although association with complete absence of stretch reflexes may already be noted in infancy. The motor handicap becomes clearer as the child struggles to sit upright, or attempts to stand. Nystagmus and/or esotropia may also be present. The *non-progressive cerebellar form* or "cerebellar palsy" presumably present from birth, and unaccompanied by other CNS findings, is considered very uncommon. A primary degeneration of the granular layer of the cerebellum has been identified.

There may be a case for describing the mildest form of ataxic CP as *apraxic* when coordination is appraised as normal during standardized neurological examination, although there is impairment in the ability to carry out purposeful gross motor acts such as hopping or skipping. Subsequent difficulties with fine motor activities such as writing or doing up buttons may follow.

On the other hand, a high familial incidence of the ataxic syndrome associated with prenatal hydrocephalus has been described in Sweden (Hagberg et al., 1974). Of eight ataxics at birth, they recorded five as of hereditary origin. Amidst 188 patients with non-progressive ataxic syndromes, ten families were also described as containing two to three siblings affected with both CP and mental retardation. They considered autosomal recessive inheritance as the main genetic factor, with especial application to what they proposed as the Dysequilibrium Syndrome. The Joubert syndrome is included amongst other recessively inherited ataxic disorders (Bolthauser et al., 1981).

## Other Genetically-Determined Cerebellar Type Ataxias

This group is not valid to our differential diagnosis because they do not appear until late in childhood or more often in adolescence. Included are:

1. that of **Fraser, Sanger-Brown and Marie**, transmitted as a mendelian dominant trait, in which the legs are more affected than are arms and tongue. Optic atrophy, strabismus and characteristic pyramidal signs also present in some families. A relationship is therefore suggested with familial spastic paraplegia of Strümpet-Lorain.

2. **Lafora: Familial progressive myoclonic epilepsy and ataxia**
   There will only be brief reference to this cerebellar type of ataxia since it first becomes manifest at a mean age of 14 years. Its pathological involvement of basal ganglia is also of special interest.

It is transmitted as an autosomal recessive trait and in the associated epileptic form, manifestations are of both petit and grand mal forms. Optic atrophy also co-exists in some cases as in the first group, along with deafness. The large round basophilic "Lafora" inclusion bodies are found in the neuronal cytoplasm, with a predilection for the dentate nucleus, substantia nigra and other basal ganglia.

3. **Strümpel-Lorain Familial Paraplegia**
   This is an inherited neuronal atrophy of either autosomal dominant or recessive type. A bipyramidal syndrome, it only appears in later childhood and very slowly progresses over years, also embodying cerebellar ataxia and mild sensory loss. One of the parents may also reveal a slight difficulty in walking.

A problem in differential diagnosis as to whether this disorder represents a classical ataxic CP or is a specific genetic entity depends on whether the spastic paraparesis is stable or progressive. This may have to be reserved for a long time, the slow progression identifying a genetic background. Such a significant sequence marks (a) certain examples of Pelizaeus-Merzbacher and other types of sudanophilic leukodystrophies, or (b) the familial spastic paraplegia with leukodystrophy of Poser et al. (1957) or the familial spastic paraplegia linked to dementia documented by McKusick (1956) and in other forms of familial spastic paraplegia.

4. **Familial Ataxic Diplegia**
Another similar entity is also attended by deficient cellular immunity (Hagberg et al., 1970). The ataxia in hereditary metabolic disorder is also typically accompanied by *myoclonus* as a major clinical feature as well as by seizures of minor motor, generalized or multifocal type, such as in Bielschowsky's disease. The ataxia and seizures may be ascribed to the *intention myoclonus* (astatic seizures) or to the cerebellar basis.

## Periodic Ataxia (of dominant inheritance)

A challenging practical therapeutic measure has been presented by Greggs and colleagues (1978) in the dominantly inherited form of periodic ataxia. They found that *acetazolamide* was specifically capable of suppressing the paroxysmal attacks of ataxia.

## Ataxia associated with Hydrocephalus

Another ataxic syndrome may complicate hydrocephalus (Hagberg and Sjogram, 1966), with or without spina bifida. Most forms of prenatal hydrocephalus are associated with periventricular or intraventricular haemorrhage, but infections may also be implicated involving meningo-encephalopathy such as may derive from mumps or secondary to resorption of damaged nervous tissue. The intercurrent infection may complicate the last trimester of pregnancy to produce a membraneous *aqueductal stenosis* as a source of such hydrocephalus and even of hydrancephaly or holoprosencephaly. Another relatively frequent cause is the *aqueductal stenosis* underlying *familial X-linked hydrocephalus*. In the Bickers and Adams type, prenatal compression of the mesencephalon by dilated lateral ventricles is held to be responsible.

## Oculo-Dento-Digital Dysplastic Syndrome (Judisch et al., 1979)

Neurological dysfunction is mainly reflected in *ataxia*, and hyperactive deep tendon reflexes sometimes associated with *hypertonicity* of mild degree in the legs characterizes this autosomally dominant syndrome immediately distinguished by microphthalmos and microcornea, accompanied by short and small palpebral fissures. The nose is also conspicuously thin with hypoplastic alae nasi and small nares. *Hypoplasia of the dental enamel*, which may account for premature dental loss, and the fine, dry, sparse and slow-growing hair are other particularly notable features. Hands and feet display syndactyly, and there is midphalangeal hypoplasia or aplasia of one or more of their fingers and toes.

## Cockayne Dwarf Syndrome

*Ataxia* may be apparent early, accompanied by *intention tremor* and *titubation*. A *spastic tetraplegia* and extensor plantar responses may develop. On the other hand, the tendon reflexes may be sluggish, and evidence of peripheral neuropathy reflected in slow velocities of nerve conduction. Sural nerve biopsies have also revealed segmental demyelination.

With time there is loss of independent mobility. Deep tendon reflexes disappear. Neuropathic findings are those of an *extensive demyelinating disease* especially prominent in the cerebellum. Patchy demyelination is also found in the cerebrum, brain stem and spinal cord, as well as cerebral atrophy reflected in ventricular enlargement. Dense calcifications are seen in the basal ganglia and elsewhere. There is also evidence of pancreatic islet hyperplasia as well as of inactivity of the adrenal cortices.

Their combination of profound microcephalic dwarfism, with photosensitivity from infancy or early childhood expressed in scarring of their atrophic skin and unusual facial features with sunken eyes and large bat ears, retinitis pigmentosa and nerve deafness, is associated with grossly delayed psychomotor development and progressive mental and motor decline. Intracerebral calcifications, as revealed on radiography or CAT scans, are also characteristic, although predominantly affecting basal ganglia. Their IQ will ultimately be below 30. The stunting of growth is not usually appreciated until the third or fourth year, and the severe truncal dwarfism is characterized by relative or disproportionately long limbs marked by large extremities.

Their diffuse cerebral and cerebellar involvement is reflected in ataxia, tremor and, occasionally in *athetosis*, seizures and bilateral *pyramidal dysfunction*. But in addition signs of peripheral neuropathy sometimes complicate the clinical picture, with tendon reflexes abolished, amyotrophy and lowered conduction velocities.

452

Aetiology is unknown but the hyper-B-lipoproteinaemia and hyperinsulinism together with consistent glucose intolerance (Russell, 1962; Cotton et al., 1970) are of challenging interest. Defective repair of DNA after UVL radiation of cultured fibroblasts (Andrews et al., 1976) which showed a greater reduction in the ability to form colonies after UV irradiation (Robbins et al., 1976) also demands further in-depth study.

# Alper's Syndrome or
# Progressive Degeneration of Cerebral Grey Matter

It probably embodies several different sporadic and familial neurologic disorders of unknown aetiology characterized by intractable seizures and *myoclonus*. The underlying cortical damage with diffuse non-specific destruction of neurones sometimes earning the label of *spongy neuroglial dystrophy*, is analogous with that in the anoxic, ischaemic or postictal encephalopathies that have been closely associated with cerebral palsy. Another label, of "progressive infantile poliodystrophy", has also been applied, although true progressivity is difficult to demonstrate in the slow steady evolution of an encephalopathy marked by frequent generalized or multifocal seizures, even if sometimes exploding into status epilepticus.

Psychomotor development is slow and myoclonic jerks emerge either in early infancy, or typically during the second or third year of life. *Incoordination of movements* as a clinical expression of ataxia does intensify, and both mental and motor deterioration advances, with optic atrophy and blindness frequent. In some familial cases, damage has been more specifically focussed upon the thalamus and dentate nucleus, in addition to widespread cortical pathology. Late in the disease, evidence of liver pathology may also emerge, whether secondary to malnutrition or to anti-epileptic drugs, or as part of the primary disorder - especially likely in some of the familial examples.

# Hartnup Disease

Its autosomal recessive basis is a defect in renal tubular reabsorption and intestinal transport of a group of monoamino-carboxylic amino acids leading to a constant aminoaciduria, and to intestinal malabsorption and retention of these aminoacids, including tryptophan.

Reversible episodes of cerebral and cerebellar dysfunction most often include *cerebellar type ataxia* and psychological derangement, whilst a *pellagra-like skin rash* is characteristically the first obvious manifestation. In late infancy, or even in early infancy, the *red scaly rash* appears over face, neck, hands and legs and is accentuated by exposure to infra red rays or sunlight. Neuropsychiatric upset including emotional lability or inexplicable anxieties and fear or violent temper tantrums, etc., is precipitated by inadequate diet, or exposure to sunlight, fever or sulfonamide therapy. It

453

probably reflects defective absorption of tryptophan and other amino acids. *Cerebellar ataxia* is still the most prominent neurological sign. Asynergia, intention tremor and dysarthria may be severe but are always reversible. Vertigo and slumping, or "fainting attacks", are other occasional clinical features.

The free amino acids excreted in excess include alanine, serine, threonine, asparagine, glutamine, valine, leucine isoleucine, phenylalanine, tyrosine, tryptophan, histidine and citrulline, indican and indoleacetic acid appear in the urine, particularly after tryptophan loading. Dramatic improvement in the dermatitis and major neuropsychiatric manifestation can be achieved by daily nicotinamide therapy.

## Batten-Bielchowsky-Jansky Disease (BBJD): (Late Infantile Amaurotic Idiocy or Myoclonic Variant of Cerebral Lipidosis, Ceroid Lipofuscinosis)

An autosomal recessive disease of unknown cause. Potent neurological symptoms includes onset between 2 and 4 years of rapidly intensifying generalized or akinetic-myoclonic *seizures*, and *myoclonic jerks*, as well as a combination of intention tremor, myoclonus and cerebellar type *ataxia*. Generalized incoordination and tremor eventually ensue, followed by mental deterioration accompanying the frequently associated microcephaly emerging in rapid sequence. Its first manifestation is usually in the form of seizures of several forms, grand mal, petit mal and minor motor, including staring spells, and the akinetic or myoclonic seizures already referred to. These are often associated with irregular asymmetric generalized myoclonic jerks.

The course of the disease ranges from 4 to 8 years. Signs of corticospinal involvement are usually already evident, with *motor* disability particularly marked in due course. Speech becomes thick and slurred, and profound psychic regression proceeds towards dementia and mutism. The EEG displays a characteristic pattern of non-periodic diffuse bursts of spikes and slow waves induced by slow low frequency photic stimulation, and disorganized background activity. To explain the progressive visual failure, macular degeneration embodies varying types of discolouration and hyperpigmentation, sometimes akin to retinitis pigmentosa. In other cases, the picture resembles retinitis pigmentosa with chorio-retinal atrophy and attenuated vessels. Degeneration of rods and cones and pigmented neuroepithelium have also been recorded. "Atrophy" associated with degenerative changes or impaired growth, involves both brain and cerebellum, and embodies severe neuronal "loss" in cortex, basal ganglia, thalamus and cerebellum (granular and Purkinje cells). Relative microcephaly is thus to be expected, being associated with the impaired or arrested brain growth or "atrophy", accompanied by evidence thereof on ultrasonographic scanning.

Apart from the typical ultrastructural visualization of intraneurone inclusions, of diagnostic help in many are the findings in peripheral blood of translucent vacuoles in 10-30% of lymphocytes, azurophilic hypergranulation in a high proportion of neutrophils, as well as ultrastructural cell changes revealing typical neuronal and other cellular inclusion bodies in biopsies of conjunctiva, skin, muscle and peripheral nerves.

The course of the disease ranges from 4-8 years. The brain, and especially the cerebellum, is atrophic, with severe loss of neurones in cerebral cortex, basal ganglia, thalamus, and in the granular and Purkinje cells of the cerebellum.

In the *juvenile form of Spielmeyer-Vogt-Sjogren*, first manifest between 5 and 12 years, loss of sight associated with pigmentary macular degeneration is followed by impaired performance at school and a motor triad syndrome wherein *ataxia* is coupled with *polymyoclonia*, and *extrapyramidal rigidity* (a so-called "amyostatic parkinsonian state").

## Marinesco-Sjögrens Ataxic Syndrome

*Ataxia* of cerebellar type is linked to nystagmus, with the underlying neurodegenerative process especially severe in the cerebellar cortex. It is also associated with dysarthria and general motor impairment leading to severe delay and difficulty in walking. Muscular weakness occurs *with* or *without hypotonia*. The co-existing bilateral congenital cataract is a distinguishing feature. Mental retardation is associated with moderate growth deficiency.

## Biemonds Syndrome

*The cerebellar type of ataxia* is linked to nystagmus in this ataxic syndrome associated with brachydactyly. Other related anomalies are limited to short fourth metacarpals and third metatarsals.

## Congenital Hypothyroidism

Already treated or hitherto unrecognized congenital hypothyroidism may be the source of long-term neurological aberrations relevant to this differential diagnosis, including:

1. *permanent residual disturbance of motor function* (gross motor problems, disturbed fine motor skills, poor fine motor coordination and overall clumsiness), or

2. of *tone* (spasticity linked to hyperreflexia), or
3. of *movement* (intermittent choreiform), and
4. of *balance* (cerebellar ataxia).

The lack of $T_3$-triodothyronine, the active thyroid hormone may itself stem from primary thyroidal defects, whether of *embryogenesis*: agenesis, hypoplasia or ectopic dysgenesis; or of *atrophy* (possibly autoimmune), or *when goitre is associated* due to familial dyshormonogenesis, or iodine deficiency, or exposure to goitre genes. The relative frequency of some of these categories was estimated by Price (1981) to be athyrosis in 25%, ectopias 29%, goitres 29% and hypoplasia s (17%).

*Secondary* or *tertiary* forms derive from pituitary or hypothalamic sources respectively.

Of common long-term neuropathic sequelae of neonatal if not prenatal hypothyroidism, there is an increased incidence of spasticity as well as of intermittent choreiform and tremor. These manifestations are especially seen amongst those with significantly lowered IQ. But even irrespective of IQ, true cerebellar ataxia and other cerebellar disorders are frequent (Hagberg and Westphal, 1970)

# References

Abe K, Okamo M, Sasaki H. (1980) Phenytoin in elimination kinetics. Eur J Pediat 135: 69

Adams RD, Lyon G. (1982) Neurology of Hereditary Metabolic Diseases of Childhood. Hemisphere Publishing Corporation, McGraw-Hill Book Co., Washington, New York, London. pp 233

Anderson RM. (1973) Hypertrophic interstitial polyneuropathy in infancy. J Pediat 82: 619-624

Andrews AA, Barrett SF, Robbins JH. (1976) Relation of DNA repair processes and pathological aging of the nervous system in xeroderma pigmentosa. Lancet 1: 1318-1320

Barde YA et al. (1987) Brain-derived neurotrophic factors. Prog Brain Res 71: 185-189

Bolthausser E, Herdan M, Dumermuth G, Isler W. (1981) The Joubert syndrome. Neuropediatria 12: 181-191

Blass JP, Avigan J, Uhlendorf BW (1970) A defect in pyruvate decarboxylase in a child with intermittent movement disorder. J Clin Invest 49: 423-432

Brown GK, Hunt SM, Scholem R et al. (1982) B-hydroxyisobutyryl CoA deacylase deficiency: a defect in valine metabolism associated with physical malformation. Pediatrics 70: 532-538

Burck V et al. (1981) Neuromyopathy and vitamin E deficiency in man. Neuropediat 12: 267-278

Burri BJ, Sweetman L, Nyhan WL. (1981) Mutant holocarboxylase synthetase. Evidence for enzyme defect in early infantile biotin-responsive multiple carboxylase deficiency. J Clin Invest 68:

Clark JB, Heyes D, Buyrne F, Morgan-Hughes JA. (1983) Mitochondrial myopathies: defects in mitochondrial metabolism in human skeletal muscle. Biochem Soc Trans 11: 626

Coker SB, Melnyk AR. (1991) Rett syndrome and mitochondrial enzyme deficiencies. J Child Neurol 6: 164-166

Cotton RB, Keats ME, McCoye E. (1970) Abnormal blood glucose regulation in Cockayne Syndrome. Pediatrics 46: 54-60

Engerstrom Ingegerd W. (1990) Rett syndrome in Sweden. Neurodevelopment disability pathophysiology. Department of Pediatrics II, Gotteberg, Sweden

Greggs RC, Muxley RT, Lafiance RA, McQuillan J. (1978) Hereditary paroxysmal ataxia. Response to acetazolamide. Neurology 28: 1259-1264

Guggenheim MA, Ringel SP, Silverman A, Grabert BE. (1982) Progressive neuromuscular disease in children with chronic cholestasis and vitamin E deficiency.

Diagnosis and treatment with α-tocopherol. J Pediat 100: 51-58

Hagberg B, Sjogram L. (1966) The chronic brain syndrome of infantile hydrocephalus. Am J Dis Child 112: 189-196

Hagberg B, Westphal O. (1970) Ataxic syndrome in congenital hypothyroidism. Acta Paediat Scand 59: 323-327

Hagberg B et al. (1970) Familial ataxic diplegia with deficient cellular immunity. Acta Paediat Scand 59: 545

Hagberg B, Sanner B, Stern M. (1974) The dysequilibrium syndrome in cerebral palsy. Acta Paediat Scand, suppl. 226

Hagberg B, Aicardi J, Dias K, Ramos O. (1983) A progressive syndrome of autism, dementia, ataxia and loss of purposeful hand use in girls: Retts syndrome. Report of 35 cases. Ann Neurol 14: 471

Hardinge E, Matthews S, James S et al. (1985) Spino-cerebellar degeneration associated with a selective defect of Vitamin E absorption. New Engl J Med 313: 32-35

Heckmatt J, Keir G, Baudouin C, Orme RL'E. (1993) A metabolic cause of ataxic cerebral palsy. Abst. 19th Ann Meeting, Br Paediatr Neurol Ass, Institute of Child Health, London. p. 65

Hyman SL, Batshaw ML. (1986) A case of ornithine transcarbamylase deficiency with features of Rett syndrome. Am J Med Genet: suppl 1

Jacobs C, Sweetman L, Nyhan WL, Packman S. (1984) Stable isotope dilution analysis of 3-hydroxy isovaleric acid in amniotic fluid. Contribution to the prenatal diagnosis of inherited disorders of leucine metabolism. J Inherited Metab Dis 7: 15

Jaffe R, Crumrine F, Hashida Y, Moser HW. (1982) Neonatal adrenoleukodystrophy. Clinical, pathological and biochemical delineation of a syndrome affecting both males and females. Am J Pathol 108: 100

Judisch GF et al. (1979) Oculodentodigital dysplasia. Arch Ophthalmol 97: 878

Lapresie I, Salisachs P. (1973) Onion bulb in a nerve biopsy from an original case of Roussy-Levi disease. Arch Neurol 29: 346-348

Leonard JV, Seakins JWT, Bartlett K, Hyde J, Wilson J, Clayton B. (1981) Inherited disorders of 3-methylcrotonyl CoA carboxyl CoA carboxylatin. Arch Dis Child 56: 53

Levi-Montalcini R. (1987) The nerve growth factor. Thirty-five years later. EMBO J 6: 1145-1154

McKusick V. (1956) Hereditable Disorders of Connective Tissue. Mosby, St. Louis

Martin, Hurley. (1977) Am J Clin Nutrition 30: 1629

Matalon R, Michaes K, Stimpf D, Goodman S, Parks J. (1982) Lactic acidosis due to lipoamide dehydrogenase (LAD) deficiency. Improvement after oral lipoic acid. Am J Hum Genet 33: 48a

Morris A, Taylor R, Birch-Machin M, Turnbull DM. (1993) Neonatal Fanconi syndrome and lactic acidosis due to deficiency of complex III of the respiratory chain. Proc 65th Ann Conf BPA, Coventry. p. 85

Norman RM, Tingey AH. (1963) Sudanophil leukodystrophy and Pelizaeus-Meizbacher disease. In: J. Folchi-Pi and H. Bauer (Eds) Brain Lipids Lipoproteins and Leukodystrophies. Elsevier, Amsterdam. pp 169-184

Nyhan WL, Sakath NO. (1987) Diagnosis and Recognition of Genetic Disease. Lea and Febiger, Philadelphia. p. 223

Packman S et al. (1982) Prenatal treatment of biotin-responsive multiple carboxylase deficiency. Lancet 1: 1435

Poser CM, De Wolf A, Van Bogaert L. (1957) Atypical cerebellar degeneration associated witih leukodystrophy. J Neuropathol Exp Neurol 16: 209-237

Price DA, Ehlich RM, Walfish PG. (1981) Congenital hypothyroidism: Clinical and laboratory characteristics in infants detected by neonatal screening. Arch Dis Child 56: 845-851

Rayner RJ, Doron R, Roussomis SH. (1993) Isolated vitamin E deficiency and progressive ataxia. Arch Dis Child 69: 602-603

Robbins JH, Kraemer KH, Andrews AD. (1976) Inherited DNA repair defects in homo sapiens. In: Biology of Radiation Carcinogenesis. Eds. Yuhas JM, Tennant RW and Regan JD. Raven Press, New York. pp 115-127

Robinson BH, Sherwood WG. (1984) Lactic acidaemia: the prevalence of pyruvate decarboxylase deficiency. J Inherited Metabolic Dis

Rush A, Kurczynski TW, Velaseeo ME. (1989) Mitochondrial alteration in Rett syndrome. Pediat Neurol 5: 320-323

Russell A. (1962) Consistent glucose intolerance in the Cockayne-Neil dwarf syndrome. Derived from unpublished data. Subjects of Neill and Dingwall, Archs Dis Child (1950) 25, 123, 213-221

Russell A, Levin B, Oberholzer VG et al. (1962) Hyperammonaemia: instance of an inborn enzymatic defect of the biosynthesis of urea. Lancet ii: 699-700

Russell A, Green S. (1991) A rare presentation of two sisters suffering from Rett syndrome of differing intensity. Unpublished observations

Russell A, Levin B. (1967) Treatment of hyperammonemia. Am J Dis Child 113: 142

Russell A, Lingam S. (1992) Hereditary cerebellar ataxia with pathology identifiable in atrophy of the vermis by CT scanning. Unpublished data

Schwarz WJ, Hutchinson AT, Berg BO. (1981) Computerized tomography in Leigh's disease. Ann Neurol 10: 268

Shih VE, Efron ML, Moser HW. (1969) Hyperornithinemia and homocitrullinuria with ammonia intoxication, myoclonic seizures and mental retardation. Am J Dis Child 17: 83-92

Singh L, Moser HW, Moser AB, Kishimoto Y. (1981) Adrenoleucodystrophy: Impaired oxidation of long chain fatty acids in cultured skin fibroblasts and adrenal cortex. Biochem Biophys Res Commun 102: 1223

Shimasaki M et al. (1978) Three cases of De Sanchs-Cacchione syndrome with endocrinological abnormalities. Acta Paediatr Jap 20: 100

Sjögren T, Larsson T. (1957) Oligophrenia in combination with congenital ichthyosis and spastic disorders. Acta Psychiatr Scand 32: suppl 113; 1

Spielberg SP, Gordon GB, Blake DA. (1981) Predisposition of Phenytoin hepatotoxicity assessed in vitro. New Engl J Med 305: 722

Tada K, Ito H, Wada Y, Arakawa T. (1963) Congenital tryptophanuria with dwarfism. Tohoku J Exp Med 80: 118

Thomas S, Hyelon M, Oberholzer V, Brett EM, Wilson J. (1987) Retts syndrome and OTC deficiency. Lancet 2: 1330-1331

van Bogaert L. (1970) Familial type orthochromatic leukodystrophies. In: PJ Vinken and CW Bruyn (eds) Handbook of Clinical Neurologgy. N. Holland, Amsterdam. Vol. 10, pp 120-128

Wagner HN Jr. (1986) Rett syndrome. Positron Emission Tomography (PET) studies. Am J Med Genet suppl 1: 211

Wanders RJA et al. (1987) X-linked adrenoleukodystrophy:defectiveperoxisomal oxidation of very long-chain fatty acids but not of very long-chain fatty acid CoA-esters. Clin Chim Acta 165: 321-329

Wolf B et al. (1981) Multiple carboxylase deficiency. Clinical and biochemical improvement following neonatal biotin treatment. Pediatrics 68: 118

Wolf B et al. (1983) Phenotype variation in biotinidase deficiency. J Pediat 103: 233

Yatziv S, Erickson RP, Epstein CJ. (1977) Mild and severe Hunter syndrome (NPS II) within the same sibships. Clin Genet 11: 119

# 20

# SPASTICITY OR HYPERTONICITY, AND RIGIDITY

# AS A PRESENTING OR PREDOMINANT MANIFESTATION

[Although associated with Ataxia or
Choreo-athetosis in some metabolic situations]

### Infantile and Early Childhood:
### Progressive Genetic Encephalopathies

**General Introduction**

**Neonatal Hypertonicity**

**Nutritional: Initial or Persistent Hypertonicity, Hyperkinesia and Seizures**

Iodine-deficient Endemic Cretinism
Pyridoxine Dependency

## Early Spasticity with Ataxia Superadded Later

Late Onset Maple Syrup Urine Disease
Methylene Tetrahydrofolate Reductase Deficiency (McKusick 23625)

## Initial Transient Hypotonia, then Classical Spasticity and Occasional Athetosis and Tremor

Phenylketonuria

## Initial Hypotonia or Hypertonicity, then more Intensive Spasticity with Classical Signs

Hyperphenylalaninaemic Variants
Hyperammonaemia in the Urea Cycle Defects

## Early Hypertonicity/Spasticity with Pyramidal Involvement including Hyperreflexia, Clonus, Jaw Tremor, etc

Farber's disease (Lipogranulomatosis)
Early Infantile Gaucher
Organic Acidaemias
*Propionic acidaemia*

## Initial Hypotonia, then Severe Hypertonicity (Spastic Tetraplegia), and sometimes even Tremor and Rigidity

Krabbe's Globoid Leukodystrophy
*Initial hypotonia in Type I*
*Early rigidity or hypertonicity in Type II*
*Slow evolution of spastic weakness in Type III*
Purine Nucleoside Phosphorylase (PNP) Deficiency associated with
Immunodeficiency
Wilson's Disease (Hepato-lenticular degeneration) in Association with Tremor and
Stiffness
"Stiff Baby-like" Syndrome with Severely Diminished GABA in CSF

## Initial Hypertonia followed by Hypotonia

Trisomy 4p Syndrome

## Hypertonicity alongside a constellation of more Conspicuous Clinical Features

Hunter Syndrome (Mucopolysaccharidosis)
De Lange Syndrome
Sjögren-Larrson Syndrome
Smith-Lemli-Opitz Syndrome
Trisomy 18
Weaver Syndrome
Gillian Turner, or Fragile or X-linked Mental Deficiency Syndrome
Sturge-Weber Syndrome
Trisomy 13
X-linked Hydrocephalus Syndrome

## Developmental Regression, Degenerative, Anatomic or Other Disorders of Unknown or Uncertain Aetiology

Polycystic White Matter Degeneration
Severe hypertonicity associated with Callosal agenesis and Choroidal lacunae
      (Aicardi Syndrome)
        *Hypertonicity associated with Intracerebral Calcification*
           *(Aicardi-Goutieres Syndrome)*
Early Hypertonicity plus Optic Nerve Hypoplasia, Agenesis of Septum
      Pellucidum and Hypothalamic-Pituitary Insufficiency
      (Septo-Optic Dysplasia)
Kinky Hair Disease (Menkes Steely Hair Syndrome)
Alexander's disease (Leukodystrophy with Rosenthal fibre formation)

## Spasticity in Association with Multifocal and Polymyoclonic Seizures

Ohtahara Syndrome

## References

# 20

## GENERAL INTRODUCTION

Clinical *metabolic* entities in which spasticity and hypertonia are prominent clinical features at some stage during the first five to seven years of their natural history, are therefore relevant to the differential diagnosis of spastic diplegic or tetraplegic cerebral palsy. They are separable by their progressivity and other more specific clinicopathological criteria.

## NEONATAL HYPERTONICITY

Extensor hypertonus is the neonatal response to various types of cerebral and systemic insult. Apart from germinal matrix, PV and IV haemorrhage, and hypoxic/ischaemic damage, this may be a product of birth asphyxia, subarachnoid haemorrhage or raised intracranial pressure. Although clinical expression of metabolic upset such as hypoglycaemia or hypocalcaemia must be kept in mine, especially if accompanied by repetitive clonic movements with or without altered consciousness, more subtle or other manifestations of seizure activity such as eye movements and apnoea. It will be reflected in overaction of neck extension and head retraction. Other hypertonic sequelae include extensor-adduction of limbs, accompanying the hyperirritability, extensor tendon reflexes are exaggerated, and spontaneous or elicited clonus is sustained.

A range of metabolic disorders leading to early spasticity and hypertonicity which are progressive will be outlined in sequence. The possible maximal focus in such metabolic *simulation* of spastic CP with episodes of opisthotonus and even transient evidence of decerebrate rigidity has been suggested as mainly involving the brain stem in the hyperammonaemia attending inborn urea cycle defects.

# NUTRITIONAL: INITIAL OR PERSISTENT HYPERTONICITY, HYPERKINESIA AND SEIZURES

## Iodine-deficient Endemic Cretinism

A triad of spasticity (spastic diplegia), deaf-mutism and mental retardation. In this syndrome of organic neurological damage occurring in association with endemic goitre (Stanbury, 1972), severe mental retardation associated with deaf mutism and strabismus characterizes the *spastic diplegia* completing the clinical pattern of endemic cretinism attributed to deficiency of maternal iodine during human pregnancy. Its prevalence increased sharply in 1955 in the Jimi Valley, New Guinea. The meticulous experimental studies of Behnaw-Rassoli et al. (1991) exploiting prophylthiouracil (PTV) which blocks synthesis of T4, and extrathyroidal conversion of T4 to T3, demonstrated the profound effect of pre and postnatal differentiation and maturation in hypothyroidism upon the early growth of the neocortex in the rat pup. They were able to show that propylthiouracil treatment during pregnancy *reduced the normal increase in the volume of the neocortex and in particular of the neuropile,* as well as significantly reducing the numbers of both neurones and glial cells. Indeed the neuropile embodies the axons, dendrites, terminal processes and myelin sheaths of the neurones, so that the implication is that its reduced foetal volume on PTU treatment of the mother is an expression of inhibited arborization as well as of general maturation of neurones (Numez, 1984). Supplementation with T4 partially reversed this effect.

More specifically, parameters of cerebral functional development including subsequent assessments of motor and cognitive function, were positively influenced by *maternal T4* although not by T3. Iodine supplementation afforded by a single slow-release injection of iodine *before conception* would have prevented cretinism in the progeny. But its prevention cannot be achieved by iodine supplementation later in pregnancy, which indicates that *development of the foetal cerebral cortex is dependent upon maternal iodine status* via T4 synthesis in the mother, before *foetal* thyroidal function takes over. In exploring other members of an affected family or pedigree, cardinal manifestations of the syndrome without spastic diplegia or goitre may be detectable, especially deaf mutism and mental retardation.

Experimental results in normal rats also suggested that the initial population of neurons is established as early as day 5 after birth, so that a partial recovery in neuronal number had remained possible.

## Pyridoxine Dependency

In this vitamin dependency situation, adequate amounts of ingested and circulating Vitamin $B_6$ fail to function as a co-factor in the relevant metabolic pathway. Of especial significance is its influence in the intra-uterine phase. Convulsions may thus arise in utero, and at birth there is then otherwise unexplained evidence of intra-uterine distress in the shape of meconium staining. The more usual situation is an initial manifestation during the first few postnatal days by a triad of seizures, hyperkinesia and *hypertonicity*. Indeed, a *generalized spasticity* may be residual in later childhood. Movements may be jittery or tremulous, and hyperaceusis is excessive. Both the seizures and EEG abnormality can dramatically respond to $B_6$ administration at a 50-100 mg dosage level. As $B_6$ is a co-factor in more than 25 biochemical reactions, it is difficult to unearth the basic metabolic reaction responsible in this instance. But only 10-15% instead of 50% of $B_6$ is excreted as *4-pyridoxic acid* after a large dose of $B_6$, and recent evidence supports the thesis that *insufficient formation of δ-aminobutyric acid (GABA)*, the inhibitory cerebral neurotransmitter is the basic defect. The apo-enzyme, glutamic acid decarboxylase, appears to be abnormal and inadequate unless a large supplement of $B_6$ is administered. As much as 100 mg/day of Vitamin $B_6$ would be advisable if intra-uterine convulsions begin.

# EARLY SPASTICITY, WITH ATAXIA SUPERADDED LATER

## Late Onset Intermittent Maple Syrup Urine Disease (Branched chain ketoaciduria)

There is underlying defect of the branched chain ketoacid dehydrogenase, the second step on the catabolic pathway and major route for disposal of the 3 branch chain amino acids. As a result of enzymatic blockage, these keto acids accumulate to induce the encephalopathy.

*Spasticity* may be recognizable as early as five days of life (Russell and Statter, 1982) although this had led to equally early identification of the pathognomonic maple syrup odour of the sweat. A similar odour of urine as well as of the skin itself is well known. The condition is confirmed by urinary and blood excess of specific metabolite precursors of the branched-chain amino acids: leucine, isoleucine and valine.

During recovery from an acute episode of mental confusion, lethargy or coma, accentuated by repeated vomiting, *ataxia* is often pronounced. Some attacks are milder, with little more than a brief episode of irritability and ataxia. Such mild ataxia, however, may persist for several months.

During the attacks, leucine, isoleucine, valine and their ketoacids accumulate in blood and urine wherein the DNPH (Dinitrophenylhydrazine) urinary reaction is positive. A low leucine diet - once the plasma leucine concentration falls below 800 umol/l - can improve the otherwise persistent neurologic and mental signs. In dietetic monitoring, the goal is to keep this plasma leucine between 200-700 $\mu$mol/l.

Other inherited disorders of branched chain amino acid catabolism may produce, in addition to the neonatal dysfunction, intermittent episodes of metabolic acidaemia with striking neurological dysfunction expressed in *ataxia* and involuntary movements. Complications during acute episodes of hyperglycinaemia include methylmalonic aciduria. The "sweaty feet" odour of urine will emerge during attacks of isovaleric aciduria, B-methylcrotonyl glycinuria and propionic acidaemia (propionyl-CoA carboxylase deficiency). This is also termed ketotic hyperglycinaemia and tends to occur later in life. *Neutropenia* is also frequent.

Hyperglycinaemia is detected especially in propionic acidaemia and methyl malonic aciduria (*ketotic* hyperglycinaemia). The excess of specific organic acid and short chain fatty acids are detectable only by gas chromatography or mass spectrometry.

## Methylene Tetrahydrofolate Reductase Deficiency
### (McKusick 23625)

This deficiency is an example of interference with remethylation of homocysteine by 5-methyl tetrahydrofolate. Its clinical severity correlates with the level of enzyme activity in outlined fibroblasts. The most severely affected succumb in early infancy to convulsions and profound neurological involvement, hypotonia merging with severe spasticity. Mental retardation and spasticity also mark the less severe examples, who tend to die of thrombo-embolic complications, possibly as a sequel to the element of homocysteinuria. In the late onset form, a schizophrenia-like psychosis may predominate. ly affected. Indeed the clinical severity corresponds with the degree of decrease in methylene tetrahydrofolate reductase activity in cultured fibroblasts. Death may be the product of thromboses, probably related to the associated homocysteinuria.

# INITIAL TRANSIENT HYPOTONIA, THEN CLASSICAL SPASTICITY AND OCCASIONAL ATHETOSIS AND TREMOR

## Phenylketonuria

In this well-known inborn deficiency of hepatic phenylalanine hydroxylase whereby phenylalanine cannot be converted to tyrosine, the mental retardation and *initial "floppiness" or hypotonia*, is associated with blondness of hair, fairness of skin, and intense vomiting in early infancy, even to a degree simulating pyloric stenosis.

Another odour is characteristic of this disorder, this time "musty" or "mousey" and is derived from phenylacetic acid. An eczematoid rash is also consistent from an early stage in these irritable whining babies. Although neurological manifestations other than the mental retardation are not considered to be particularly prominent, it is nonetheless noteworthy that a third or more of the child subjects of this inborn error of metabolism have been described as manifesting "all the signs of cerebral palsy". *About 5% certainly show hypertonicity* and *a classical spastic picture* linked to pyramidal signs of hyperreflexia and bilaterally positive Babinski. This can be conspicuous enough to warrant a careful differential diagnosis. Another 5% solely produce mild neurological signs such as an unilateral Babinski or briskly hyperactive deep tendon reflexes. Seizures also occur in about 25% of these children, some of "Salaam" character.

Hyperactivity and behaviour problems are common, also marked by purposeless movements, rhythmic rocking and stereotypy. More precise *athetosis* and *tremors* have emerged in some cases.

# INITIAL HYPOTONIA OR HYPERTONICITY, THEN MORE INTENSIVE SPASTICITY WITH CLASSICAL SIGNS

## Hyperphenylalaninaemic Variants

There has so far been definition of at least three of these variants of hyperphenylalaninaemia which derive from inadequate availability of tetrahydro biopterin $BH_4$ resulting:

(a) in two variants stemming from defective synthesis of this co-factor in which there is a tendency to low birth-weight; or

(b) defective recycling because of deficiency of dihydropteridine reductase.

Their progressive cerebral deterioration is accompanied by a much *more pronounced neurological disorder of movement and tone* than typically characterizes phenylketonuria.

Mild *hypotonia* or *hypertonia* tends to present after 2 to 3 months of normal development. The onset of a progressive neurologic "degenerative" disorder or developmental regression is *typically heralded by loss of head control* or a decline in activity, or convulsions recurring from 3 months of age.

There is *hypertonicity*, especially in the lower extremities. Even a rare episodic manifestation of *"lead-pipe" rigidity* has been claimed (Kaufman et al., 1978). Concurrently, there is *extensor posturing of the extremities* and *opisthotonic arching* of the back. Babinski responses are positive and clonus is often elicited. Dystonic movements may occur, and the seizures are predominantly myoclonic.

The simplest mode of diagnosis of these variants is informative in terms of a therapeutic trial of tetrahydro biopterin, administered at a dosage level of 2 mg/kg or 7.5 mg/kg. A prompt fall to normal of phenylalanine distinguishes them from PKH. In an early preventive approach, it is now proposed to assay biopterin, dihydropheridine, as well as phenylalanine, on spots of dried bloods on the cards used for neonatal screening.

Those with defects in $BH_4$ metabolism are to be treated with $BH_4$, using a regimen of biogenic amine precursors, including 5-hydroxytryptophan, DOPA and carbidopa, which do not require hydroxylation whilst the carbidopa inhibits their peripheral decarboxylation. Some children have been treated effectively with $BH_4$ alone. Even without $BH_4$, the combined form of therapy outlined above has led to progressive and exciting improvement. In particular, the myoclonus and involuntary movements have disappeared, and of even more dramatic import, their associated tetraplegia has been overcome. Concurrent monitoring of the CSF for neurotransmitter metabolites, and for the pterins including $BH_4$, could be a usefully objective method for assessing the efficacy of such therapeutic programmes.

## Congenital Hyperammonaemia in the Urea Cycle Defects

Its acute neonatal presentation with poor feeding and vomiting is especially characterized by lethargy. *Hypotonia* or *spasticity* may be cardinal signs from the outset. The irritability and twitching may culminate in convulsions followed by stupor to come, after misinterpreted as "collapse". Migraine-like headache, lethargy, seizures and periods of coma may also mark the more chronic courses, which may sometimes be interrupted by pulmonary or gastric haemorrhage, possibly precipitated by a high protein meal.

Within this group of inborn urea cycle enzymes, arginase deficiency runs an exceptional course... Although there may be a five-fold increase in plasma arginine, its urinary excretion is very variable, and may even be normal. Initially, in infancy, only minor symptoms of irritability and mild developmental delay may present, but over subsequent years *progressive spasticity* of the lower limbs and a mixed pattern of tremor, ataxia, choreo-athetosis takes over, linked to severe mental retardation. This intense although belated progressive simulation of CP is attributed mainly to the direct effects of the considerably raised arginine rather than to hyperammonaemia which appears to be the principal damaging factor in all these urea cycle defects, other than in arginase deficiency. Its deficiency in erythrocytes is still a valid diagnostic procedure.

Unlike citrullinaemia, argininosuccinic acidaemia or arginaemia wherein urinary or plasma excess of the corresponding amino acid can be diagnostic, recognition of carbamyl phosphate synthetase or of ornithine carbamyl transferase deficiency usually hinges upon finding hyperammonaemia and raised urinary or plasma glutamine. Elevated pyrimidine in the usrine, associated with an inhibited or blocked uptake into RNA (Statter and Russell, 1978) which serves to distinguish OCT deficiency from carbamyl phosphate synthetase deficiency and from N-acetyl glutamate synthetase deficiency.

Hyperammonaemia is found incidentally in a high proportion of neonates with a birth-weight below 2500g. That these are believed to be ostensibly asymptomatic should be regarded with caution since hyperammonaemia is also commonly a product of perinatal asphyxia, or even of some infections. Its later association with liver disease, Reye's syndrome, and many of *the organic acidaemias*, especially propionic acidaemias in which urinary orotic acid and uridine levels would be normal. Within each of these organic acidaemias, one should recall that hyperammonaemia arises within the first week or so.

Recent advances in prenatal diagnosis are of special moment in the OCT disorder. Probes for regions of the X-chromosone adjacent to the ornithine carbamyl transferase gene can now provide an early diagnostic technique by analysis of restriction fragmail length polymorphism.

# EARLY HYPERTONICITY/SPASTICITY WITH PYRAMIDAL INVOLVEMENT INCLUDING HYPERREFLEXIA, CLONUS, JAW TREMOR, ETC.

## Farber's Disease or Lipogranulomatosis

Histiocytic granulomas containing macrophages filled with PAS-positive material infiltrate joints, subcutaneous tissues and various viscera as a result of this inborn error of sphingolipid metabolism. The stored material is believed to consist essentially of ceramide which accumulates even in neurons, and is attributed to a deficiency in ceramidase (Sugita et al., 1972). Initial presentation is with *swelling and sensitivity of hands and feet* in the first few weeks or months of life, attended typically by a hoarse cry. Severe progressive arthropathy supervenes, with ankylosis as the end-point. Characteristic *subcutaneous nodules* embodying these histiocytic granulomata mark the dorsal surface. Dysphonia, derived from immobilization of laryngeal cartilage, appears either as early as the first month of life, or in late infancy. The laryngeal and pulmonary infiltration may extend later, however, to evoke severe dyspnoea.

Their hyperirritability and paucity of movement, considered to have a neurological source, may in part be traceable to the painful joints. But *signs of pyramidal involvement* with *hypertonicity* and *hyperreflexia* are typical, whilst severe motor and mental deterioration is a constant component, leading on to death within the first 2 years.

## Early Infantile Gaucher

This early neurological syndrome is due to a deficiency of glucocerebrosidase, leading to the accumulation of glucosylceramides (glucose-containing cerebrosides) in liver and spleen - producing the characteristically distinctive hepato-splenomegaly - as well as in other tissues including cerebral, leading to diffuse destruction of neurones. Psychomotor deterioration is soon followed by spasticity, neck retroflexion, dysphagia and oculomotor paralysis.

## Organic Acidaemias

In propionic acidaemia and other disorders of organic acid metabolism, apart from the Maple Syrup Urine Disease already outlined, *hypertonia* evidences within the first week or so of life, *but is accompanied by vomiting* and *lethargy which may progress to coma* associated with the severe ketoacidosis. *Hypertonus* may actually be the presenting feature in infants and children who have already displayed failure to thrive and occasional seizures. The influence of an *hyperammonaemic component* in this and related organic acidaemias, possibly superadding a characteristic hypertonic clinical expression, may also be integral to the urea cycle defects.

### Propionic Acidaemia

Propionate derives from several sources, about 50% from breakdown of the amino acids, isoleucine, valine, methionine and threonine. The mechanisms include about 20% derived from anaerobic bacterial fermentation in the gut, and about 20-30% from catabolism of odd chain fatty acids. Propionate production from the gut can be reduced by metronidazole, *removal of the propionyl groups* being augmented by forming propionyl carnitine with administration of L-carnitine orally or intravenously at a dosage level of 100 mg/kg/day.

Recurrent episodes of ketosis and acidosis associated with the lactic acidaemia typical of the organic acidaemias, lead to severe vomiting and dehydration. These are often heralded by ketonuria leading on to coma which is not infrequently lethal, and are the cardinal clinical expressions of propionic acidaemia. The underlying enzymatic deficiency is of propionyl CoA carboxylase.

*Osteoporosis* may incur pathological fractures. *Neutropenia* is regularly found, and stubborn moniliasis may also characterize this syndrome, as it does in methylmalonic acidaemia. The neurological impact may be considerable. *Intense hyperreflexia* is impressive alongside sustained *ankle clonus*. In one patient, clonus could be readily elicited by tapping the patella. This *spread of excitability* could

also be illustrated by clonus of the jaw on eliciting the knee jerk... Even *spontaneous tremor* of the jaw may be noted. The EEG is also abnormal, with bursts of slow activity and sharp waves. Mental retardation and microcephaly are apparent. Apart from *propionyl CoA accumulation*, ketotic or non-ketotic hyperglycinaemia is frequently associated. An unusual metabolite - *methylcitrate* - may be a reliable indicator of this disorder.

There is restriction of the intake of all amino acids, the metabolism of which takes them through propionyl CoA to the amounts required for growth and normal development. Addition of carnitine to their therapy at a dosage level of 100-200 mg/kg/day to overcome their carnitine depletion, has had a major impact on management. It reduces propensity for ketogenesis, and concomitantly better tolerates the catabolism of infections. Acetyl CoA, deprived of a substrate with which to condense to form citrate, would condense with itself to form acetoacetate. This could suggest another therapeutic tool, this time *aspartate*.

# INITIAL HYPOTONIA, THEN SEVERE HYPERTONICITY (SPASTIC TETRAPLEGIA), AND SOMETIMES EVEN TREMOR AND RIGIDITY

## Krabbe's Globoid Leukodystrophy

Association of this symptom with optic atrophy, deafness, and pseudobulbar palsy characterizes the rapidly progressive degenerative disease of the central nervous

system, due to a deficit in galactosyl ceramide ß-galactosidase. It is marked by *extensive demyelination of the central* and *peripheral nervous system* and is accompanied by heavy infiltration of multinucleated globoid cells within the demyelinated areas, the histological hallmark of this disorder. Extreme hardness or sclerosis of the white matter is the end-result. Spastic tetraplegia is the outstanding clinical manifestation. But three syndromes have been defined within *a cardinal clinical constellation of spastic tetraplegia, blindness linked to optic atrophy, deafness* and *pseudobulbar palsy* more or less rapidly supervening:

1. One manifest from the first weeks of life, is marked by hyperirritability, persistent and inexplicable crying, vomiting and persistent anorexia, whilst clenching of the hands or "fisting" is continuous, and the body stiffens whenever the infant is held. Seizures may be clearly myotonic. Brain and skull growth is diminished so that *microcephaly* supervenes. The initial *hypotonia* gives way to *spasticity*.

2. *The second syndrome* manifests later in the first year. After initially normal development, hyperirritability again becomes prominent with bouts of inexplicable crying or screaming emerging at about 4 months of age. Loss of head control becomes conspicuous, alongside *diminished movement and alertness,* also accompanied by *frequent vomiting.* Characteristically universal rigidity of the muscles then manifests, although in some infants this may have been subtly evident from birth. It intensifies progressively in limbs, trunk and neck, punctuated by tonic spasms typically provoking opisthotonic curvatures of trunk and neck. Indeed complete lack of head control develops. Vomiting is frequent, and aspiration pneumonia may result. Initially, pyramidal involvement is also exhibited in terms of the hyperreflexia and positive Babinski and Rossolino reflexes. The stiff lower limbs usually hyperextend in a scissor position with initially hyperreactive reflexes. But this is gradually supplanted by depression of the reflexes until they are absent, and in association with unmistakable reduction in nerve conduction velocities. The spasticity also lessens. Meanwhile, amongst early evidence of visual failure are pendular nystagmus and squints, with optic atrophy and blindness later in the disease. By 9 to 12 months, the child has become decerebrate, flaccid and hypotonic.

3. In the third variant, after several years of ostensibly normal neuro-development a slowly evolving spastic weakness of the extremities as well as pseudobulbar palsy are superimposed. Another expression of the slow involvement is the postponement of intellectual deterioration until after the seventh to eighth year.

CSF protein will be found to be particularly high any time from birth, ranging from 70 to 450 mg per 100 ml. Like metachromatic leukodystrophy, inclusions occur in Schwann cells on peripheral nerve biopsy. Partly in reflection of this, slowing of conduction in the peripheral nerves (Hogan et al., 1969) is characteristic.

## Purine Nucleoside Phosphorylase (PNP) Deficiency

This disorder of purine metabolism excreting urinary excess of purine nucleoside, is associated with an immunodeficiency embodying a milder form of T-cell dysfunction. Nonetheless, enhanced susceptibility to viral disease, particularly vaccinia, constitutes a constant threat. The basic deficiency of purine nucleoside phosphorylase (PNP) results in virtually absent uric acid production, with serum urate levels as low as 1 mg/dl. A comparable suppression of renal tubular reabsorption of urate and hypouricaemia is seen in xanthinuria, and also after excessive ingestion of drugs such as chlorprothixine. *Spastic tetraparesis* was the consequence in one such patient (Stoop et al., 1977).

## Wilson's Disease (Hepato-lenticular Degeneration) in Association with Tremor and Stiffness

In this autosomal recessive disorder of copper metabolism, the age of onset of symptoms is highly variable, although neurological manifestations do not usually emerge until the second decade of life. Most develop symptoms in adolescence or early adulthood. Nevertheless, symptoms may on occasion first appear as early as 4 years of age.

The elevated copper level in brain tissue presents essentially as a progressive Parkinsonian syndrome, so that of the two major groups of symptoms, gross postural and intention tremor is eventually conspicuous. The second major expression is a generalized rigidity predominately in the facio-oro-pharynx.

*Rigidity*, as an extreme form of hypertonicity, is thus classically associated with Wilson's Disease although its earliest manifestation is deferred until 7 to 10 years of age. *Flapping tremors of wrist and shoulders* are usually the major disabling symptoms, the rigidity and spasticity being relatively less marked, although certainly manifests in the young adult, alongside drooling of saliva, dysarthria and dysphagia. It was nonetheless considered appropriate to add this clinical outline. The selective tissue accumulation of copper, although decreased levels in serum related to deficiency of caeruloplasmin is concentrated in the lenticular nuclei, is also found in the substantia nigra, dentate nuclei, cerebellar cortex and in thalamic and mesencephalic nuclei. The pathognomonic clinical sign of the Kayser-Fleischer Corneal Rings, visible on slit-lamp microscopy from the earliest stages, made up of corneal copper salt deposition visible is a golden brown outer ring in the lamina propria of Descemet's membrane within the cornea, may be absent in childhood, and the accumulation of copper particles in the vitreous may not yet be visible.

Although neurological manifestations of this widespread deposition do not become apparent before 7 to 10 years of age, the clinical correlationships are of special

473

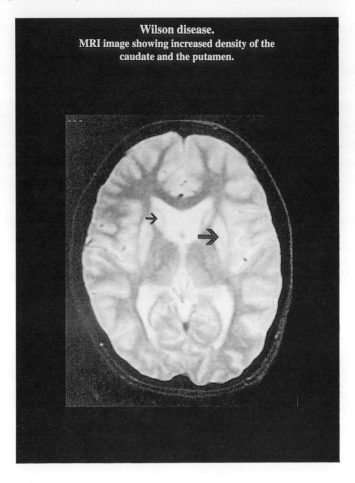

**Wilson disease.**
**MRI image showing increased density of the**
**caudate and the putamen.**

interest in this context. In the more rapidly evolving "Wilsonian" form of the disease, a facio-linguo-pharyngeal rigidity causes facial masking, dysarthria, dysphagia and *rigidity* of the limbs as the earliest motor signs. Where the disease is of slow evolution (the Strompell-Westphall pseudosclerotic form), tremor of one arm when the limb is used voluntarily or is held in a particular posture, is often the first sign. But as the disease progresses well beyond the age period relevant to this text, the rigidity becomes generalized and accentuated, with the extra-pyramidal syndrome expressed intermittently by tonic spasms, bizarre dyskinesias resulting in unnatural postures of the limbs which tend to disable, walking being difficult and falling frequent.

Peripheral nerve involvement is associated, with markedly slowed conduction velocities.

Although serum ceruplasmin levels and total serum copper levels are low, both copper levels in urine and in biopsied liver tissue are exceptionally high. Yet the precise metabolic defect is still unknown. But the locus of the disease has been mapped to Chromosome B13q14-q21. In consequence, it is now possible to identify the disease before the onset of clincial manifestations.

# "Stiff-Baby-like" Syndrome
## with Severely Diminished GABA in CSF

Although the dominantly inherited stiff baby syndrome is marked by muscle rigidity from birth, the ultimate outcome is good. It is analagous to the sporadic stiff man syndrome in adults due to autoimmune antibodies against glutamic acid decarboxylase which were not detected in the infant examples.

The muscle stiffness is accompanied by a fixed stare, flexion of forearms and legs, tightly closed fists, and myoclonic jerks. Sensory deafness and severely disturbed peripheral sensory pathways were defined neurophysiologically.

Extremely low levels of free GABA were exposed in the CSF (0 to 3, controls 30-40 nmol/l). Attempts to potentiate GABA transmission were unsuccessful.

Regardless of the system of physical therapy, a careful evaluation of primitive reflexes is an essential pre-requisite for facilitation/inhibition leading to enhancement of motor function.

# INITIAL HYPERTONIA
# FOLLOWED BY HYPOTONIA

## Trisomy 4p Syndrome

This trisomy for the short arm of Chromosome 4 is reflected in growth deficiency of prenatal onset with tendency towards obesity, is consistently associated with severe mental deficiency and disproportionate retardation of speech development.

The microcephaly also displays prominence of forehead, glabella and supraorbital ridges. The nose is bulbous with a depressed nasal bridge. There is macroglossia, a small pointed mandible. The ears are often enlarged with abnormal helix and antihelix, and the neck is short.

Camptodactyly of fifth fingersis accompanied by hypoplastic finger and toenails. Hypogenitalism is also evident with microphallus, hypospadias and cryptorchidism. The neuropathy follows an unusual course with hypertonia during infancy being followed by hypotonia. Seizures, with abnormal EEG readings, recur. An occasional cerebral anomaly may be agenesis of the corpus callosum, and there may be associated talipes equino varus and other anomalies of foot position together with pre-axial polydactyly.

# HYPERTONICITY
# ALONGSIDE A CONSTELLATION
# OF MORE CONSPICUOUS CLINICAL FEATURES

## Hunter Syndrome (Mucopolysaccharidosis)

The growth deficiency in this X-linked syndrome of iduronidase deficiency, and other now classical features, are first appreciated from 2 to 4 years including the gradual evolution of mental and neurological deterioration. Deafness is often undeniable by 2 to 3 years. Eventually, the spasticity is a recognizable component in this phase alongside mental deficiency and aggressive hyperkinesia. By then, the coarsening of the facial features, full lips and macrocephaly will be established, as well as the claw hand due to the excessive mucopolysaccharide infiltration of phalanges and the partial contractures and stiffness of joints, the inguinal herniation, hepatosplenomegaly, and even nodular skin lesions over the scapular area. My colleagues (Yatziv et al., 1977) have shown how both mild and severe examples of this clinical phenotype have appeared within the same sibship.

## De Lange Syndrome

Initial hypertonicity linked to prominent musculature is an unusual feature of this syndrome of severe psycho-motor retardation, with hypertonia sometimes severe enough to interfere with feeling. Microbrachycephaly is associated with short stature already evident at the time of birth, along with subsequent delay in bone maturation linked to some distinctive facial features such as the bushy eyebrow and synophrys, the long curly eyelashes, hypertelorism, anti-mongoloid slant, the small nose, anteverted nares, long or protruding philtrum and characteristic thin downturning upper lip plus micrognathia. Other stigmata include the hirsutism, the hypoplastic nipples, micromelia of hands and arms (69%) and of feet (99%), phocomelia and oligodactyly, the clinodactyly, and proximal implantation of thumbs (in 81%). Broad tubular bones are also characteristic, and flexion contraction of elbows occurs in 84%. The association with a Chromosome 3 duplication was described by Wilson, Hieber and Schmickel in 1978.

## Sjögren-Larrson Syndrome

Although the slowly progressive spastic paraplegia in this autosomal dominant syndrome first reported in a large Swedish pedigree (Sjögren-Larsson, 1957) is most marked in the lower extremities as in spastic diplegia, a subtle hypertonic element in the upper extremities would justify categorization as mild tetraplegia. The associated mental retardation is severe with IQs of 30 to 60, accompanied by dysarthria or monosyllabic speech, if any. But the most characteristic sign is the erythema of skin in early infancy progressing through scaling and hyperkeratosis to produce a *generalized ichthyosis*, except of the face. The lichenification with thickened ridged skin is most obvious in the axillae and neck folds.

## Smith-Lemli-Opitz Syndrome (Garcia et al., 1973)

A variable pattern of hypertonicity is associated in this syndrome, with moderate to severe mental deficiency linked to deficiency of growth already evident at birth. The narrow frontal area of the microcephaly with keeling and upheaping of the metopic sutures giving rise to a trigonocephalic pattern is especially characteristic alongside auricles which are slanted and low set, inner epicanthal folds, ptosis and strabismus. The nasal tip is unusually broad, nares are anteverted, and micrognathia is associated. At the genital level, there is hypospadias and cryptorchidism, and apart from a Simian crease, syndactyly of second and third toes is typical. The metopic craniostensosis has been especially emphasized in what has been described as the "Opitz Trigonocephalic Syndrome" (Cohen, 1986), when hypotonia was included.

## Trisomy 18 Syndrome

The *hypertonicity* is definable after the neonatal period in this second most common malformation syndrome. The incidence is around 0.3 per 1000 newborn, but it may already be expressed in the foetus by feeble activity. Polyhydramnios, a small placenta and poor growth at birth are further evidence. The significant degree of hypoplasia of skeletal muscle, subcutaneous and adipose tissue are supportive features of this syndrome (Butler et al., 1965). Craniofacially, there is microcephaly with a wide fontanelle (in 10-50%), the frontal diameter is narrow whilst the occiput is prominent. The papebral fissures are short, the ears low set and poorly formed. Micrognathia is associated with a small oval opening.

The clenched hand, with overlapping of the index finger over the third, fifth finger over the fourth, is a well known characteristic. Inguinal or umbilical herniation and/or diastasis recti appear, as well as a small pelvis. Equinovarus and rocker-bottom feet also appear in a definite proportion (10-50%).

In a smaller proportion, other significant neuropathy has been identified which might well have some bearing upon on the characteristic hypertonicity: paucity of myelination, microgyria, cerebellar hypoplasia and defect of the corpus callosum, apart from facial palsy.

## Weaver Syndrome (Weaver et al., 1974)

The hypertonic component is mild in this pattern of macrosomia or overgrowth, but delayed developmental progress is also involved here. The acceleration of growth and of bone maturation is of prenatal onset. The bifrontal diameter of the cranium is large, but the occiput is flat. Hypertelorism is associated, and the ears are also large. The philtrum is long and there is relative micrognathia. The element of limited elbow and knee extension can be differentiated from the hypertonicity.

Camptodactyly, broad thumbs, as well as broadness of the distal femurs and ulnae, and clinodactyly of toes are amongst other characteristic anomalies.

# Gillian Turner,
## or Fragile or X-linked Mental Deficiency Syndrome
### (Turner et al., 1980)

Increased reflexes in the lower limbs and the associated element of hypertonicity have been observed only as occasional abnormalities. The marker of the X chromosome on a fragile site at Xq27 is associated with another macrosomic syndrome, the birth-weight being already increased and the rate of growth accelerated in the early years. The head size is also above the 50th centile, and the shape is dolichocephalic. The early features can therefore suggest acromegalo-gigantism. A degree of prognathism is also consistent. Broadening of the nasal bridge extends down to the nasal tip, the large ears are characteristic, and likewise, the testes are especially large (macro orchidism) but with only a slight increase of testicular volume prepuberally.

## Sturge-Weber Syndrome (Chao, 1959)

This syndrome is made up of an unduly conspicuous compound of aberrant vasculature in facial skin apart from eyes and meningeal sites. The defect in a trigeminal facial distribution may certainly be harshly conspicuous. The ocular involvement may be of the choroid, with secondary buphthalmos and/or glaucoma. The arachnoid and pia mata, especially in occipital, temporal and frontal areas, are the main locations of the intracranial haemangiomata, which are strikingly demonstrable on radiography by their "double-contour" calcification which becomes visible by late infancy. The secondary cerebral atrophy also contributes to the recurrent seizures and the *spastic paresis* in over 30% of cases.

## Trisomy 13 Syndrome

Reference has already been made to this chromosomal syndrome under the heading of hypotonia (Chapter 18). It is true, however, that in a proportion of cases, less than 50%, hypertonicity either diplegic or tetraplegic may be an unequivocal feature.

## X-Linked Hydrocephalic Syndrome (Fried, 1973)

Spasticity, especially of the lower extremities is associated with this X-linked recessive syndrome. Whilst spastic diplegia is the principal mode of presentation, some more or less slight degree of hypertonicity of the upper limbs coexists, so that a mild tetraplegia could be the correct designation.

The underlying cerebral defect includes aqueductal stenosis as the basis of the hydrocephalus of prenatal onset, which may be so severe as to impede delivery. But other major defects may be superadded: fusion of thalami, small pons, absence of septum pellucidum, absence of corpus callosum and hypoplasia of the corticospinal tracts which may contribute very significantly to the spastic presentation.

# DEVELOPMENTAL REGRESSION, DEGENERATIVE, ANATOMIC OR OTHER DISORDERS OF UNKNOWN OR UNCERTAIN AETIOLOGY

## Polycystic White Matter Degeneration

The onset of *spasticity* and weakness in the extremities at 4 to 5 years of age, followed by mental regression, was described in one family by Adams and Lyon (1982). The underlying organic basis, with *cavitation of cerebral white matter* throughout both hemispheres, strikingly recalls the cystic cavitation of periventricular leukomalacia, especially associated with cerebral palsy in preterm infants. The slow progressive natural history over many years also serves to distinguish it from the cavitation of white matter characterizing Leigh's Disease.

# Severe Hypertonicity associated with Callosal Agenesis and Choroidal Lacunae
## (Aicardi Syndrome)

The two main anatomical components of this syndrome (Aicardi et al., 1965) are of cerebral malformation, *callosal agenesis* and *choroidal lacunae*. There is no microcephaly initially, but it appears in due course in one-fifth of these children. In terms of cerebral motor dysfunction, the principal manifestations are of *hemiplegia* or *spastic diplegia*, and other organic cerebral pathology akin to that in a high proportion of cases of cerebral palsy in its association with varying gradations of ventricular dilatation. The relative prominence of such neuropathic features is illustrated by their presence in 37 cases of a series of 125. In contrast to the cerebral palsies in which there is a male preponderance, and like the Rett syndrome, it also occurs exclusively in females [other than one phenotypic exception in a male with Klinefelter syndrome documented by Hopkins et al. (1979)].

*A severe progressive form of spasticity* amongst a wide range of familial encephalopathies of infancy related to *intracerebral calcification* has recently been defined as the *Aicardi-Goutieres syndrome* (Shillito et al., 1993). It may emerge in the first weeks of life. Consistent limb spasticity is associated with marked truncal hypotonia, abnormal eye movements and the development of microcephaly. No developmental progress follows and life terminates within a few years. Characteristic abnormalities with evident leukodystrophy is linked to the basal ganglia calcification. The CSF shows a mild lymphocytosis and raised interferon level.

# Early Hypertonicity plus Optic Nerve Hypoplasia, Agenesis of Septum Pellucidum, and Hypothalamic-Pituitary Insufficiency
## (Septo-Optic Dysplasia)

This complex and wide spectrum of neuro-endocrine maldevelopment appears as a source of early hypertonicity (spasticity) with pyramidal (ONH) involvement, optic nerve hypoplasia, agenesis of septum pellucidum and hypothalamo-pituitary insufficiency [neuro-oculo-endocrine dysplasia (NOEDS)].

A developmentally regressive form of CP-like condition is exemplified in this instance. Developmental delay is the commonest basic disability but superadded blindness and severe cerebral palsy are not infrequent clinical expressions. It is the consequence of a developmental anomaly of mid-line brain structures such as the agenesis of septum pellucidum (ASP) in addition to the optic nerve hypoplasia and hypothalamo-pituitary insufficiency. Outcome of the latter may include seizures with or without hypoglycaemia and hypernatraemia, as well as hypothyroidism of hypothalamic or central origin, i.e. without elevation of thyrotrophic hormone. Diabetes insipidus and deficiencies of adrenocortical function and of growth hormone may co-exist. Other clinico-metabolic expressions can include seizures.

The congenital malformation can give rise to progressive central nervous system damage and increasing handicap. The spectrum of defects thus ranges from an isolated lesion such as developmental delay, to which may be superadded low vision, short stature associated with failure to thrive, and to the other extreme marked by a severe multiple situation with severe cerebral palsy linked to mental retardation, epilepsy and blindness.

## Kinky Hair Disease (Menkes' steely hair syndrome)

This sex-linked disorder solely presenting in boys as a result of intestinal malabsorption of copper has already been outlined in the Chapter on "Progressive and Metabolic Sources of Initial and/or Persistent Hypotonia sometimes with Associated Disorders of Movement and Balance". *Onset is in the first three months* of life. Neurodevelopmental arrest marks the onset of clinical manifestations. There is failure of acquisition or rapid loss of smiling on the generally expressionless "pudgy" face, as well as of awareness of surroundings and head control. Even recurrent hypothermia is a later manifestation. Lethargy prevails with limited spontaneous motility. *Spasticity in the presence of pyramidal signs* is characteristic.

*Seizures* are an almost constant feature and often consists of asymmetrical myoclonic jerks. The corresponding EEG shows multifocal spike and wave activity.

Pili torti, or twisting of the hair shaft confirmed microscopically, is its hallmark. Hair growth is also typically sparse from the outset, with hair shafts poor in pigment, stiff, wiry and many broken to form a short stubble. The eyebrows are also twisted, and horizontal. Presumably the hair abnormality is principally due to the underlying copper deficiency, already referred to on page    in reference to the role of kinky hair disease in the superimposed manifestation of ataxia in association with spasticity.

## Alexander's Disease
## (Leukodystrophy with Rosenthal fibre formation)

Unique neuropathology involving the astrocytes (Rosenthal fibre formation) in this rare form of psychomotor retardation is

associated with progressive *head enlargement* from early infancy, even from birth (Garret and Ames, 1976). There is concomitant

481

failure to achieve motor and mental development from early infancy, with neither head control nor sitting up ever achieved. *Bilateral spasticity* is typical although the corticospinal damage may at first appear unilaterally. Rod-shaped or round bodies staining red with haematoxylin and eosin, and black with myelin stains, permeate the cerebral cortex and white matter. They predominate in subpial subependymal and perivascular regions. They closely resemble Rosenthal fibres which reflect degenerative changes within astrocytes. The second most prominent pathological change is diffuse demyelination or arrest of myelination.

# SPASTICITY IN ASSOCIATION WITH MULTIFOCAL AND POLYMYOCLONIC SEIZURES

## Ohtahara Syndrome

A rare association of early multifocal and polymyoclonic seizures with frequent desaturation requiring ventilation, and an EEG burst suppression pattern has been identified as the *Ohtahara syndrome* (*early infantile epileptic encephalopathy*). This has been known as classically resistant to all anti-convulsants although the efficacy of Vigabatrin (50 mg/kg/day) has been reported in similar cases (Chiron et al., 1990). The first revealed atypical polymicrogyria, and in the second similar child extensor hypertonus was evident at six months.

### References

Adams RD, Lyon G. (1982) In: Neurology of Hereditary Metabolic Diseases of Children. McGraw Book Co., 194-195

Aicardi J, Lefebre J, Lerique-Koechlin H. (1965) A new syndrome of spasms in flexion, callosal agenesis and ocular abnormality. Electroencephalographr Clin Neurophysiol 19: 600-610

Behnaw-Rassoli M, Herbert LC, Howard V, Pharoah POD, Stanistreet M. (1991) Effect of prophylthiouracil treatment during prenatal and early postnatal development on neocortex of rat pups. Neuroendocrinol 53: 321-327

Butler LJ, Snodgrass AJA, France NE, Sinclair L, Russell A. (1965) No E (16-18) trisomy syndrome: Analysis of 13 cases. Arch Dis Child 40: 600

Chao DH-C. (1959) Congenital neurocutaneous syndromes of childhood. III. Sturge-Weber disease. J Pediat 55: 635

Chiron C, Dulac O, Luna D, Palacias C, Mondragon S, Beaumont D, Mumford JP. (1990) Vigabatrin in infantile spasms. Lancet 335: 363-364

Cohen MM (1986) Craniosynostosis, Diagnosis, Evaluation and Management. Raven Press, New York.

Fried K. (1973) X-linked mental retardation and/or hydrocephalus. Clin Genet 3: 258

Garcia CA et al. (1973) Neurological involvement in the Smith-Lemli-Opitz syndrome. Dev Med Child Neurol 15: 48

Garret B, Ames RP. (1976) Alexander's disease. Archs Pathol 38: 379

Hogan GR, Guttman L, Chon Sin. (1969) Peripheral neuropathy in Krabbe's globoid leuko ursti. Neurol (Minneapolis) 19: 1094-1100

Hopkins IJ et al. (1979) The Aicardi syndrome in a 47 XXY male. Aust Paediat J 15: 278-280

Kaufman S et al. (1978) Hyperphenylalaninemia due to a deficiency of biopterin. New Engl J Med 299: 673

Numez J. (1984) Effects of thyroid hormones during brain differentiation. Mol Cell Endocrinol 37: 125-132

Russell A, Statter M. (1982) Maple syrup disease: presentation in the neonate. Unpublished observation

Shillito P, Stephenson J, Tolmie J, Hughes-Benzies R, Lebon P. (1993) Aicardi-Goutieres syndrome - two unrelated sporadic cases. Abst. XIXnth Annual Meeting of British Paediatric Neurology Assoc. Inst of Child Health, London. p.51

Sjögren T, Larsson T. (1957) Oligophrenia in combination with congenital ichthyosis and spastic disorders. Acta Psychiatr Scand 32: suppl 113; 1

Stanbury JB. (1972) Familial goiter. In: JB Stanbury, JB Wyngaarden, DS Fredrickson (Eds) The Metabolic Basis of Inherited Disease 3rd Edition. McGraw-Hill, New York. p 233

Statter A, Russell A. (1978) Competitive interrelationships between lysine and argenine in rat liver under normal conditions and in experimental hyperammonaemia. Life Sci 22: 2097-2102

Stoop JW et al. (1977) Purine nucleoside phosphorylase deficiency associated with selective cellular immunodeficiency. New Engl J Med 296: 651-655

Sugita M, Kulaney JT, Moser HW. (1972) Ceramidase deficiency in Farber's disease. Science 178: 1100-1102

Turner G, Daniel A, Frost M. (1980) X-linked mental retardation, macro-orchidism and the Xq27 fragile site. J Pediat 96: 837

Weaver DD et al. (1974) A new overgrowth syndrome with accelerated skeletal maturation, unusual facies and camptodactyly. J Pediat 84: 547

Yatziv S, Erickson RP, Epstein CJ. (1977) Mild and severe Hunter syndrome (NPS II) within the same sibships. Clin Genet 11: 119

# 21

# CHOREO-ATHETOSIS: DEFINITION, EARLY DIAGNOSIS AND NEUROPHYSIOLOGY

## General Introduction

## Progressive Disorders with Chorea, Athetosis or Choreo-athetosis as Cardinal Presenting Features

Congenital Lactic Acidosis

## Choreo-athetosis following Initial Hypotonia

Adenic phosphoribosyl transferase (APRT) deficiency
Dihydrolipoyl transacetylase deficiency

## Athetosis or Choreo-athetosis associated with One Other Disorder of Tone and Balance including Dystonia

Glutaric Acidaemia (Type 1) and Medium and Long Chain Acyl-CoA
       Dehydrogenase Deficiencies
Sulfite Oxidase or Specific Metalloenzyme Deficiency
Xeroderma pigmentosa
Syndrome of Choreo-athetosis, Dystonia and Pillidal Atrophy
Progressive Athetosis with Skeletal Dysplasia and Keraton Sulfaturia
Fahr's Encephalopathy or Familial strio-cerebellar calcinosis

# Choreo-athetosis superimposed on Hypertonicity or Hypotonicity and Mental Retardation

Familial Striatal Necrosis
Primary Degeneration of Corpus Luysi
Status Dysmyelinisatus Vogt

# References

# 21

# GENERAL INTRODUCTION

The positive symptom of involuntary irregular and arrhythmic movements may involve all muscles, although most affected are in the arms, neck, face and tongue. There is a profusion of such movement, even though alongside a relative immobility and impairment of postural control of the trunk.

Although there is evidence of *direct* damage of basal ganglia components, important *indirect influences* may stem from undamaged an uninhibited areas of the central nervous system, presumably from the cortex or other as yet undefined foci. Hence these abnormal movements are absent in early infancy before maturation of cortical function, or rather before myelinogenesis of the cortical-basal ganglia control loops is completed. Lack of inhibition from damaged components of the motor ganglia may then come into play. *The dyskinetic elements tend to appear first in toes and fingers*. These movements are most evident in supine or vertical positions and less evident when prone. They may be absent in repose, or when attention is deeply held, being accentuated by emotion, insecurity, startle effects or the desire to perform a voluntary act as in feeding.

Conversely, the child may remain motionless when they are in complete postural equilibrium. If not, there is often overactivity of tonic neck and labyrinthine reflexes. *Therapy could thus be focussed on defects of postural fixation.* Since they also remain motionless when their attention is fully engaged in watching television, one wonders to what extent intermittent video and teaching periods could be exploited during the daily programming of the Petö-inspired or other neuro-habilitative method.

The slow writhing fluctuant movement of athetosis, and the jerking involuntary movements of chorea, may each occur in relatively pure form in several metabolic encephalopathies, or there may be "fragments" of chorea and athetosis combined in more complex movement disorders. This metabolic category is rarely encountered before the end of the first year of life, mainly through 12 to 18 months of age. Probably this is mainly because the process of myelinization of basal ganglia circuits, and of their loops of cortical and cerebellar control interconnections, does not appear to reach completion until well into the second year of life.

# PROGRESSIVE DISORDERS WITH CHOREA, ATHETOSIS OR CHOREO-ATHETOSIS AS CARDINAL PRESENTING FEATURES

Whatever the category of cerebral palsy, a metabolic or degenerative basis or certain specific entities of unknown genesis would become suspect once it becomes clear that the cerebral dysfunction is *progressive* and is combined with other neuropathic manifestations.

*Kernicterus*, in which choreo-athetosis is one of the major neuropathic manifestations, was once one of the commonest causes in the West of the non-progressive state of cerebral palsy. Hypoxic-ischaemic or viral or other infective encephalopathy are displacing it, although hyperbilirubinaemic encephalopathy of other causation is still a threat. Whenever athetosis or choreo-athetosis occur without evidence of such antecedents, and is one component of a progressive disorder, a *metabolic* basis remains a possibility. *The Lesch-Nyhan syndrome* (congenital hyperuricaemia), in which ataxia may also be a feature, is a metabolic source which must always be considered in the presence of *typical auto-mutilations*. But these do not usually appear before the third year. There should, in any case, be an earlier overview in this perspective of all examples of choreo-athetosis in young boys or adolescents. Leigh's disease, some types of *familial striatal degeneration, Pelizaeus-Merzbacher, juvenile Nieman-Pick* and *Kuf's* form of *ceroid lipofuscinosis* can all induce choreo-athetosis in childhood and adolescence but *not* without other accompanying neurological signs, including ataxia...

The whole litany of progressive disorders simulating the choreo-athetoid category of cerebral palsy in some part of their clinical course has been listed and will be clinically outlined below. In each there will be specific emphasis upon the timing of onset, and duration of their clinical component of choreo-athetosis.

## Congenital Lactic Acidosis

This situation can be the result of a variety of genetically-determined enzymatic deficiencies with one common denominator theme, *chronic metabolic acidosis associated with hyperlacticacidaemia*. These include deficiencies of pyruvate carboxylase and decarboxylase, as well as Leigh's disease. The disorder may be acute or chronic in its course, with hyperventilation related to the metabolic acidosis. There is invariable association with neuropathy, mainly comprising seizures superimposed upon generalized *hypotonia underlying ultimate choreo-athetosis.*

Again, *consciousness is impaired*, especially during episodic exacerbations. Severe mental and developmental motor retardation is progressive, *and permanent choreo-athetosis may ultimately manifest*. In some infants, microcephaly is established, statural growth as well as head growth, being stunted. So much so, that *adiposity* may supervene because of a combination of inactivity and overfeeding. In addition to lactic acidaemia, associated *pyruvic acidaemia and hyperalaninaemia* have been reported. *Hypoglycaemic episodes* have appeared where there is coexistent fructose-1,6-diphosphate deficiency or even pyruvate carboxylase deficiency. Overall *failure to thrive* may ensue in some cases. The significance remains to be resolved of such an association of undoubtedly specific neurometabolic disturbance with one or more profoundly neuropathological structural patterns. These include:

1. *Symmetrical periventricular cysts in the lateral walls of the lateral ventricles* and near the fourth ventricle, adjacent to the hilum of the dentate nucleus.

2. *Spongy demyelination around the cysts* within the central white matter in both cerebrum and cerebellum.

3. *Seriously retarded myelination.*

4. *Pallidal necrosis*, which was superadded in two cases.

Excessive parietal wormian bone formation is also characteristic, apart from scurvy-like changes in the long bones. *Distinctive tortuosities* also mark the cerebral vessels, as revealed by angiography, as well as in some vessels of the limbs and trunk in which arterial occlusions have sometimes been found. Both *brain and cerebellum are atrophic,* and the brain shows *diffuse and focal lesions of ischaemic necrosis.* Atrophy in the cerebellum is of the granular layer. The *optic nerve is demyelinated* probably accounting for the clinical impression of blindness without obvious fundal changes. Whether these neuropathic changes are partly due to perfusion failure secondary to arterial changes, or to deficiency of copper and cytochrome oxidase remains to be determined (Danks et al., 1972). The very low copper content of brain and liver, but high in the duodenal mucosa, is in support of a basic copper malabsorption.

# CHOREO-ATHETOSIS FOLLOWING INITIAL HYPOTONIA

## Adenine Phosphoribosyltransferase (APRT) Deficiency

Marked *hyperlaxity of joints* with *muscular hypotonia* still manifest towards the end of his second year of life are the presenting features requiring differentiation from CP. Inability to walk without support continued until 2½ to 3 years of age when the hypotonia gradually lessened until by 2½ to 3 years walking without support may have been achieved. Otherwise, this recessively transmitted disorder is relatively benign except for urinary tract calculi composed of the very sparingly soluble products of adenine metabolism, 2,8-dihydroxyadenine. The gravel crystal and small calculi in urine may be identified from birth, and after nine months of age frequent episodes of renal colic are associated with dysuria and urethral pain.

Allopurinol 20 mgs/kg/24 hours (Barratt et al., 1979) proved to be effective in substantially reducing the excretion in the urine of 2,8-dihydroxyadenine, i.e. to about one third. In combination with a low purine diet, this succeeded in virtually eliminating 2,8-dihydroxyadenine from the urine.

## Dihydrolipoyl Dehydrogenase Deficiency

This so-called $E_3$ enzyme, *dihydrolipoyl dehydrogenase*, is associated with combined deficiencies of PDH, of 2-oxoglutarate dehydrogenase, and of branched-chain keto acid dehydrogenase, all three enzymes sharing the same $E_3$ enzyme. Such patients present within the first few months of life with delayed physical and mental development. A few examples have emerged with deficiency of the $E_2$ enzyme of the complex, dihydrolipoyl transacetylase. Severe mental and growth retardation becomes conspicuous by later childhood (Cederbaum et al., 1976). *Flexion deformities of the hands* were conspicuous, whilst *choreoathetoid movements* and occasional dystonia were also manifest. On a high carbohydrate diet, they may develop life-threatening acidosis.

# ATHETOSIS OR CHOREO-ATHETOSIS WITH ONE OTHER DISORDER OF TONE AND BALANCE INCLUDING DYSTONIA

## Glutaric Acidaemia (Type I) and Medium and Long Chain Acyl CoA Dehydrogenase Deficiencies

Glutaryl-CoA dehydrogenase and the three fatty acyl-CoA dehydrogenases (short, medium and long chain) are grouped amidst at least eight mitochondrial flavin-requiring dehydrogenases. (The others are specific for isovaleryl-CoA, isobutyryl and 2-methylbutyryl-CoA, Sarcosine and dimethyl glycine.) Their flavin electrons move to *electron transfer flavoprotein* (ETF) thereby reducing the heterodimers' single flavin to the semiquinone. In turn ETF reduces *ETF dehydrogenase*, an iron-sulphur flavo-protein incorporated within the inner mitochondrial membrane from which electrons pass on to co-enzyme O.

Glutaric acidaemia Type II or multiple acyl CoA dehydrogenase deficiency, rapidly fatal in the neonate is dealt with elsewhere under severe hypotonic manifestations.

It is not yet understood why such apparently specific degeneration of neurones in this disorder is confined to the striatum or the nuclei, but its implications are of vital importance. Firstly, Stocke, Goodman and Moe (1976) suggested that glutarate and glutaconate and ß-hydroxy glutarate are competitive inhibitors of neuronal glutamate decarboxylase, and secondly, that the concentration of glutaric acid, etc., in the brain of affected children approximates its $K_1$ on this enzyme within rat brain (Leibel et al., 1980) may also be a valid basis. Other possibilities are worthy of exploration:

1.  That glutaric acid may also inhibit the synaptic high-affinity uptake of glutamic acid; or

2.  That deficiency of the enzyme concerned may crucially interfere with the normal function of a specific population of neurones.

That the destructive effects may already be operative at *a very early prenatal stage* may also have wide significance in these progressive metabolic encephalopathies. It is important to realise that toxic changes were already identified (Goodman et al., 1980) in the striatum of an affected abortus at 22 weeks gestation.

The characteristic large head was already evident at or shortly after birth in 9 of the 11 patients studied and can be diagnosed prenatally. It preceded the subsequent neuropathic manifestations such as the acute illness resembling encephalitis which emerged in 7 of these children (Hoffman et al., 1991) after a period of normal development. All nine displayed athetotic features believed to reflect disorder of the basal ganglia, and two more specifically dystonic movement. Despite the macrocephalus, there was underlying generalized severe cerebral atrophy predominantly of the frontal and temporal lobes. This was clearly demonstrable in ten of the children through the medium of both computed tomography and MRI. The considerable total body production of glutaric acid expressed in the excessive plasma levels and excretion in urine and cerebral spinal fluid, and severe secondary deficiency of carnitine marked all these children. It has been claimed that a low protein diet complemented by formulae low in lysine and tryptophan, with supplements of riboflavin and L-carnitine, together initiated once the diagnosis has been made, can arrest further deterioration. Vigorous management of acute intercurrent infections also appears to reduce the frequency and intensity of recurring acute episodes. Patchy success has also followed restriction an intake of *glutarigenic amino acids*, e.g. lysine, tryptophan and hydroxylysine. Certainly this has reduced glutaric acid excretion, although the whole clinical course was scarcely influenced, probably because the existing cerebral damage appears to be irreversible.

A few children have nevertheless demonstrated remarkable improvement (Brandt et al., 1979) after a combination of riboflavin and lioresal (the parachlorphenyl analogue of gamma-amino butyric acid [GABA]), apparently attended by enhanced enzyme activity.

## Sulphite Oxidase or Specific Metalloenzyme Deficiency

This syndrome is worthy of note diagnostically even though extremely rare, because it represents another new category of neuro-metabolic disease expressed in choreo-athetosis. The high level of sulphite in blood is due to deficiency of sulphite oxidase. Combined deficiency with xanthine oxidase is somewhat more common (Johnson et al., 1980; Wadman et al., 1983) and is the result of a deficiency in a specific pterin (Molybdenum co-factor) essential for these molybdo-metalloenzymes. The clinical features of sulphite oxidase deficiency overshadow those of the xanthine oxidase defect. Manifestation *as early as the neonatal period* (Mudd et al., 1967) could be with feeding difficulties and a reduced level of responsivity, interrupted intermittently by seizures or muscular spasms culminating in opisthotonic contractures of the neck and trunk. Dysmorphic features are characteristic with slight abnormality of head shape and appear related to the co-existing cerebral and cerebellar atrophy. *Mental retardation* subsequently evolves. *Generalized hypertonicity* gradually becomes apparent although hypotonicity may less commonly prevail instead.

Another group of cases was reported by Shih a decade later (1977) with already established features: myoclonic jerks punctuating retardation of cognitive development, as well as episodic stupor and confusion. Even more significantly, *choreo-athetosis was superimposed. Subluxation of the lens* is also identifiable, as seen in homocysteinuria. Its neuropathology is characterized by cerebral atrophy with widespread *destruction and cavitation of white and grey matter* including that of the cerebral *cortex, basal ganglia* and *cerebellar nuclei.* Cystic lesions in the basal ganglia were indeed revealed at autopsy as long ago as 1955 (Harvey, Haworth and Lorber) or in 1968 (Rosenblum), although little attention has been paid to eliciting the mechanism of this specifically localized pathology, and the overt connection to be expected with the choreo-athetosis.

Both sulphite oxidase deficiency, and its combination with xanthine oxidase, are detectable by the urinary excretion of the hitherto unknown amino acid, *S-sulfocysteine* (1-7 mmol/g creatinine), normally neither detectable in blood nor urine. It is formed by interaction of sulphite with cysteine. Moreover its level in the CSF is virtually two-thirds of that in blood. *Plasma uric acid* and *cysteine levels* are very low but urinary taurine is increased. Over 50% of the sulphur in urine was in the form of *inorganic sulphate* (normally 75-95% in this form).

The high level of sulphite in blood is traceable to a deficiency of sulphite oxidase, one of the known *molybdo-enzymes* in humans which are dependent upon a molybdenum *co-factor.* Activities of both sulphite oxidase and xanthine dehydrogenase were undetectable in liver biopsy material. Not yet known, however, is whether this is due to inadequacy of dietary molybdenum, defective synthesis of the enzyme protein, or a specific intestinal malabsorption. In Mudd's child of early neonatal onset, it is significant that this enzyme deficiency was more complete. In therapy, two options may be accessible, either to increase the intake of molybdenum or lower the sulphur amino acids. Sulphite oxidase is measurable in cultured amniotic fluid cells so that primarily preventive prenatal diagnosis should be practicable.

## Xeroderma Pigmentosa (Hebra-Kaposi Disease)

The homozygotes present with unusually thin or atrophic skin, displaying hyperpigmentation, and a predisposition to keratosis and skin cancers (Cleaver and Bootsma, 1975). This has been ascribed to a freckling defect and deficiency of hexokinase required in the excision and repair of DNA damaged by UV irradiation. It is in the first years of life that actinic exposure produces an abnormal erythematous response of the skin culminating in blistering, and also of the conjunctiva leading to erythema and photophobia.

Clinical expression of the degeneration of the nervous system, as reflected in only one of five types, comprise *choreo-athetosis* and *motor incoordination* expressed as *ataxia*. Eventually corticospinal or pyramidal deteriorations manifest in *tetraparesis with spasticity*, and *extensor plantar* responses, paralleled this progressive development, including evidence of mental retardation. The EMG reveals denervation atrophy. Therefore, there may be some differential confusion with the various entities of CP, quite apart from the distinctive skin lesions.

## Syndrome of Choreo-athetosis, Dystonia and Pallidal Atrophy

This rare familial disorder characteristically (van Bogaert, 1946) begins between the ages of 5 and 15 years and manifests a mixed pattern upon which dystonic *torsion spasms* and *choreic movements are superimposed upon the athetosis*. Initially unilateral, it subsequently generalizes.

As in torsion dystonia, the facial grimacing and contortions of the mouth accompany the dysarthria and dysphagia. Gradual progression terminates in death after 5 to 10 years.

The underlying lesions are confined to the globus pallidus, with the pallidal atrophy attended by loss of efferent nerve fibres.

## Progressive Athetosis with Skeletal Dysplasia and Keraton Sulfaturia

This familial disorder affecting both sexes, has a slowly progressive athetosis to abnormalities of the vertebrae and femoral heads and corneal opacities identifiable

493

under slit-lamp microscopy. Urinary excretion of keraton sulphate is also found. As a result, the first signs are *kyphosis* and *limited mobility of the axofemoral joints*, but soon followed, certainly by the age of 5 to 7 years, by athetosis. The involuntary movements increase progressively and soon involve the facial musculature. It was presented as a new form of mucopolysaccharidosis by Maroteaux (1973).

The bony abnormalities comprise a platys spondylisis of vertebrae with occasional anterior beaking at the thoracolumbar junction and irregular flattening of the femoral heads.

## Fahr's Encephalopathy or Familial Strio-cerebellar Calcinosis

A group of slowly progressive familial encephalopathies are represented in Fahr's syndrome. These are expressed by various timings of onset of mixed patterns of movement disorder which have included *intermittent dystonia*, *cerebellar ataxia*, *chorea* and *athetosis*.

Calcification of the basal ganglia, in particular of lenticular and dentate nuclei, had been described well before Fahr's presentation (Foley, 1951). It has been regarded especially integral to Fahr's syndrome although it may also be found in certain calcium metabolic disorders of mitochondrial encephalomyopathy. In a comprehensive overview of 14 examples of such calcification by Billard and his colleagues in 1989, they categorized them into four groups of sporadic or familial basis:

1. In this group, the encephalopathy is accompanied first by microcephalic dwarfism as well as retinal degeneration linked to optic atrophy with a basic cerebral lesion in symmetrical patchy demyelination which has undergone calcification.

2. In this group, the children suffer from a congenital encephalopathy or cerebral palsy without the ocular and other abnormalities listed in (1) above. A sporadic non-progressive anoxic-ischaemic, or viral prenatal disease, without known genetic basis is proposed in explanation.

3. In this group, encephalopathy is also associated with microcephaly, but with another special feature, persistent cerebral spinal fluid lymphocytosis.

4. An autosomal dominant basis characterizes this fourth group which may occur with or without neuropathy.

# CHOREO-ATHETOSIS SUPERIMPOSED ON HYPERTONICITY OR HYPOTONICITY AND MENTAL RETARDATION

## Familial Striatal Necrosis

This progressive disorder first presented in five children between 2 to 6 years of age. First manifest by a gait distorted by rigidity of the limbs and pyramidal signs in some, athetosis follows, modified by superimposed dystonia linked to dysarthria and dysphagia. Important findings at autopsy were the necrotic lesions strictly confined to the caudate nucleus and putamen. In other sporadic examples in children and adolescents, a rapidly progressive neurological disorder with involuntary movements has been reported by Hawke and Donahue (1950) and by Bargeton-Frakas (1964) as the clinical expression of such exclusively *striatal* pathology.

## Primary Degeneration of Corpus Luysi

Bilateral choreo-athetosis with elements of ballismus were observed in two such cases of 5 and 6 years of age by Melamud and Demmy (1960). Mental regression and emotional lability intensified. At autopsy a selective degeneration of each Corpus Luysi was identified. In addition, a Wernicke-like spongy degeneration in the periaqueductal region and mammillary bodies was described, the pathology being postulated by them as a form of subacute necrotizing encephalomyelopathy or Leigh's disease.

## Status Dysmyelinisatus Vogt

Developmental delay and seizures followed by early manifestation of athetosis were first reported by Vogt and Vogt (1920). In two related children, one born at 7 months gestation the other at 8 months, profound atrophy of both pallidum and Corpus Luysi was found in both, attended by loss of medullated striopallidae and pallido-luysian fibres.

# References

Bargeton-Frakas E et al. (1964) Encephalopathie infantile familose avec necrose bilaterale et symetrique des corps stries. J Neurol Sci 1: 429-445

Barratt TM et al. (1979) Complete deficiency of adenosine phosphoribosyl transferase. Arch Dis Child

Brandt NJ et al. (1979) Treatment of glutaryl CoA dehydrogenase deficiency (glutaric aciduria): experience with diet of riboflavin and GABA analogue. J Pediat 94: 669-673

Cederbaum SD, Blass JP, Minkoff N, Brown WJ, Cotton ME, Harris SH. (1976) Sensitivity to carbohydrate in a patient with familial intermittent lactic acidosis and pyruvate dehydrogenase deficiency. Pediat Res 10: 713-720

Cleaver JE, Bootsma D. (1975) Xeroderma pigmentosum: Biochemical and genetic characteristics. Ann Rev Genet 9: 19

Danks DM, Cartwright E, Stevens BJ, Townley RRW (1972) Menkes' kinky hair disease: a further definition of the defect in copper transport. Science 179: 1140-1141

Foley J. (1951) Calcification of the corpus striatum and dentate nuclei. J Neurol Neurosurg 14: 251

Goodman SI, Gallegos DA et al. (1980) Antenatal diagnosis of glutaric acidaemia. Am J Hum Genet 33: 695-699

Harvey CC, Haworth JC, Lorber J. (1955) A new heredofamilial neurological syndrome. Arch Dis Childh 19: 96

Hawke WA, Donohue WK. (1950) Bilateral symmetrical nerosis of corpora striata: report of fatal case and reference to a possible syndrome of corpora striata. J Nerv Ment Dis 113: 20-39

Hoffman GF, Trefz FK, Barth PG et al. (1991) Glutaryl coenzyme A dehydrogenase deficiency: a distinct encephalopathy. Pediatrics 88: 1194-1203

Johnson WL, Waud WR, Rajagopalan KV, Duran M, Beemer FA, Wadman SK. (1980) Inborn errors of molybdenum metabolism: combined deficiencies of sulfite oxidase and xanthine dehydrogenase in a patient lacking the molybdenum cofactor. Proc Nat Acad Sci USA 77: 3715-3719

Leibel RL, Shih VE et al. (1980) Glutaric acidaemia: a metabolic disorder causing progressive choreoathetosis. Neurology 30: 1163-1168

Maroteaux P. (1973) Un nouveau type de mucopolysachoridose avec athetose et elimination de keratan sulfate. Nouv Presse Med 2: 975-979

Melamud N, Demmy N. (1960) Degenerative disorder of the subthalamic nodes. J Neuropathol Exp Neurol 19: 96

Mudd SH, Irrevere F, Laster L. (1967) Sulfite oxidase deficiency in man: demonstration of an enzymatic defect. Science 156: 1599-1602

Rosenblum WJ. (1968) Neuropathological changes in a case of sulfite oxidase deficiency. Neurology 18: 1187-1196

Shih VE, Abrams IF, Johnson JL, Mudd SH. (1977) Sulfite oxidase deficiency. New Engl J Med 297: 1022-1028

van Bogaert L. (1946) Aspects cliniques et pathologiques des atrophies pallidales et pallidoluysiennes progressives. J Neurol Neurosurg Psychiatry 9: 125-157

Vogt C, Vogt O. (1920) Zur Lehre der Erkramkungen des Striaren systems. J Psychol Neurol 25: 631

Wadman SK, Duran M, Beemer FA, Cats BP, Johnson JL, Rajagopolan KV, Krywawych S. (1983) Absence of hepatic molybdenum cofactor: an inborn error of metabolism leading to combined deficiency of sulphite oxidase and xanthine dehydrogenase. J Inherit Metab Dis 6: suppl 1, 78-83

# References

Abe K, Okamo M, Sasaki H. (1980) Phenytoin in elimination kinetics. Eur J Pediat 135: 69

Abrahams P, Burkitt BFE. (1976) Hiatus hernias and gastro-oesophageal reflux in children and adolescents with cerebral palsy. Aust Paediat J 26: 41-46

Adams RD, Lyon G. (1982) Neurology of Hereditary Metabolic Diseases of Children. Hemisphere Publishing Corporation, McGraw-Hill Book Co., Washington, New York, London.

Adlard BP et al. (1973) Effect of undernutrition in early life on glutamate decarboxylase activity. Biochem J 130: 12p

Ahman PA, Lazzara A, Dykes FD. (1980) Intraventricular haemorrhage in high risk preterm: Incidence and outcome. Ann Neurol 7: 118-124

Aicardi J. (1991) The argyria-pachygyria complex: a spectrum of cortical malformation. Brain Dev 13: 1-8

Aicardi J, Lefebre J, Lerique-Koechlin H. (1965) A new syndrome of spasms in flexion, callosal agenesis and ocular abnormality. Electroencephalographr Clin Neurophysiol 19: 600-610

Akopian AV, Pshel'la V, Khobba VD. (1988) Characteristics of cerebral blood flow in children with cerebral palsy during the dynamics of treatment. Zh Nevropatol psikhiat 88: 50-53

al-Rajeh S et al. (1991) Cerebral palsy in Saudi Arabia: a case-control study of risk factors. Dev Med Child Neurol 33: 1048-1052

Alberman ED. (1963) Birthweight and length of gestation in CP. Dev Med Child Neurol 5: 388-394

Alberman E. (1991) Personal communication.

Altman DS, Volpe JJ. (1987) Cerebral blood flow in the newborn infant: Measurement and role in the pathogenesis of PV and IV haemorrhage. Adv Pediat 34: 111-138

Amin-Zaki L et al. (1974) Intra-uterine methyl mercury poisoning in Iraq. Pediatrics 54: 587-595.

Ampola MG, Mahoney MJ, Nakamura E, Tanaka K. (1975) Prenatal therapy of a patient with Vitamin B12-responsive methylmalonic acidemia. New Engl J Med 293: 313-317

Andermann E, Palmini A et al. (1992) Familial bilateral congenital perisylvian syndrome: a localized neuronal migration disorder. Neurology 42: suppl 3, 354

Anderson JC, Mawk JR. (1988) Intrauterine arterial duplex Doppler wave form analysis in infants. Childs Nerv Syst 4: 144-148

Anderson LT, Dancis J, Alpert M, Herrmann L. (1977) Punishment learning and self-mutilation in Lesch-Nyhan. Nature (London) 265: 461-463

Anderson RM. (1973) Hypertrophic interstitial polyneuropathy in infancy. J Pediat 82: 619-624

AndreThomas AJ, Chesni Y, Dargassies SA. (1960) The neurological examination in the infant. Little Club Clin Dev Med 1. No. 1 (London) Medical Adviser Committee of National Spastics Committee

Andrews AA, Barrett SF, Robbins JH. (1976) Relation of DNA repair processes and pathological aging of the nervous system in xeroderma pigmentosa. Lancet 1: 1318-1320

Anthony MY, Levene MI. (1993) Neonatal cranial ultrasound. In: Recent Advances in Paediatrics. Churchill Linvingstone, Edinburgh, London 6: 85-102

Arens LJ, Molteno CD. (1989) A comparative study of postnatally acquired cerebral palsy in Cape Town. Dev Med Child Neurol 31: 246-254

Arens LJ, Molteno CD, Marshall SR, Robertson WI, Rabkin J. (1978) Cerebral palsy in Cape Town - a comparative 12-year retrospective study. S Afr Med J 53: 319-324

Ashkenazi CMV, Russell A, Zadik Z. (1972) Prevalence of cytomegalovirus complement fixing antibodies in Jerusalem and Rechovat Arcas. Proc Israel Paediat Soc. XVth Nattional Scientific Congress, Beir Harojeh. pp 12-13

Atkinson S, Stanley FJ. (1983) Spastic diplegia among children of low and normal birthweight. Dev Med Child Neurol 25: 693-708

Ayres AJ. (1985) Sensory Integration and the Child. Western Psychological Services, Los Angeles

Baker AW, Duncan SP. (1985) Child sex abuse: a study of prevalence in Great Britain. Child Abuse Negl 3: 565-575

Baker SP. (1979) Motor vehicle occupant deaths in young children. Pediatrics 64: 860-861

Barbeau A. (1984) Manganese and extrapyramidal disorders. Neurotoxicol 5: 13-36

Barde YA et al. (1987) Brain-derived neurotrophic factors. Prog. Brain Res 71: 185-189

Bargeton-Frakas E et al. (1964) Encephalopathie infantile familose avec necrose bilaterale et symetrique des corps stries. J Neurol Sci 1: 429-445

Barratt TM et al. (1979) Complete deficiency of adenosine phosphoribosyl transferase. Arch Dis Child

Bax M. (1990) Motor delay and cerebral palsy. Dev Med Child Neurol 32: 283-284

Bayley N. (1969) Manual for the Bayley Scale of Infant Development. Psychological Corporation, New York

Behnaw-Rassoli M, Herbert LC, Howard V, Pharoah POD, Stanistreet M. (   ) Effect of prophylthiouracil treatment during prenatal and early postnatal development on neocortex of rat pups. Neuroendocrinol 53: 321-327

Benson JWT, Drayton MR, Hayward J et al. (1986) Multicentre trial of ethamsylate for prevention of PVH in very low birth weight infants. Lancet 2: 1297-1299

Bennett FC, La Veck B, Sells CJ. (1979) The Williams' elfin facies syndrome. Pediatrics 61: 303

Beverley DW, Chance D. (1984) Cord blood gases, birth asphyxia, and intraventricular haemorrhage. Arch Dis Child 59: 384-386

Billard C et al. (1989) Encephalopathy with calcification of the basal ganglia in children: A reappraisal of Fahr's syndrome with respect to 14 new cases. Neuropediat 20: 12-19

Bishop DVM (1983) The test for reception of grammar. University of Manchester

Blair E, Stanley FJ. (1982) An epidemiological study of cerebral palsy in Western Australia. III: Postnatal aetiology. Dev Med Child Neurol 24: 575-585

Blair E, Stanley F. (1988) Intrapartum asphyxia: a rare cause of cerebral palsy. J Pediat 113: 420

Blair E, Stanley F. (1990) Intra-uterine growth and spastic cerebral palsy. I: Association with birth weight for gestational age. Am J Obstet Gynecol 162: 229-237

Blair E, Stanley F. (1992) Intrauterine growth and spastic cerebral palsy. II. The association with morphology at birth. Early Hum Dev 28: 91-103

Blashke TF, Birk PD et al. (1974) Crigler-Naggar syndrome: an unusual course with neurological damage at age eighteen. Pediat Res 8: 573-590

Blass JP, Avigan J, Uhlendorf BW (1970) A defect in pyruvate decarboxylase in a child with intermittent movement disorder. J Clin Invest 49: 423-432

Blass JP, Kark RAP, Menon NK. Low activities of the pyruvate and oxoglutarate dehydrogenase complexes in 5 patients with Freidreich's ataxia. New Engl J Med 295: 62-67

Bliss CK (1965) Semantography - Bliss Symbolics. Semantography Publications, Sydney

Bodensteiner T, Gay CT. (1990) Colpocephaly: Pitfalls in the diagnosis of a pathological entity. J Child Neurol 5: 166-168

Boesch C et al. (1989) Magnetic resonance imaging of brain in congenital cytomegalovirus encephalopathy. Pediat Radiol 19: 91-93

Bolthausser E, Herdan M, Dumermuth G, Isler W. (1981) The Joubert syndrome. Neuropediatria 12: 181-191

Booth JW. (1992) Silent gastro-oesophageal reflux: how much do we miss? Arch Dis Child Annot 67: 1325-1326

Bowley AH, Gardner L. (1980) The child with hearing loss. In: The Handicapped Child. Churchill Livingstone, Edinburgh

Bozynski ME et al. (1988) Cranial ultrasonography and the prediction of cerebral palsy in infants weighing less than or equal to 1200 gms at birth. Dev Med Child Neurol 30: 542-548

Brandt NJ et al. (1979) Treatment of glutaryl CoA dehydrogenase deficiency (glutaric aciduria): experience with diet of riboflavin and GABA analogue. J Pediat 94: 669-673

Breakey AS. (1955) Ocular findings in cerebral palsy. Arch Ophthalmol 53: 85

Breg WR et al. (1970) The cri-du-chat syndrome in adolescents and adults. J Pediat 27: 782

Brorson LO, Wranne L. (1987) Long term prognosis in childhood epilepsy: survival and seizure prognosis. Epilepsia 28: 324-330

Brown GK, Hunt SM, Scholem R et al. (1982) B-hydroxyisobutyryl CoA deacylase deficiency: a defect in valine metabolism associated with physical malformation. Pediatrics 70: 532-538

Bruininks RH. (1978) Bruininks-Oberetsky Test. Examiners Manual, Circle Pines, American Guidance Service

Burck V et al. (1981) Neuromyopathy and vitamin E deficiency in man. Neuropediat 12: 267-278

Burri BJ, Sweetman L, Nyhan WL. (1981) Mutant holocarboxylase synthetase. Evidence for enzyme defect in early infantile biotin-responsive multiple carboxylase deficiency. J Clin Invest 68:

Burstein J, Papile I, Burstein R. (1979) IVH and hydrocephalus in premature newborns: a prospective study with CT. Am J Roentgenol 132: 631-635

Butler LJ, Snodgrass AJA, France NE, Sinclair L, Russell A. (1965) No E (16-18) trisomy syndrome: Analysis of 13 cases. Arch Dis Child 40: 600

Byrne P, Welch R, Johnson MA, Darrah J, Piper M. (1990) Serial magnetic resonance imaging in neonatal hypoxic-ischaemic encephalopathy. J Pediat 117: 694-700

Campbell S et al. (1986) Qualitative assessment of uteroplacental blood flow: early screening test for high risk pregnancies. Obstet Gynecol 68: 493-506

Canadian Preterm Labor Investigators Group (1992) Treatment of preterm labor with the beta-adrenergic agonist Ritodrine. New Engl J Med 327: 308-312

Caraceni T, Broggi G, Avanzini G. (1974) Familial idiopathic basal ganglia calcification exhibiting features of DMD. Neurology 12: 357-359

Carlson DE. (1988) Maternal diseases associated with intrauterine growth retardation. Semin Perinatol 12: 17-22

Carr LJ et al. (1991) Evidence of bilateral innervation of homologous motor neurone pools in man. J Physiol 446: 567

Catto-Smith AG, Yu VYH, Bajuk B, Orgill AA, Astbury J. (1985) Effect of neonatal periventricular haemorrhage on neuro-developmental outcome. Arch Dis Child 60: 8-11

Cederbaum SD, Blass JP, Minkoff N, Brown WJ, Cotton ME, Harris SH. (1976) Sensitivity to carbohydrate in a patient with familial intermittent lactic acidosis and pyruvate dehydrogenase deficiency. Pediat Res 10: 713-720

Cepeda EE et al. (1987) Reduced frequency of intraventricular haemorrhage in the infants of drug-addicted mothers. Acta Paediat Scand 76: 16

Chamberlain A et al. (1984) Issues in fertility control for mentally retarded female adolescents. 1. Sexual activity, sexual abuse and contraception. Pediatrics 73: 445-450

Chan J et al. (1991) Idiopathic cervical dystonia. Movement Disorders 6: 119-126

Chao DH-C. (1959) Congenital neurocutaneous syndromes of childhood. III. Sturge-Weber disease. J Pediat 55: 635

Childs B, Evans PR. (1954) Birthweight of children with CP. Lancet 1: 642-645

Chimura T. (1992) Clinical studies of Imipenem/Cilastatin sodium in the early therapy of preterm premature rupture of the membrane or threatened abortion and premature delivery. Jap J Antibiotics 45: 1023-1028

Chiron C, Dulac O, Luna D, Palacias C, Mondragon S, Beaumont D, Mumford JP. (1990) Vigabatrin in infantile spasms. Lancet 335: 363-364

Chiswick ML, Wynn J, Toner N. (1982) Vitamin E and IVH in the newborn. Ann NY Acad Sci 393: 109-118

Chiswick ML, Johnson M, Woodhall C. (1983) Protective effect of Vitamin E against IVH in premature babies. Br Med J 287: 81-84

Churchill JA. (1958) The relationship of Little's disease to premature birth. Am J Dis Child 96: 779-786

Cioni L et al. (1992) Neuroimaging and functional outcome of neonatal leukomalacia. Behav Brain Res 49: 7-19

Clark DL et al. (1977) Vestibular stimulation influence on motor development in infants. Science 196: 1228-1229

Clark JB, Heyes D, Buyrne F, Morgan-Hughes JA. (1983) Mitochondrial myopathies: defects in mitochondrial metabolism in human skeletal muscle. Biochem Soc Trans 11: 626

Cleaver JE, Bootsma D. (1975) Xeroderma pigmentosum: Biochemical and genetic characteristics. Ann Rev Genet 9: 19

Coffin GS, Siris E. (1970) Mental retardation with absent fifth fingernail and terminal phalanx. Am J Dis Child 119: 433

Cohen HL, Haller JO, Pollark A. (1990) Ultrasound of the septum pellucidum. Recognition of evolving fenestrations in the hydrocephalic infant. J Ultrasound Med 9: 377-383

Cohen MM (1986) Craniosynostosis, Diagnosis, Evaluation and Management. Raven Press, New York.

Cohen et al. (1991) Reorganisation in motor pathways following a large congenital hemispheric lesion in man: different ipsilateral motor representation areas for ipsi- and contralateral muscles. J Physiol 438: 33

Coker SB, Melnyk AR. (1991) Rett syndrome and mitochondrial enzyme deficiencies. J Child Neurol 6: 164-166

Collaborative European Multicentre Study Group (1988) Surfactant replacement therapy for severe neonatal respiratory distress syndrome: an international randomised clinical trial. Pediatrics 82: 683-691

Collaborative Group of Antenatal Steroid Therapy. (1981) Effect of antenatal dexamethasone in the prevention of respiratory disress syndrome. Am J Obstet Gynecol 141: 276-286

Conlon RA Jr. (1981) Outcome of intraventricular haemorrhage in the neonate based on CT scan and/or post mortem grading. In: Am Soc Pediat Neurosurg Concepts, Vol 1, pp 148-173. New York, S Karger

Cooke RWI, Morgan MEL. (1984) Prophylactic ethamsylate for periventricular haemorrhage. Arch Dis Child 59: 82-83

Costa LD, Scarola LM, Rapin I. (1964) Purdue pegboard scores for normal grammar school children. Perceptual Motor Skills 18: 748

Costeloe K, Rolfe P. (1989) Techniques for studying cerebral perfusion in the newborn. In: Perinatal Brain Lesions. Eds. KE Pape and JS Wiggleworth. Blackwell Scientific Publications, Oxford, London.

Cotton RB, Keats ME, McCoye E. (1970) Abnormal blood glucose regulation in Cockayne Syndrome. Pediatrics 46: 54-60

Cussen GH, Barry JF, Moloney ME, Buckley NM, Crowley M, Daly C. (1978) Cerebral palsy - a regional study. J Irish Med Assoc 71: 568-572

500

Crawford, Michael (1992) Personal communication. Institute of Brain Surgery. Proc Br Assoc Sci Festival, Southampton University

Crepel F, Delhaye-Bouchaud N, Guastavino JM, Sampaio I. (1980) Multiple innervation of cerebellar Purkinje cells by climbing fibres in staggerer mutant mouse. Nature 283: 483-484

Crothers B, Paine RS. (1959) Disorders of the nervous system in childhood. In: The Natural History of Cerebral Palsy. Cambridge Press, London. p 299

Crothers B, Paine RS. (1988) Effects of growth retardation and aswphyxia on brain electrolytes. Paediat Res 7: 494-499

D'Amato CJ, Hicks SP. (1978) Normal development and post-traumatic plasticity of corticospinal neurons in rats. Exp Neurol 60: 551-569

Danks DM, Cartwright E, Stevens BJ, Townley RRW (1972) Menkes' kinky hair disease: a further definition of the defect in copper transport. Science 179: 1140-1141

de Long GR. (1993) Effects of nutrition on brain development in humans. Am J Clin Nutr 57: 2865-2905

de Vries LS, Dubowitz LMS, Dubowitz V, et al. (1985) Predictive value of cranial ultrasound: a reappraisal. Lancet ii: 137-140

de Vries LS, Eken P, Dubowitz LMS. (1992) The spectrum of leucomalacia using cranial ultrasound. Behav Brain Res 49: 1-6

de Vries LS, Eken P, Pierrat Y, Daniels H, Cassaer P. (1992) Prediction of neurodevelopmental outcome in the preterm infant: short term latency somatosensory evoked potentials compared with cranial ultrasound. Arch Dis Child 67: 1177-1181

de Vries LS, Regev R, Pennock JM, Wigglesworth JS, Dubowitz LM. (1988) Ultrasound evolution and later outcome of infants with periventricular densities. Early Hum Dev 16: 225-233

Denays R et al. (1989) Brain single photon emission computed tomography in neonates. J Nuclear Med 30: 1337-1341

Denays R et al. (1990) Cerebral palsy: initial experiences with Tc-99m HMPAO SPECT of the brain. Radiology 175: 111-116

Dennis M. (1976) Impaired sensory and motor differentiation with corpus callosum agenesis. Neuropsychologist 14: 455-469

Dennis M. (1981) Language in a congenitally acallosal brain. Brain Lang 12: 33-53

Denny-Brown DE. (1949) Interpretation of the electromyogram. Arch Neurol Psychiat 61: 99-128

Denhoff E, Robinauth IP. (1960) Cerebral Palsy and Related Disorders. McGraw-Hill Book Co., New York

Diamond CJ, Jaudes PK. (1983) Child abuse in a CP population. Dev Med Child Neurol 25: 169-174

Dobyns WB. (1989) The neurogenetics of lissencephaly. Neurol Clinics 7: 89-105

Dolfin T et al. (1983) Incidence, severity and timing of subependymal and intraventricular haemorrhage in preterm infants as detected by serial real-time ultrasound. Pediatrics 71: 541-546

Donat JP, Okazaki H, Kleinberg F, Reagan JS. (1978) Intraventricular hemorrhage in full-term and premature infants. Mayo Clin Proc 53: 437-441

Donn SM, Roloff DW, Goldstein GH. (1981) Prevention of intraventricular haemorrhage in preterm infants by phenobarbitone: a controlled trial. Lancet 1: 215-217

Donner M, Rapola J, Somer H. (1975) Congenital muscular dystrophy: a clinico-pathological and follow-up study of 15 patients. Neuropädiatrie 6: 239

Doran L. (1992) Periventricular leukomalacia. Neonat Net 11: 7-13

Douglas AA. (1961) Ophthalmological aspects. In: JL Henderson (Ed) Cerebral Palsy in Childhood and Adolescence. Edinburgh, Livingstone.

Dowding VM, Barry C. (1988) Cerebral palsy: changing patterns of birth weight and gestational age (1976-81). Br Med J 81: 25-29

Dubowitz LMS, Bydder GM, Muskin J. (1985) Developmental sequence of periventricular leukomalacia correlation of ultrasound, clinical and nuclear magnetic resonance function. Arch Dis Child 60: 349-355

Dubowitz LMS, Bydder GM. (1990) Magnetic resonance imaging of the brain in neonates. Sem Perinatol 14: 212-223

Dubowitz LMS, Rutherford MA, Bouza H, Acolet D, Pennock JM, Bydder GM (1993) Early diagnosis of congenital hemiplegia: Prospective study of five full-term neonates. Proceedings 19th Annual Meeting, British Paediatric Neurology Association, Institute of Child Health. p.8

Dubowitz V. (1985) Muscle Biopsy. A practical approach. 2nd Ed. Balliere Tindall, London

Dubowitz V, Davies K. (1991) Pontocerebellar hypoplasia. Neuromuscular Dis 1: 81

Dunsdon MI. (1952) The educability of cerebral palsied children. Newness, London. 170, 92

Drillien CM. (1972) Abnormal neurological signs in the first year of life in low birth-weight infants: possible prognostic significance. Dev Med Child Neurol 14: 575

Drillien CM, Drummond MB. (1977) Neurodevelopmental Problems in Early Childhood. Blackwell Scientific Publications Oxford. pp 243-245

Edvinsson L, Lou HC, Tvede K. (1986) On the pathogenesis of regimal cerebral ischaemia in intracranial hemorrhage: a causal influence of potassium. Pediat Res 20: 478-480

Edwards MJ. (1969) Congenital defects in guinea pigs. Prenatal retardation of brain growth of guinea pigs following hyperthermia during gestation. Teratology 2: 239

Eldjarn L et al. (1966) Dietary effects upon serum phytanic acid levels and clinical manifestations. Lancet 1: 691-693

Ellenberg JH, Nelson KB. (1979) Birth weight and gestational age in children with cerebral palsy or seizure disorder. Am J Dis Child 133: 1044

Eldridge R. (1970) The torsion dystonias. Literature review and genetic and clinical studies. Neurology (Minneapolis) 20: 1-78

Embil JA et al. (1970) Congenital cytomegalovirus in two siblings. J Pediat 77: 417-423

Engerstrom Ingegerd W. (1990) Rett syndrome in Sweden. Neurodevelopment disability pathophysiology. Department of Pediatrics II, Gotteberg, Sweden

Enhorning G, Shennan A, Possmayer F, Dunn M, Chen CP, Milligan T. (1985) Prevention of neonatal respiratory distress by tracheal instillation of surfactants. Pediatrics 76: 145-153

Erdlinger G et al. (1972) Agenesis of the corpus callosum: a behavioural investigation. Brain 95: 327

Evrard P. (1988) Les troubles du developpment pernatal du cortex cerebral humain. Bull Med Acad R Med Belg 143: 356-368

Evrard P, Lyon G, Gadisseux JF. (1984) Les processus destructifs agissant durant la seconde montré de la grossesse, durant la période de croissance et la differenciation du tissu nerveux. Progrés en Neonatologie, Vol 4, pp 85-106. Basel, New York, Karger

Fahn S. (1976) Biochemistry of the basal ganglia. Adv Neurol 14: 59-85

Fahn S, Eldridge R. (1976) Definition of dystonia and classification of the dystonic state. Adv Neurol 14: 1-5

Farmer SF et al. (1991) Plasticity of central motor pathways in children with hemiplegic cerebral palsy. Neurology 41: 1505-1510

Feldman HM, Scher MS, Kemp SS. (1990) Pediat Neurol 6: 276-302

Fenichel GM. (1983) Myasthenia gravis. In: Emery AEH, Rimoin DI (Eds) Principles and Practice of Medical Genetics. Churchill Livingstone, Edinburgh. Ch. 34

502

Ferehmin PA, Eberovic VA, Caputto R. (1970) Studies of brain weight and RNA content after short periods of exposure to environmental complexity. Brain Res 20: 49-57

Fernell E, Hagberg B, Hagberg G, Hult G, von Wendt L. (1988) Epidemiology of infantile hydrocephalus in Sweden. Current aspects of the outcome in preterm infants. Neuropediat 19: 143-145

Ferrari F, Cioni G, Prechtl HF. (1990) Qualitative changes of general movement in preterm infants with brain lesions. Early Hum Dev 23: 193-231

Finlay BL, Slattery M. (1983) Local differences in the amount of early cell death in neocortex predict adult local specialization. Science 219: 1349-1351

Finlay KH. (1958) Postencephalitis manifestation of viral encephalitis. In: WS Fields, RJ Blattner (Eds) Viral Encephalitis. Springfield, Illinois, CC Thomas. pp 69-94

Fisch L. (1957) Hearing impairment and cerebral palsy. Speech 21: 43

Fisher DA, Dussault JH, Sack J, Chopra IJ. (1977) Ontogenesis of hypothalamic-pituitary-thyroid function and metabolism in man, sheep and rat. Rec Prog Norm Res 33: 59-116

Fitz C. (1989) Computed tomography: state of the art. In KE Pape, JS Wigglesworth (Eds) Perinatal Brain Lesions. Blackwell Scientific Publications, Boston, London. pp 25-53

Fitzhardinge PM, Flodmark O, Fitz CR, Ashby S. (1982) The prognostic value of computed tomography of the brain in asphyxiated premature infants. J Pediat 100: 476-481

Flanagan A, Harris E. (1969) Differentiation and degeneration in the motor horn of the foetal mouse. J Morphol 129: 281-306

Flodmark D, Scott G, Harwood-Nash DC. (1981) Clinical significance of ventriculomegaly in children after perinatal asphyxia. J Comput Assist Tomogr 5: 663-673

Friedl HP, Smith DJ et al. (1990) Ischaemia reperfusion in humans. Appearance of xanthine oxidase activity. Am J Pathol 136: 491-495

Foley J. (1951) Calcification of the corpus striatum and dentate nuclei. J Neurol Neurosurg 14: 251

Foley J. (1977) Visual defects. In: CM Drillian, MB Drummond (Eds) Neurodevelopmental Problems in Early Childhood. Oxford, Blackwell Scientific Publications

Foley J. (1992) Dyskinetic and dystonic cerebral palsy and birth. Acta Paediat 81: 57-60

Ford FR. (1973) Diseases of the Nervous System in Infancy, Childhood and Adolescence. CC Thomas, Springfield. 3,6,37,41,49,53,60

Fowler KB et al. (1992) The outcome of congenital cytomegalovirus infections in relation to maternal antibody studies. New Engl J Med 326: 663-667

Freud S. (1968) Infantile cerebral palsies. Translation: LA Russin. University of Miami Press, Miami

Fried K. (1973) X-linked mental retardation and/or hydrocephalus. Clin Genet 3: 258

Friede RL. (1989) Dysplasias of cerebral cortex. In: Developmental Neuropathology. Springer, Vienna. pp 330-346

Gaddes WH, Crockett DJ. (1975) The Spreen-Benton aphasia tests: normative data as a measure of language development. Brain Language 3: 257-280

Garcia CA et al. (1973) Neurological involvement in the Smith-Lemli-Opitz syndrome. Dev Med Child Neurol 15: 48

Garg BK, Srivastava JR. (1965) Cerebral palsy - a clinical study of 124 cases with a review. Indian Pediat 2: 195-208

Garret B, Ames RP. (1976) Alexander's disease. Archs Pathol 38: 379

Gibbin KP (1992) Paediatric cochlear implantation. Arch Dis Child 67: 669-671

Gibson KM, Sweetman L, Nyhan WL, Page TM, Green C, Cann HM. (1982) 3-hydroxy-3 methyl glutaric aciduria. A new assay of 3-hydroxy-3 methylglutarye CoA lyase. Clin Chim Acta 126: 171

Gibson NA, Graham M, Levene MI. (1992) Somatosensory evoked potentials and outcome in perinatal asphyxia. Arch Dis Child 67: 393-398

Gizelmann R, Steinmann B. (1978) Non-ketotic hyperglycinaemia treated with strychnine: a glycine receptor antagonist. Helv Paediat Acta 32: 517-525

Gluckman PD, Williams EB, Guan J. Neuronal rescue after hypoxic-ischaemic injury (HI) using insulin-like growth factor 1.

Goldblatt J, Ballo R, Sachs B, Moosa A. (1989) X-linked spastic paraplegia: Evidence for homogeneity with variable phenotype. Clin Genet 35: 116-120

Goldman PS, Lewis ME. (1978) Developmental biology of brain damage and experience. In: Neuronal Plasticity. Ed. Cotman CKI. New York, Raven Press. pp 291-310

Goldstein G, Donn S, Roloff D. (1982) Further observations on the use of phenobarbital to prevent neonatal intracranial haemorrhage. In: J Lucey (Ed) Second Special Ross Conference on Perinatal Intracranial Haemorrhage. Columbus, Ross Labs. pp 810-815

Goodman SI et al. (1975) Glutaric aciduria. A "new" disorder of amino acid metabolism. Biochem Med 12: 12

Goodman SI, Gallegos DA et al. (1980) Antenatal diagnosis of glutaric acidaemia. Am J Hum Genet 33: 695-699

Gornall P, Hitchcock AHS, Kirkland IS. (1975) Stereotaxic neurosurgery in the management of cerebral palsy. Dev Med Child Neurol. 17: 279-286

Graham M, Levene MI, Trounce JQ, et al. (1987) Prediction of cerebral palsy in very low birth weight infants: prospective ultrasound study. Lancet 2: 593-595

Grant A et al. (1989) Routine formal fetal movement counting and risk of antepartum late death in normally formed singletons. Lancet ii: 345-349

Greenough A, Wood S, Morley CJ, Davis JA. (1984) Pancuronium prevents pneumothorax in ventilated premature babies. Lancet i: 1-3

Greggs RC, Muxley RT, Lafiance RA, McQuillan J. (1978) Hereditary paroxysmal ataxia. Response to acetazolamide. Neurology 28: 1259-1264

Gross SJ, Oehler JM, Eckerman CO. (1983) Head growth and developmental outcome in very low birth-weight infants. Pediatrics 71: 70-75

Guerrini R et al. (1992) Epilepsy and focal gyral anomalies detected by MRI: electroclinico-morphological correlations. Dev Med Child Neurol 34: 706-718

Guggenheim MA, Ringel SP, Silverman A, Grabert BE. (1982) Progressive neuromuscular disease in children with chronic cholestasis and vitamin E deficiency. Diagnosis and treatment with α-tocopherol. J Pediat 100: 51-58

Guthrie RD et al. (1971) The 4p-syndrome. Am J Dis Child 122: 421

Guzzetta FF, Shackelford GD, Volpe S, Perlman JM, Volpe JJ. (1986) Periventricular intraparenchymal echodensities in the premature newborn. Critical determinant of neurologic outcome. Pediatrics 78: 995-1006

Hagberg BA. (1972) The Dysequilibrium syndrome in cerebral palsy. Acta Paediat Scand: suppl 226

Hagberg B et al. (1970) Familial ataxic diplegia with deficient cellular immunity. Acta Paediat Scand 59: 545

Hagberg B, Aicardi J, Dias K, Ramos O. (1983) A progressive syndrome of autism, dementia, ataxia and loss of purposeful hand use in girls: Retts syndrome. Report of 35 cases. Ann Neurol 14: 471

Hagberg B, Hagberg G, Glow I. (1975) The changing panorama of cerebral palsy in Sweden 1954-1970. Analysis of the general changes. Acta Paediat Scand 64: 187-192

Hagberg B, Hagberg G, Olow I. (1975) The changing panorama of cerebral palsy in Sweden 1954-1970. II. Analysis of the various syndromes. Acta Paediat Scand 64: 193-200

Hagberg B, Hagberg G, Olow I, Von Wendt I. (1989) The changing panorama of CP in Sweden in the birth year period 1979-1982. Acta Paediat Scand 78: 283-290

Hagberg B, Hjalmarson O, Lindstedt S, Ransnas L, Steen G. (1983) 3-methylglutaconic aciduria in two infants. Clin Chim Acta 134: 59

Hagberg B, Hultquist G, Ohman R, Jvennerholm L. (1965) Congenital amaurotic idiocy. Acta Paediat Scand 54: 116-130

Hagberg B, Kyllerman M, Steen G. (1979) Dyskinesia and dystonia in neurometabolic disorders. Neuropädiat 10: 305-320

Hagberg B, Sanner B, Stern M. (1974) The dysequilibrium syndrome in cerebral palsy. Acta Paediat Scand, suppl. 226

Hagberg B, Sjogram L. (1966) The chronic brain syndrome of infantile hydrocephalus. Am J Dis Child 112: 189-196

Hall BD et al. (1974) Langer-Giedion syndrome. Birth Defects 10: 147

Hall DM et al. (1989) Birth asphyxia. Br Med J 299: 272-282

Hallman A, Merritt A, Jarvenfaa F, et al. (1985) Exogenous human surfactant for treatment of severe respiratory distress. J Pediat 106: 963-965

Halpern IM, Jolly SE, Johnson DG. (1991) Gastrooesophageal reflux: a significant association with central nervous system disease in children. J Pediat Surg 26: 171-173

Hamano S, Nara T, Nizaki H, Fukushima K, Imai M, Kumagai K, Maekawa K. (1991) Crossed cerebellar diaschisis demonstrable by SPECT in hemiplegic children. No To Hattatsu 23: 58-64

Hambleton G, Wigglesworth JS. (1976) Origin of intraventricular haemorrhage in the preterm infant. Arch Dis Child 5: 651-659

Hansen TWJ, Tydal T, Jorgensen H et al. (1985) Effect of bilirubin on uptake of 5-HT and Dopamine in rat brain synaptosomes. Pediat Res 19: 390A

Hardinge AE, Matthews S, Jones S et al. (1985) Spino-cerebellar degeneration associated with a selective defect of Vitamin E absorption. New Engl J Med 313: 32-35

Harvey CC, Haworth JC, Lorber J. (1955) A new heredofamilial neurological syndrome. Arch Dis Child 19: 96

Haworth JC, Perry TL, Blass JP, Hansen S, Urquhart N. (1976) Lactic acidosis in three siblings due to defects in both pyruvate dehydrogenase and α-ketoglutarate dehydrogenase complex. Pediatrics 58: 564-574

Hawke WA, Donohue WK. (1950) Bilateral symmetrical nerosis of corpora striata: report of fatal case and reference to a possible syndrome of corpora striata. J Nerv Ment Dis 113: 20-39

Hayashi M, Satoh J, Saramoto K, Morimatsu Y. (1991) Clinical and neuropathological findings in severe athetoid cerebral palsy: a comparative study of globo-Luysian and thalamo-putaminal groups. Brain Dev 13: 47-51

Heckmatt J, Keir G, Baudouin C, Orme RL'E. (1993) A metabolic cause of ataxic cerebral palsy. Abst. 19th Ann Meeting, Br Paediat Neurol Assoc, Institute of Child Health, London. p. 65

Heimkes S, Stotz S, Heid T. (1992) Pathogenesis and prevention of spastic hip dislocation. Orthop Ihre Grenzgeb 130: 413-418

Herrman J, Opitz JM. (1974) Naming and nomenclature. Birth Defects 10(7): 69

Herrman J et al. (1975) The Stickler syndrome of hereditary arthro ophthalmopathy. Birth Defects 11: 76

Heuman D, Leuba G. (1983) Neuronal death in the development and aging of the cerebral cortex

Radiol 4: 28-37

Kennara MA. (1938) Reorganisation of motor function in the cerebral cortex of monkeys deprived of motor and premotor areas in infancy. J Neurophysiol 1: 477-496

Kenny DJ, Casas MJ, McPherson KA. (1989) Correlation of ultrasound imaging of oral swallow with ventilatory observations in the cerebral palsied. Dysphagia 4: 112-117

Kerrigan JF, Chugani HT, Phelps ME. (1991) Regional cerebral glucose metabolism in clinical subtypes of cerebral palsy. Pediat Neurol 7: 415-425

Kirk SA, McCarthy JJ, Kirk WD (1968) The Illinois Test of Psycholinguist Abilities. University of Illinois

Kitchen WH et al. (1990) 5-year outcome of infants of birth-weight 500-1500gms; relationship with neonatal ultrasound. Am J Perinatol 7: 60-65

Koeda T, Suganuma I, Kohno Y, Takamatsu T, Takashita K. (1990) MR imaging of spastic diplegia: comparative study between preterm and term infant. Neuroradiol 32: 187-190

Koeda T, Watanabe N, Kimura M, Nishi N, Takeshita K. (1990) Disturbances of visual perception and the lesions in spastic diplegia. No-To-Shinkel 42: 759-763

Koike K, Hamada M, Tanaka N, Otsuka K, Ogashara K, Koike M. (1974) Properties and sabunit composition of the pig heart 2-oxoglutarate dehydrogenase. J Biol Chem 249: 3836-3842

Kok O, Bruyn GW. (1962) An unidentified hereditary disease. Lancet 1: 1359

Konishi Y, Kuriyama M, Hayakaior K et al. (1990) Periventricular hyperintensity detected by magnetic resonance imaging in infancy. Pediat Neurol 6: 229-232

Kondo K, Tsubaki T, Sakamoto F. (1970) The Ryukyuan muscular atrophy. J Neurol Sci 11: 359

Krageloh-Mann I et al. (1992) Bilateral spastic cerebral palsy - pathogenetic aspects from MRI. Neuropaediat 23: 46-48

Kreusser KL, Tarby TJ, Kovnar F. (1985) Serial lumbar punctures for at least temporary amelioration of neonatal post-haemorrhage hydrocephalus. Pediatrics 75: 719-724

Kuban KC et al. (1992) Maternal toxaemia associated with reduced incidence of germinal matrix haemorrhage in premature babies. J Child Neurol 7: 70-76

Kulakowski S, Larroche JC. (1980) Cranial computerized tomography in cerebral palsy. Neuropadiat 11: 339-353

Kwong MS, Egan EA. (1986) Reduced incidence of hyaline membrane disease in extremely premature infants following delay in delivery in mothers with preterm labour. Use of ritodrine and betamethasone. Pediatrics 78: 767-774

Lademann A. (1978) Postnatally acquired cerebral palsy. Acta Neurol Scand: suppl. 65, 3

Landmesser L. (1981) Pathway selection by embryonic neurons. In: Studies in Developmental Neurobiology. Ed. Cowan WM. New York, Oxford University Press. pp 53-73

Laplaza F, Janvier F, Root L, Tassanawipas A, Cervera P. (1992) Cerebral palsy in twins. Dev Med Child Neurol 34: 1053-1063

Lapresie I, Salisachs P. (1973) Onion bulb in a nerve biopsy from an original case of Roussy-Levi disease. Arch Neurol 29: 346-348

Largo RH, Molinari L, Pinto LC, Weber M, Duc G. (1986) Language development of term and preterm children during first 5 years of life. Dev Med Child Neurol 28: 333-350

Largo RH et al. (1990) Neurological outcome in high risk weight appropriate for gestational age in preterm children at early school age. Europ J Pediat 149: 835-844

Lecky BRF et al. (1986) Congenital myasthenia: Further evidence of disease heterogeneity. Muscle Nerve 9: 233-242

Lee FA. Isaacs H Jr, Strauss J (1972) The "camptomelic" syndrome. Am J Dis Child 124: 485

Lee LV et al. (1976) Torsion dystonia in Panay. Adv Neurol 14: 137-150

Lees JA, Neville BGR. (1990) Acquired aphasia in childhood: case studies in five children.

Aphasiology 4: 463-478

Leibel RL, Shih VE et al. (1980) Glutaric acidaemia: a metabolic disorder causing progressive choreoathetosis. Neurology 30: 1163-1168

Lejeune J et al. (1963) Trois cas de deletion partielle du bras court d'un chromosome 5. CR Acad Sci(D) Paris 257: 3098

Leonard JV, Seakins JWT, Griffin NK. (1979) ß-hydroxy-ß-methylglutaric aciduria presenting as Reye's syndrome. Lancet 1: 680

Leonard JV, Seakins JWT, Bartlett K, Hyde J, Wilson J, Clayton B. (1981) Inherited disorders of 3-methylcrotonyl CoA carboxyl CoA carboxylatin. Arch Dis Child 56: 53

Levene MI (1981) Measurement of the growth of the lateral ventricles in preterm infants with real-time ultrasound. Arch Dis Child 56: 900-904

Levene MI, Fawer CL, Lamont RF. (1982) Risk factors in the development of intraventricular haemorrhage in the preterm neonate. Arch Dis Child 57: 410-417

Levene MI, Starte DR. (1981) A longitudinal study of post-haemorrhagic ventricular dilatation in the newborn. Arch Dis Child 56: 905-910

Levi-Montalcini R. (1987) The nerve growth factor. Thirty-five years later. EMBO J 6: 1145-1154

Levine RL, Ferericks AB, Rappaport SL. (1982) Entry of bilirubin into the brain due to opening of the blood-brain barrier. Pediatrics 69: 255-259

Leviton A, Paneth N. (1990) White matter damage in preterm newborn - an epidemiological perspective. Early Hum Dev 24: 1-22

Little J, Bryan E. (1986) Congenital anomalies in twins. Semin Perinatol 10: 50-64

Longo LD et al. (1973) An anaerobic glycogen-dependent transport of amino acids by the placenta. Nature

Lou HC, Phibbs RH, Wilson SL, Gregory GA. (1982) Hyperventilation at birth may prevent early periventricular haemorrhage. Lancet 1: 1407

Lucas A, Morley R, Cole TJ. (1988) Adverse neurodevelopmental outcome of moderate neonatal hypoglycaemia. Br Med J 297: 1304-1308

Lumley JTA, Wood C. (1967) Influence of hypoxia on glucose transport across the human placenta. Nature 216: 403-404

McCarthy GT et al. (1981) The Physically Handicapped Child: Interdisciplinary Approach to Management. Faber and Faber, London

McCord FB, Curstedt T, Halliday HL, McClure G, Reid MMc, Robertson B. (1988) Surfactant treatment and incidence of IV haemorrhage in severe respiratory distress syndrome. Arch Dis Child 63: 10-16

McIlwaine GM et al. (1979) Scottish perinatal mortality study. Br Med J 8: 1103-1106

McKusick V. (1956) Hereditable Disorders of Connective Tissue. Mosby, St. Louis

McMenamin JB, Shackleford GD, Volpe JJ. (1984) Outcome of neonatal intraventricular haemorrhage with periventricular echodensities. Ann Neurol 15: 285

Maher P, Lane B, Ballard R, Piecuch R, Clyman RI. (1985) Does indomethacin cause extension of intracranial haemorrhages: a preliminary study. Pediatrics 75: 491-499

Mari G et al. (1989) Doppler assessment of the fetal and uteroplacental circulation during Nifedipine therapy for preterm labor. Am J Obstet Gynecol 161: 1514-1518

Marlin AE. (1980) Protection of the cortical mantle in premature infants with posthaemorrhagic hydrocephalus. Neurosurg 7: 464-471

Maroteaux P, Lang M, Robert JM. (1967) Le nanisme thantophere. Presse Med 75: 2519

Maroteaux P et al. (1971) Le syndrome campomelique. Presse Med 79: 1157

Maroteaux P. (1973) Un nouveau type de mucopolysachoridose avec athetose et elimination de keratan sulfate. Nouv Presse Med 2: 975-979

Setzer ES, Morse BM, Goldberg RN, Smith M, Bancalari E. (1984) Prophylactic indomethacin and intraventricular haemorrhage in the premature. Pediat Res 18: 345

Shankaren S et al. (1976) Antenatal phenobarbitone for the prevention of intracranial hemorrhage. Am J Obstet Gynecol 154: 53-57

Shanks DC, Wilson WC. (1988) Lobar holoprosencephaly presenting as spastic diplegia. Dev Med Child Neurol 30: 383-386

Sharav T. (1991) Aging gamete in relation to incidence, gender and twinning in Down syndrome. Am J Med Genet 39: 116-118

Shaw E, Steinbach HL. (1968) Aminopterin-induced fetal malformation. Am J Dis Child 115: 477

Shields JR, Schifrin BS. (1988) Perinatal antecedents of cerebral palsy. Obstet Gynecol 71: 899-905

Shih VE, Abrams IF, Johnson JL, Mudd SH. (1977) Sulfite oxidase deficiency. New Engl J Med 297: 1022-1028

Shillito P, Stephenson J, Tolmie J, Hughes-Benzies R, Lebon P. (1993) Aicardi-Goutieres syndrome - two unrelated sporadic cases. Abst. XIXnth Annual Meeting of British Paediatric Neurology Assoc. Inst of Child Health, London. p.51

Shimasaki M et al. (1978) Three cases of De Sanchs-Cacchione syndrome with endocrinological abnormalities. Acta Paediat Jap 20: 100

Shortland D, Levene MI, Trouncer J, Ng Y, Graham M. (1988) The evolution and outcome of cavitating periventricular leukomalacia in infancy: a study of 46 infants. J Perinatal Med 16: 241-247

Shprintzen RJ et al. (1981) The velo-cardio-facial syndrome: a clinical and genetic analysis. Pediat 67: 167

Shuman RM, Selednik LJ. (1980) Periventricular leukomalacia. Arch Neurol 37: 231-235

Siegel ML, Shakelford GP, Perlman JM, Fulling KH. (1984) Hypoxic-ischemic encephalopathy in term infants. Diagnosis and prognosis evaluated by ultrasound. Radiology 24: 418

Singer SR, Crooks LE. (1983) Nuclear magnetic resonance blood-flow measurements in the human brain. Science 221: 654-656

Singh L, Moser HW, Moser AB, Kishimoto Y. (1981) Adrenoleucodystrophy: Impaired oxidation of long chain fatty acids in cultured skin fibroblasts and adrenal cortex. Biochem Biophys Res Commun 102: 1223

Sinha SK, Davies JM, Sims DG, Chiswick ML. (1985) Relation between periventricular haemorrhage and ischaemic brain lesions diagnosed by ultrasound in very premature. Lancet 2: 1154-1156

Sinha SK, D'Souza SW, Rivlin E, Chiswick ML. (1990) Ischaemic brain lesions diagnosed at birth in preterm infants: clinical events and developmental outcome. Arch Dis Child 65: 1017-1020

Sjögren T, Larsson T. (1957) Oligophrenia in combination with congenital ichthyosis and spastic disorders. Acta Psychiatr Scand 32: suppl 113; 1

Skullerud K, Westre B. (1986) Frequency of prognostic significance of germinal matrix haemorrhage, PVL and Pontosubicular necrosis in preterm neonates. Acta Neuropathol (Berlin) 70: 257-261

Smithells RW, Sheppard S, Schorah CJ, Seller MJ, Nevin NC, Harris R, Reid AP, Fielding DW. (1981) Parent prevention of neural tube defects by periconceptional vitamin supplementation. Arch Dis Child 56: 911-918

Speer ME, Blifield C, Rudolph AJ. (1984) IVH and Vitamin E in very low birthweight infants: evidence for efficacy of early intramuscular Vitamin E. Pediatrics 74: 1107-1112

Sperry RW. (1963) Chemoaffinity in the orderly growth of nerve fibre patterns and connections. Proc Natl Acad Sci USA 50: 703-710

Spielberg SP, Gordon GB, Blake DA. (1981) Predisposition of Phenytoin hepatotoxicity assessed in vitro. New Engl J Med 305: 722

Spiro AJ, Fogelson MH, Goldberg AC. (1967) Microcephaly and mental subnormality in chronic progressive spinal muscular atrophy of childhood. Dev Med Child Neurol 9: 594

Srivastava VK, Laisram N, Srivastava RK. (1992) Cerebral palsy. Ind Paediat 29: 993-996

Staino A, Cuechiara SH, Del Giudice E et al. (1991) Disorders of oesophageal motility in children with psychomotor retardation. Eur J Pediat 150: 638-644

Staller SJ, Dowell RC, Beiter AL, Brimacombe JA. (1991) Perceptual abilities of children with the nucleus 22 channel cochlear implant. Ear Hear 12: suppl.

Stanbury JB. (1972) Familial goiter. In: JB Stanbury, JB Wyngaarden, DS Fredrickson (Eds) The Metabolic Basis of Inherited Disease 3rd Edition. McGraw-Hill, New York. p 233

Stanley FJ. (1979) An epidemiological study of CP in Western Australia: changes in total incidence. Dev Med Child Neurol 21: 701-713

Stanley FJ. (1981) Spastic cerebral palsy - changes in birthweight and gestational age. Early Human Dev 5: 167-178

Stanley FJ. (1987) The changing face of cerebral palsy. Dev Med Child Neurol 29: 263-265

Stanley F, Blair E. (1984) Postnatal risk factors among the cerebral palsy. In: F Stanley, E Alberman (Eds) The Epidemiology of the Cerebral Palsies.

Stanley FJ, Blair E. (1991) Why have we failed to reduce the frequency of cerebral palsy. Med J Aust 154: 623-626

Stanley FJ et al. (1985) A Cerebral Palsy Register Methodology: The Western Australian experience. Neuro-epidemiol 4: 146-160

Stanley FJ, English DR. (1986) Prevalence of an risk factors for cerebral palsy in a total population cohort of low-birthweight (<2000 g) infants. Dev Med Child Neurol 28: 559-568

Stanley FJ, Watson L. (1988) The cerebral palsies in Western Australia trends 1968-1981. Am J Obstet Gynecol 158: 89-93

Statter A, Russell A. (1978) Competitive interrelationships between lysine and argenine in rat liver under normal conditions and in experimental hyperammonaemia. Life Sci 22: 2097-2102

Steele RJC, Little K. (1983) Effect of seat-belt legislation. Lancet 2: 341

Steinlin M, Dirr R, Marlin E, Boesch C, Largo RH, Fanconi S, Boltshauser E. (1991) MRI following severe perinatal asphyxia. Pediat Neurol 7: 164-170

Stewart AL, Reynolds EOR. (1974) Improved prognosis for infants of very low birthweight. Pediatrics 54: 724-735

Stoop JW et al. (1977) Purine nucleoside phosphorylase deficiency associated with selective cellular immunodeficiency. New Engl J Med 296: 651-655

Sugita K et al. (1991) Magnetic resonance imaging of the brain in congenital rubella virus and cytomegalovirus infections. Neuroradiol 33: 239-242

Sugita M, Kulaney JT, Moser HW. (1972) Ceramidase deficiency in Farber's disease. Science 178: 1100-1102

Suzuki A, Iso A. (1993) Incidence rates of cerebral palsy, mental and motor retardation in Suberkan Tokyo. No To Hattatsu 26: 16-20

Szymonowicz E, Walker AM, Yu YYH, Steward ML, Cannata J, Cussea. (1990) Regional cerebral blood flow after hemorrhagic hypotension in the preterm, near term and newborn. Pediat Res 28: 361-366

Tada K, Ito H, Wada Y, Arakawa T. (1963) Congenital tryptophanuria with dwarfism. Tohoku J Exp Med 80: 118

Takahama K et al. (1982) A new type of $\alpha$-amino acid possessing bicuculline-sensitive action in the mammalian brain. Brain Res 239: 294-298